C0-AQH-854

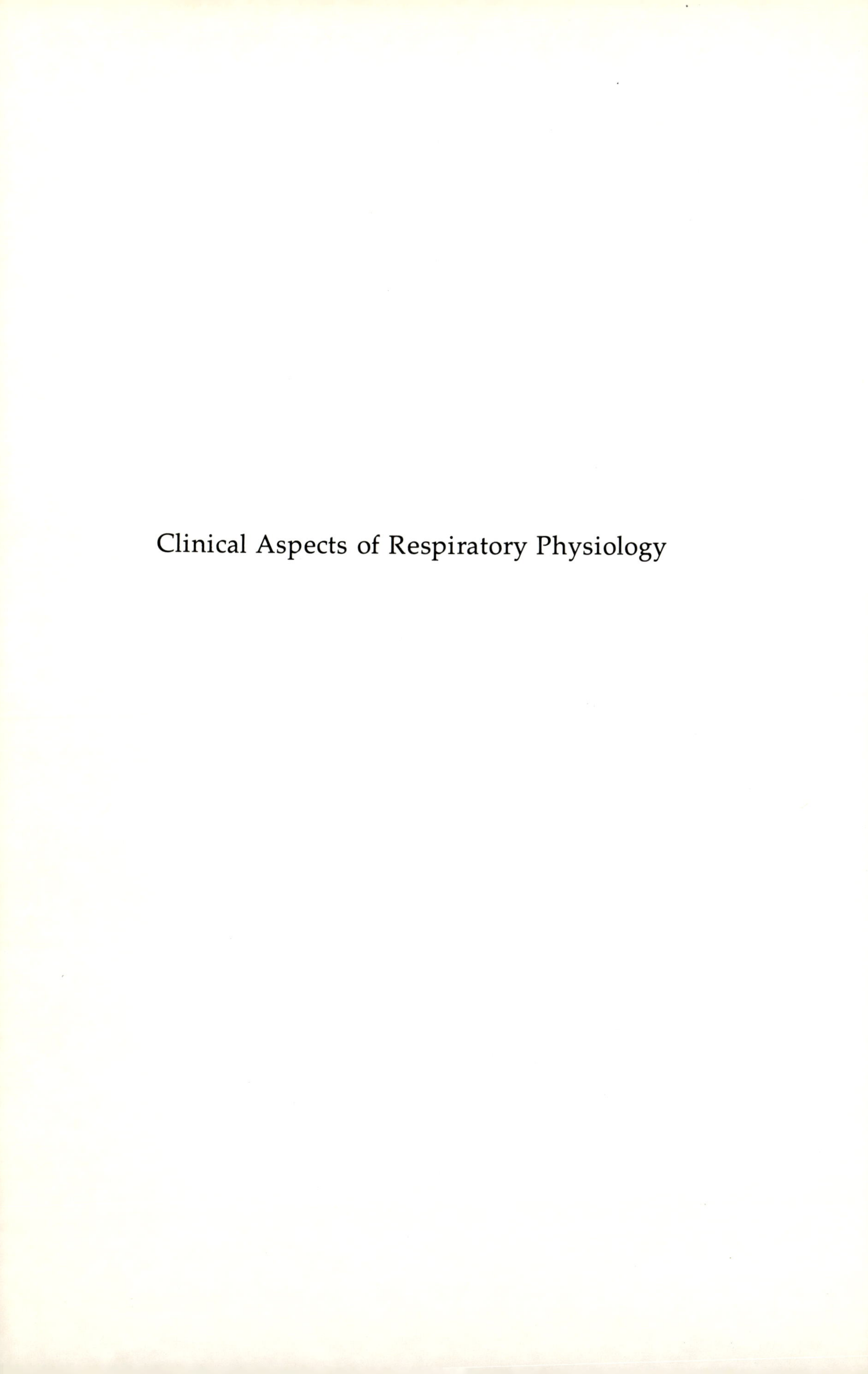

Clinical Aspects of Respiratory Physiology

Clinical Aspects of Respiratory Physiology

Clarence A. Guenter, M.D.
Professor and Head
Division of Internal Medicine
University of Calgary;
Director, Department of Internal Medicine
Foothills Provincial General Hospital
Calgary, Alberta

Martin H. Welch, M.D.
Associate Professor of Internal Medicine
Wichita State University Branch
University of Kansas School of Medicine;
Chief, Medical Service
Veterans Administration Center
Wichita, Kansas

James C. Hogg, M.D., Ph.D.
Professor of Pathology
University of British Columbia Faculty of Medicine;
Director, University of British Columbia
Pulmonary Research Laboratory
Vancouver, British Columbia

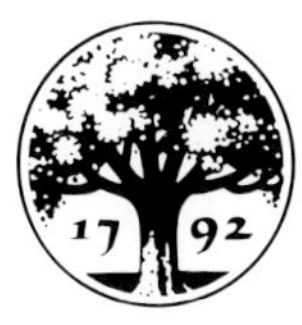

J. B. Lippincott Company
Philadelphia • Toronto

Copyright © 1978, by J. B. Lippincott Company
Copyright © 1977, by J. B. Lippincott Company

This book is fully protected by copyright, and, with the exception of brief excerpts for review, no part of it may be reproduced in any form, by print, photoprint, microfilm, or any other means, without written permission from the publisher.

This book was first published as Part 1 of *Pulmonary Medicine.*

ISBN 0-397-50400-4

Library of Congress Catalog Card Number 78-498

Printed in the United States of America

1 3 5 6 4 2

Library of Congress Cataloging in Publication Data
Main entry under title:

Clinical aspects of respiratory physiology.

Constitutes first 4 chapters of Pulmonary medicine, published in 1977.
Includes bibliographical references.
CONTENTS: Guenter, C. A. The respiratory environment. —Hogg, J. C. The respiratory airways.—Welch, M. H. Ventilatory function of the lungs.—Guenter, C. A. Respiratory function of the lungs and blood.
1. Respiratory organs—Diseases. 2. Pulmonary function tests. 3. Respiration. I. Guenter, Clarence A. II. Welch, Martin H. III. Hogg, James C. [DNLM: 1. Respiratory system—Physiology. 2. Respiratory system—Physiopathology. WF102 G927c]

Library of Congress Cataloging in Publication Data
RC734.P84P842 1978 616.2 78-498
ISBN 0-397-50400-4

Preface

This book emphasizes respiratory physiology as it is applied to clinical medicine. Written by clinical teachers with an ongoing interest in clinical investigation, the text emphasizes a critical approach to known applications of physiology, rather than intricate aspects of basic physiology. Such intriguing phenomena as metabolism of the numerous lung cell types and tissue release and uptake of biochemical substances are not included, because their clinical importance is not yet clearly defined. This material was first published as an introduction to respirology in Part I of the major work, *Pulmonary Medicine*. There, it provided the physiological basis for understanding altered lung function as it was dealt with comprehensively in the encyclopedic review of lung diseases in Part II. In response to requests by many readers who do not require the more exhaustive description of specific diseases and their management, this portion of that book is offered for medical students, nurses, respiratory therapists, and practicing physicians.

This book begins with a discussion of normal environmental gases, followed by the environmental effects of altered barometric pressures (high-altitude and underwater environments). Abnormal components of the atmospheric gases (pollutants) are reviewed with particular emphasis on common types of gaseous pollution. The next section deals with air flow in the lungs, demonstrating some of the complexities of the human airways and the factors affecting the distribution of inhaled air. Chapter 3 deals with the assessment of ventilatory function, emphasizing symptoms and bedside examination as they relate to simple as well as sophisticated laboratory tests. In Chapter 4 the role of the blood in respiration is summarized. This begins with the sampling of arterial blood and analysis for respiratory gases, and progresses through factors determining gas exchange in the lungs to a comprehensive discussion of oxygen transport from the environment to the body tissues, and carbon dioxide transport from the tissues to the lungs.

During times of rapidly expanding technology, the student is often overwhelmed by new and incompletely evaluated advances. Each student must have criteria against which to assess these advances. In these chapters the authors repeatedly emphasize the principles underlying laboratory assessment, the importance of recognizing artifact, and knowing the limitations on interpretation. As in so many clinical fields, the correlation of physical findings in the patient, with assessment of the laboratory results, must be made to ensure the validity of the laboratory measurements. These correlations have been itemized throughout.

This book will not replace the excellent in-depth treatises available in the broad field of respiratory physiology. It is written to translate those principles for bedside application and to raise the interest in the quality of patient care.

Clarence A. Guenter, M.D.
Martin H. Welch, M.D.
James C. Hogg, M.D., Ph.D.

Contents

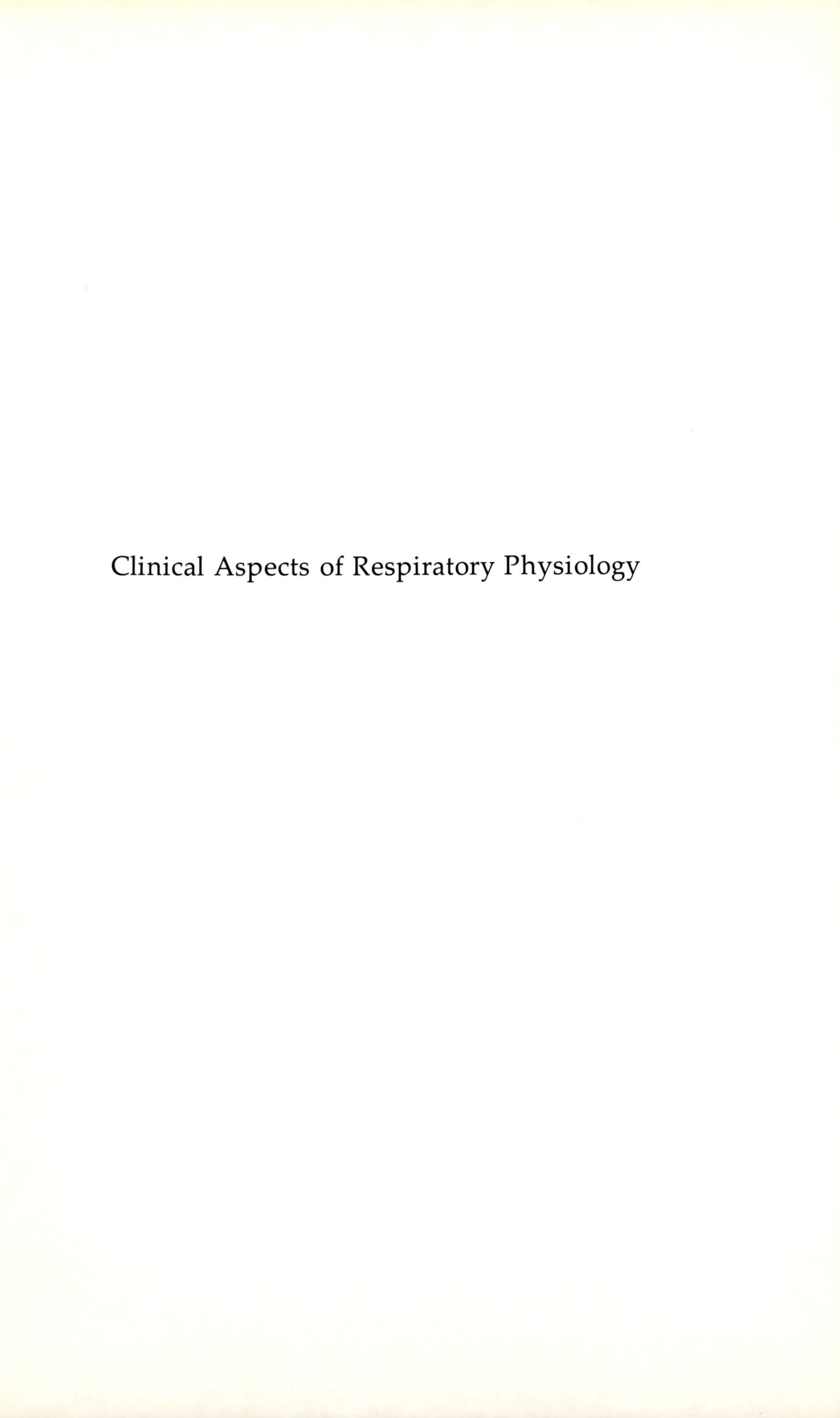

Clinical Aspects of Respiratory Physiology

1 The Respiratory Environment

Clarence A. Guenter, M.D.

GASES IN THE RESPIRATORY PATHWAY

Atmospheric Gases

The ubiquitous nature of oxygen, man's most immediately life-sustaining natural resource, may diminish the intrigue of the study of environmental gases. Curiosity is frequently stimulated by the threat of extinction of natural resources, and no satisfactory evidence can be accumulated as to a significant loss of available oxygen in our atmosphere. How the relatively constant concentration of gases (Table 1-1) is maintained in the atmosphere has not been established. Estimates indicate that the proportion of oxygen has been stable for several millennia.[2] The major source of oxygen for environmental replenishment is photosynthesis by plants. The major utilization of oxygen is by land and marine animals and by the combustion of fossil fuels. The enormous reserves of oxygen in the earth's atmosphere and in the oceans suggest that there will be no global life-limiting oxygen deficiency in the foreseeable future. A recent estimate indicated that if all the fossil fuels were completely burned instantaneously, a decrease of 3 per cent of the earth's global oxygen resources would occur. Variably contested evolutionary hypotheses attempt to explain these atmospheric conditions; however, there are major inadequacies in these hypotheses.

The convenience of unlimited oxygen reserves provides the respirologist with eternal optimism. Fortunately, the other major atmospheric gases are as conveniently arranged. Nitrogen and argon, the major inert gases, have no known biologi-

Table 1-1. Composition of Atmospheric Gas (Dry, Sea Level)

Gas	*mm. Hg*	*% Total*
Nitrogen	590	78.09
Oxygen	158	20.95
Carbon Dioxide	0.2	0.03
Other Inert Gases*	7.0	0.93
Water Vapor†	—	—
Total	760.2	100.00

*Predominantly argon.
†Water vapor pressure varies greatly with temperature (see Factors Affecting Alveolar Gas Partial Pressures, p. 5), but minimally with altitude. Although no figure is included in the above table, water vapor is never completely absent from the environment.
(Adapted from Altman, P. L., and Dittmer, D. S.: Biological Handbooks, Respiration and Circulation. Federation of the American Society of Experimental Biologists, 1971[1])

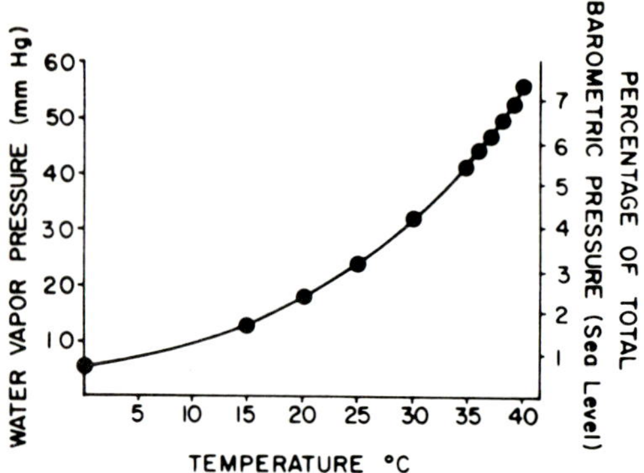

Fig. 1-1. The water vapor pressure, in mm. Hg, is plotted on the ordinate on the left, and water vapor pressure as a percentage of total barometric pressure (at sea level) on the ordinate on the right. All values are for fully saturated gas. Note that water vapor pressure in cold environments approaches zero. Sub-zero temperatures frequently encountered in winter in northern climates result in water vapor pressure of less than 5 mm. Hg, even when the atmosphere is fully saturated. As a result, warming of such air in heated buildings produces an atmosphere with a relative humidity of approximately 10 per cent. Humidification of air under these circumstances may be a major objective of inside air conditioning. Even when air that is fully saturated with respect to vapor pressure is warmed from room temperature to body temperature (approximately 20° to 37° C.), it becomes less than 50 per cent saturated. (Adapted from Altman, P. L., and Dittmer, D. S.: Biological Handbooks. Respiration and Circulation. Federation of the American Society of Experimental Biologists, 1971[3])

cal effects in concentrations that occur in the atmosphere. Carbon dioxide is suitably present in trace amounts only, permitting the metabolizing body to efficiently discharge its accumulated carbon dioxide into the atmosphere.

At sea level, the barometric pressure is about 760 mm. Hg. This pressure is comprised of the pressures of all the gases that are present in the atmosphere, regardless of temperature (see Table 1-1). (Dalton's law of partial pressures states that the partial pressure of each gas in a mixture is independent of the other gases present; therefore, the total pressure equals the sum of the partial pressures of all gases present.)

Since man's environment embraces a wide range of atmospheric pressures, functional amounts of the gases are expressed more conveniently as partial pressures than as concentrations. For example, a person traveling from sea level, at a barometric pressure of 760 mm. Hg, to a high altitude, with a barometric pressure of 380 mm. Hg, is still breathing 20.95 per cent oxygen; however, the 50 per cent decrease in available oxygen per unit of atmospheric volume is reflected in the partial pressure of oxygen (P_{O_2}), which has decreased from 160 to 80 mm. Hg.

Water vapor is a significant variable in atmospheric gas composition. Water vapor pressure (P_{H_2O}) is dependent on available water and (H_2O) capacity at fixed temperature. Thus, at 0° C., air that is fully saturated has a water vapor pressure of 4.6 mm. Hg, whereas at body temperature (37° C.), the water vapor pressure is 47 mm. Hg (Fig. 1-1). In the human body, all gases are saturated with water vapor. When dry air is inhaled, it is humidified; the increase in temperature in the body increases the capacity of the gases to carry water vapor. Water vapor is added to gases in the respiratory airways by the moist linings of the respiratory tract.

Gases in the Body

The interrelationship of atmospheric gases and, in particular, the effect of water vapor pressure on the partial pressures of the gases in the respiratory passages is demonstrated in Table 1-2. Nitrogen and oxygen are the only gases present in noteworthy concentrations in dry air; however, moist, warm tracheal air contains significant amounts of water vapor. Because the total barometric pressure is unchanged in the trachea, water vapor displaces each of the other gases, thereby decreasing their partial pressures. Thus, the partial pressure of oxygen is decreased from 159.1 to 149.2 mm. Hg, simply by the warming and humidification of air. As the gas advances to the lower respiratory tract, where gas exchange takes place, there are additional changes in its composition as indicated in the alveolar air column (Table 1-2). These changes in gas composition do

Table 1-2. Composition of Respired Gases

Gas	*Dry Air* Partial Pressure (mm. Hg)	*Dry Air* Percent Total	*Moist Tracheal Air* Partial Pressure (mm. Hg)	*Moist Tracheal Air* Percent Total	*Alveolar Air* Partial Pressure (mm. Hg)	*Alveolar Air* Percent Total
Nitrogen*	600.7	79.02	563.6	74.16	568.0	74.74
Oxygen	159.1	20.95	149.2	19.63	105.0	13.82
Carbon dioxide	0.2	.03	0.2	.03	40.0	5.26
Water vapor	0.0	0.00	47.0	6.18	47.0	6.18
Total†	760.0	100	760.0	100	760.0	100

*This value includes other inert gases separately itemized in Table 1-1.

†Values may be calculated for other altitudes by utilizing local barometric pressures (e.g., mean barometric pressure in Denver of 640 mm. Hg, or in Calgary, Alberta, 660 mm. Hg). For dry gas, the Po_2 at a barometric pressure of 660 mm. Hg: $20.95 \times 660 = 138$ mm. Hg. For saturated gas at 37° C.: $20.95 \times (660 - 47) = 128$ mm. Hg.

not merely reflect physical changes in temperature and water vapor pressure, but result from the actual uptake of oxygen from the alveolar space and the release of carbon dioxide into the alveolar space through the gas-exchanging surfaces of the peripheral lung units (see Chap. 4). Under normal circumstances, oxygen is taken up by the blood in the lungs in proportion to the utilization of oxygen by the tissues; carbon dioxide is released by the blood flowing through the lungs in proportion to the production of carbon dioxide by the tissues.

Figure 1-2 demonstrates the changes in oxygen and carbon dioxide along the entire respiratory pathway under various conditions. Each stage or physiological compartment is completely dependent on the gas pressures in the stage that precedes it and in the stage that follows it. The gases are predominantly moved by convection from the atmosphere to the alveolar space, and vice versa. Figure 1-2A illustrates the normal progression of oxygen and carbon dioxide partial pressures through the respiratory pathway.

The availability of oxygen to the blood is most immediately dependent on oxygen in the alveolar compartment; similarly, the release of carbon dioxide from the blood is most immediately dependent on the level of carbon dioxide in the alveolar compartment. Therefore, an understanding of factors that determine the partial pressures of these gases at the alveolar level is fundamental. Sequentially, the first important factor is the partial pressure of the inhaled gases. It is apparent that if the inhaled Po_2 were decreased, it would necessarily result in a decreased Po_2 of moist tracheal air. This in turn would result in a decrease in alveolar Po_2. High-altitude environments characteristically result in a decreased barometric pressure and a decreased partial pressure of inspired oxygen, compared with sea-level values.

Factors Affecting Alveolar Gas Partial Pressures

1. Inspired Po_2, Pco_2
2. Volume of oxygen uptake and carbon dioxide release in lungs
   a. Oxygen consumption and carbon dioxide production at tissue level (metabolic rate)
   b. Fuel being utilized by tissues and metabolic respiratory quotient
3. Volume of alveolar gas exchange (alveolar ventilation)

The second important factor determining the alveolar gas partial pressures is the oxygen uptake and carbon dioxide release in the lungs. It is clear that the decrease in oxygen would be precisely the same as the increase in carbon dioxide if the oxygen consumption and carbon dioxide production were equal. Although this is true under certain circumstances, the alveolar oxygen uptake and carbon dioxide release

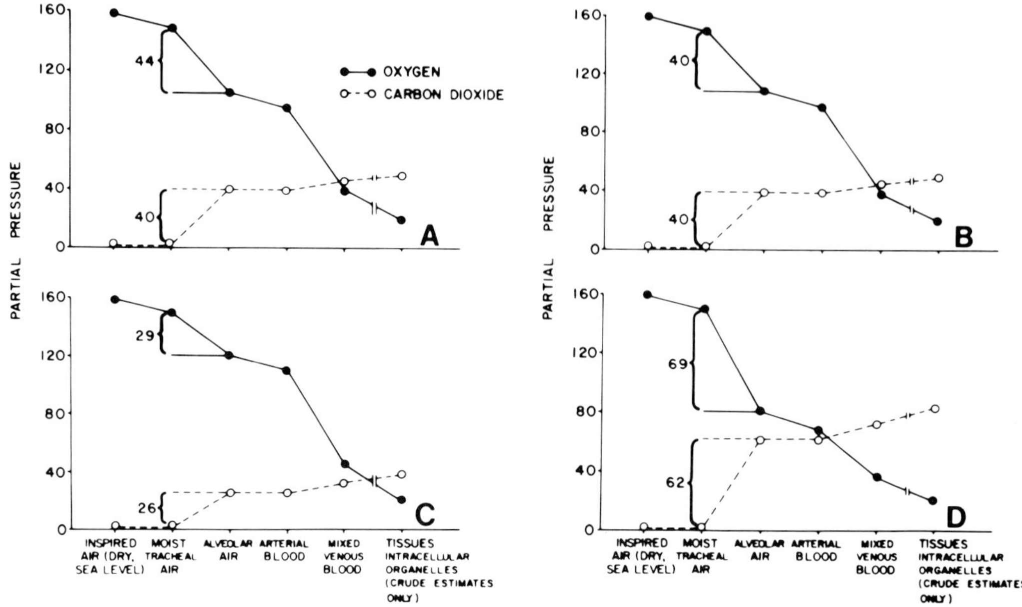

Fig. 1-2. Partial pressures of oxygen and carbon dioxide in the respiratory pathway steady-state conditions. (*A*) Normal resting. The solid line indicates the partial pressure of oxygen beginning in the inspired air on the left and progressing to the moist tracheal air, alveolar air, arterial blood, mixed venous blood, and, ultimately, tissues. The values represented indicate the average value in each region of the pathway, but are entirely speculative at the final level of the tissues. Movement of oxygen from the inspired air to the trachea, and from the trachea to the alveolar spaces is almost entirely by convection. Movement of oxygen from the alveolar spaces to the blood is by diffusion. Movement of oxygen within the arterial blood to the systemic capillaries is, again, by convection, as a result of blood flow. Movement of oxygen from the blood to the tissues is by diffusion. The interrupted line demonstrates the partial pressures of carbon dioxide in each region of the respiratory pathway; the same transport processes apply as for oxygen.

(*B*) Normal, resting, metabolic fuel—carbohydrate. The partial pressures for oxygen and carbon dioxide are again illustrated. Note that the alveolar extraction of oxygen and release of carbon dioxide are equal, thus resulting in a respiratory exchange ratio of 1.0. Thus, the alveolar ventilation and the partial pressures of carbon dioxide and oxygen become somewhat dependent on the fuel being metabolized.

(*C*) Effect of increased ventilation without increased metabolic rate. In a hyperventilating individual, the partial pressure of oxygen may be increased throughout the respiratory pathway, and the partial pressure of carbon dioxide decreased. The values illustrated apply only to an individual who has reached a steady state or equilibrium throughout the respiratory pathway.

(*D*) Effect of increased metabolic rate without increased alveolar ventilation. This illustration demonstrates the marked reduction of oxygen and the marked elevation of carbon dioxide throughout the body's respiratory pathways, as a result of the metabolic rate which is in excess of the level of ventilation.

(*B* adapted from Saltzman, H. A., and Salzano, J. V.: Effects of carbohydrate metabolism upon respiratory gas exchange in normal men. J. Appl. Physiol., *30*:228, 1971[4])

are generally not equal. As indicated in Figure 1-2A, the decrease in Po_2 of 44 mm. Hg which takes place at the alveolar level is compared with the increase in carbon dioxide of 40 mm. Hg. If oxygen uptake and carbon dioxide release were precisely equal, these changes would also be of equal value.

The obvious discrepancy between oxygen utilization and carbon dioxide production referred to above is a result of the particular fuel being metabolized. The ratio of CO_2 production to oxygen consumption has been termed the *metabolic respiratory quotient*. For example, when pure carbohydrate is metabolized, the oxidation equation may be summarized as follows: $C_6H_{12}O_6 + 6O_2 \rightarrow 6CO_2 + 6H_2O$ (+ energy).

It is apparent that when pure carbohydrate, such as glucose, is being metabolized, precisely the same amount of carbon dioxide is produced as oxygen utilized. Thus, the metabolic respiratory quotient is 1.0. Similarly, one can calculate the metabolic respiratory quotient for protein (approximately 0.8), fat (approximately 0.7), and ethanol (0.67). Therefore, the alveolar gas composition may be influenced by the fuel that the individual is metabolizing. For example, persons utilizing carbohydrate extract less oxygen in relation to the carbon dioxide production. Because the carbon dioxide controls ventilation, there is an increase in the alveolar oxygen partial pressure.[4] When the alveolar gas, blood flow, and tissue metabolism are in equilibrium, this results in an oxygen extraction from inspired air to alveolar gas of 40 mm. Hg and a carbon dioxide washout from alveolar gas to atmospheric air of 40 mm. Hg (Fig. 1-2B). The precise fuel being metabolized at any time by the body, or by specific tissues, cannot be ascertained. The oxygen extraction at the alveolar level, and the carbon dioxide washout from the alveoli, however, can be readily assessed. This indirect measurement of the average metabolic respiratory quotient has been termed the *respiratory exchange ratio* (R). It is clear that when the entire respiratory pathway is in equilibrium, this measurement accurately reflects the average of the total body metabolic respiratory quotient. Frequently, however, steady-state conditions do not prevail, and conditions such as transient hypoventilation or hyperventilation alter the respiratory exchange ratio, so that it does not reflect tissue metabolism accurately.

Several important circumstances that result in altered respiratory exchange ratios should be noted. Completely normal increases in the respiratory exchange ratio are seen at the onset and immediately following cessation of exercise. During these times, alveolar ventilation exceeds tissue metabolic requirements. This does not result in increased oxygen extraction from the alveoli, because oxygen stores cannot be significantly supersaturated. It does result, however, in depletion of carbon dioxide from tissue carbon dioxide stores. Thus, the carbon dioxide washout is greater than the oxygen consumption, and the respiratory exchange ratio may exceed 1.0. Similarly, during transient periods of metabolic acidosis, such as occur with anaerobic metabolism, the oxygen utilization may be relatively fixed, but due to circulating organic acids, body carbon-dioxide stores in the form of bicarbonate and blood carbonic acid are dissociated to H_2O and CO_2, with exhalation of the CO_2. The availability of large body-CO_2 stores thus permits temporary depletion of carbon dioxide, resulting in a respiratory exchange ratio that may exceed 1.0. This abnormal release of CO_2 has been studied as an early indication of tissue hypoxia. The level of exercise (as a determinant of the amount of metabolism) that produces such an increase in the respiratory exchange ratio has been suggested as a sensitive test for metabolic acidosis resulting from limited oxygen delivery (reflecting cardiorespiratory disease).[5] Conversely, circumstances under which ventilation is depressed and the carbon dioxide washout diminished, such as transient alveolar hypoventilation due to breath holding or sudden sedation, result in a respiratory exchange ratio less than that which would be appropriate for the fuel being metabolized at the time, e.g., < 0.70.

Figure 1-2C illustrates changes in partial pressures of oxygen and carbon dioxide in the respiratory pathway as a result of an increase in ventilation above body requirements, under steady-state conditions. Note that under these circumstances, the partial pressures of the inspired gases in moist tracheal air are unchanged. As a result of a marked increase in alveolar ventilation (hyperventilation), an increased amount of oxygen is available at the alveolar level when compared with normal conditions illustrated in Figure 1-2A. Consequently, in this example, the alveolar Po_2 is 120 mm. Hg. This permits increased oxygen availability for diffusion into the arterial blood and throughout the delivery system, with eventual increased oxygen availability at the tissue level. Carbon dioxide partial pressures are comparably affected. Due to the increase in alveolar gas exchange, the amount of carbon dioxide remaining in the alveoli is decreased. Thus, the alveolar Pco_2 is decreased to 26 mm. Hg, the arterial Pco_2 is approximately the same, and the tissue CO_2 is washed out to a somewhat lower level than indicated under normal circumstances in Figure 1-2A. Under these steady-state circumstances, the extraction of oxygen from alveolar gas results in a Po_2 decrease of 29 mm. Hg from inspired air to alveolar gas, and a Pco_2 decrease of 26 mm. Hg from the alveolar gas to the atmosphere.

The partial pressures depicted in Figure 1-2A represent approximate values seen throughout the respiratory tract, under normal resting steady-state conditions. It is quite clear that if tissue metabolism were suddenly accelerated, as during exercise, oxygen utilization and carbon dioxide production would be increased. Under these circumstances, the body generally responds by delivering more oxygen to the alveoli and by removing the carbon dioxide more rapidly by increasing alveolar ventilation. If ventilation were constant, however, the increased extraction of oxygen and production of carbon dioxide would severely alter alveolar gas levels. This situation is illustrated in Figure 1-2D, where alveolar ventilation has been held constant but the metabolic rate has increased. Note that the marked decrease in tissue oxygen tension results in increased extraction of oxygen from the blood at the tissue level, so that the mixed venous blood Po_2 is diminished. Because alveolar ventilation and, consequently, alveolar oxygen delivery are fixed, there is a decrease in alveolar Po_2. Similarly, the high metabolic rate results in a high tissue Pco_2, increased transport of carbon dioxide from the tissues, and increased mixed venous Pco_2. Because the alveolar ventilation is fixed, removal of carbon dioxide from the alveoli is inadequate, and the alveolar Pco_2 is elevated. The Pco_2 of blood leaving the alveoli (arterial blood Pco_2) is elevated. This represents an inadequate response to tissue respiratory requirements, and because the response is inadequate primarily with respect to ventilation, it is termed *alveolar hypoventilation*. Note that the alveolar extraction of oxygen results in a drop of Po_2 from inspired air to alveolar gas of 69 mm. Hg, and the washout of carbon dioxide at the alveolar level results in a decrease in Pco_2 from alveolar gas to the atmosphere of 62 mm. Hg. This, then, represents a new steady state in which inadequate alveolar ventilation is responsible for marked alterations in alveolar gas partial pressures.

In each of the above circumstances, the person has developed an equilibrium with respect to carbon dioxide and oxygen partial pressures throughout the respiratory pathway. Thus, alveolar gas exchange, blood transport of gases, and tissue metabolism reflect a continuous and stable exchange of oxygen and carbon dioxide. Within wide physiological ranges, once an equilibrium has been established, the actual rate of blood flow (cardiac output) is not a determinant of the gas levels in the alveoli or respiratory airways.

VARIATIONS IN ATMOSPHERIC CONDITIONS

Decreased Barometric Pressure

Human awareness of adverse effects of the low barometric pressure of high altitudes is recorded in literature regarding the Spanish invasion of the Western Hemisphere. As early as the 1500's, the Spanish complained of the "thinness of the air" in the high mining areas of South America. Their concern about the inability to have offspring suggested that this, too, was a result of environmental hazard. Probably, detailed analysis of folk literature from other high-lying areas in the world would produce additional historical evidence of recognition of these atmospheric problems. Acute mountain sickness, at an elevation of about 10,000 feet, was first described in 1671 by the physiologist, Borelli. Subsequently, many additional descriptions of illness were recorded, and we now recognize an entire spectrum, ranging from mild alterations in judgment at relatively low altitudes, to severe acute or chronic altitude disease at higher altitudes. Although persons with previous cardiorespiratory disease may be significantly less well at altitudes as low as 5,000 feet, more than 3,000,000 persons in South America live above 13,000 feet, and there are communities in the United States at altitudes above 7,000 feet. Furthermore, recent wars have been fought between the Indians and the Chinese at altitudes in excess of 15,000 feet.

Intriguing studies of human adaptation to high altitudes describe life on the Andean Plateau, from Colombia to Chile in South America.[6] This plateau rises above 8,000 feet and is suitable for human habitation up to the permanent snow line (17,500 feet). There are more than 10,000,000 persons living in this zone, and historical and archeological records indicate that it has been densely populated for a long time. The Inca Empire had its center in this zone, and it is clear that reproduction by the natives effectively perpetuated the race. Studies of selected communities in this area indicate that although fertility is reasonably maintained (certainly compatible with a population increase), cultural patterns favor reproductive function. The native population has a high birth rate and a high death rate, with peculiarly high prenatal and postnatal death rates for females. This results in a high ratio of males to females in the adult population. Birth weights are low, postnatal growth is quite slow relative to other populations throughout the world, and the adolescent growth spurt is less than that for other groups. Nevertheless, environmental factors appear to be less important than socioeconomic factors in determining the ability of the natives to thrive.

Effects of Altitude on Lung Function. In view of the constant concentration of oxygen in air, availability of oxygen to the individual is dependent on barometric pressure. Large changes in barometric pressure are observed with varying altitudes. Figure 1-3 demonstrates the decrease in barometric pressure and the decrease in inhaled Po_2 with increasing altitude (an exponential relationship). Thus, the inspired oxygen partial pressure may be predicted on the basis of the change in barometric pressure resulting from the altitude. Figure 1-4 illustrates the approximate values for inspired Po_2 at several different altitudes, with approximate changes in Po_2 of moist tracheal air, alveolar gas, arterial blood, mixed venous blood, and the directional changes in tissue oxygen partial pressure.

The immediate effects of a sudden change in barometric pressure have been studied in persons transported to high altitudes and have been simulated in low-pressure chambers. Among the earliest outstanding and comprehensive studies

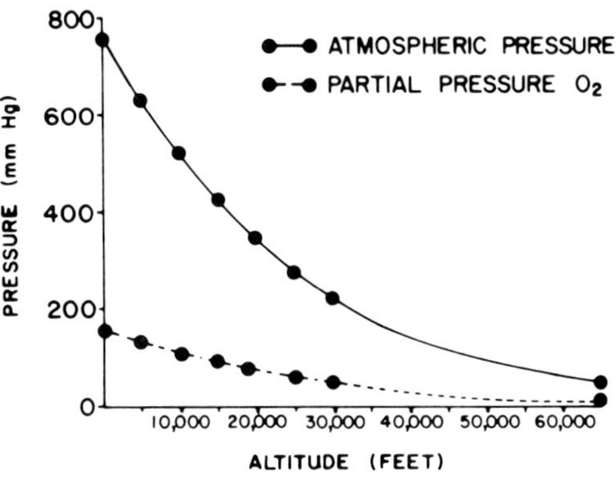

Fig. 1-3. Effect of altitude on barometric pressure and partial pressure of oxygen. The barometric pressure at various geometric elevations is plotted by the solid line. Note the exponential relationship. The partial pressure of oxygen is a fixed proportion (20.95%) of the total barometric pressure and is plotted by the interrupted line. Whereas the atmospheric partial pressure of oxygen at sea level is approximately 160 mm. Hg, it is reduced to half that value at 18,000 feet. (Adapted from Altman, P. L., and Dittmer, D. S.: Biological Handbooks. Environmental Biology. Federation of the American Society of Experimental Biologists, 1966[7])

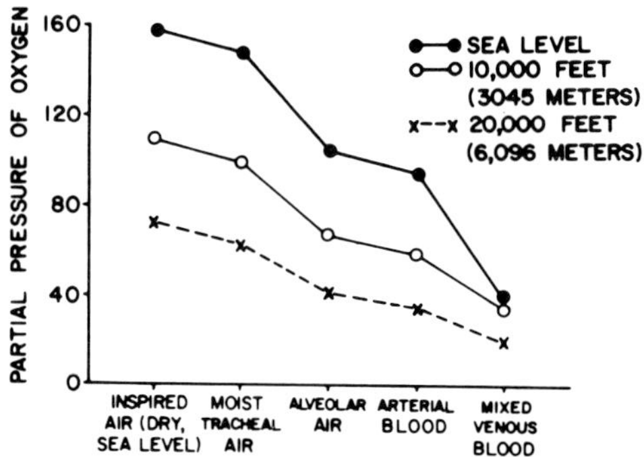

Fig. 1-4. Effect of altitude on partial pressures of oxygen in the respiratory pathway. Average values for partial pressure of oxygen have been plotted at sea level, at a 10,000-foot altitude, and at a 20,000-foot altitude. Considerable individual variation limits the precise application of this data. Note that although the partial pressure of oxygen decreases along the respiratory pathway in approximately the same fashion at higher altitude as at sea level, the adaptive mechanisms are sufficient to minimize the effect on tissue oxygenation. Thus, the mixed venous blood (and the tissues) reflect much smaller changes in partial pressure of oxygen than the arterial blood. (Adapted from Altman, P. L., and Dittmer, D. S.: Biological Handbooks. Environmental Biology. Federation of the American Society of Experimental Biologists, 1966[7])

are those of Hurtado performed in the Andes. Numerous other important contributions have clarified details of the acute physiological responses to low barometric pressures and have explored adaptive mechanisms that take place early in the sojourner, as well as some of those that appear to take place over generations in inhabitants of high-altitude regions.

Many of the physiological responses of native sea-level inhabitants to sudden exposure to higher altitude are illustrated in Table 1-3. A large number of studies with frequently conflicting results are summarized, but it is quite clear that sudden exposure to high altitude, such as occurs with rapid ascent by airplane, results in findings different than the effects of gradual ascent by climbing or slow travel.[8] In general, the effects of sudden ascent are quite comparable to exposure to low oxygen partial pressures in gas chambers. The summary data in Table 1-3 refer to responses to sudden ascent to medium altitudes (10,000 to 15,000 feet). Although the mechanisms controlling ventilation are complex, it is teleologically noteworthy that the increase in ventilation is proportional to the decrease in the density of the air. Thus, the increase in ventilation is approximately the amount required to produce equivalent delivery of oxygen to the alveolar spaces. This is achieved predominantly through the increase in tidal volume, though in certain instances the respiratory rate may also increase. This elevated minute ventilation is generally sustained throughout the period at higher altitude, although it does not reach its plateau until the second or third day there. As discussed previously and demonstrated in Figure 1-4, the arterial Po_2 is decreased as a result of the decrease in alveolar Po_2 and inspired Po_2. Although minimal alterations may occur as a result of early adaptive processes, this remains in approximately the same range throughout the time at higher altitude. The arterial hypoxia results in stimulation of the peripheral chemoreceptors in the aortic and carotid bodies, which are responsible for hypoxic control of respiration. This results in an increase in alveolar ventilation; the carbon dioxide is washed out of the alveolar spaces at a more rapid rate, and the arterial Pco_2 is decreased. These circumstances also persist throughout the exposure to higher altitude. This decrease in arterial Pco_2 results in a respiratory alkalosis. A major adaptive mechanism, however, comes into play within hours of the arrival at higher altitude, when the decreased arterial Pco_2 (and associated increase in arterial pH) stimulates the excretion of bicarbonate from the blood by the kidneys. As a consequence, during the ensuing hours to days, the blood bicarbonate is reduced, and a new level appropriate for the degree of hyperventilation is established, with a normal, or nearly normal, arterial pH. Thus, the respiratory alkalosis is compensated.

These respiratory adaptations and the bicarbonate excretion affect spinal fluid electrolyte status and alter subsequent ventilatory responses. Initially, the hyperven-

Table 1-3. Physiological Responses to High Altitude Relative to Sea-Level Control Values*

	Immediate	*Early Adaptive (72 hours)*	*Late Adaptive (2 to 6 weeks)*
Spontaneous ventilation:			
Minute ventilation	↑	↑	↑
Respiratory rate	Variable	Variable	Variable
Tidal volume	↑	↑	↑
Arterial Po_2	↓	↓	↓
Arterial Pco_2	↓	↓	↓
Arterial pH	↑	↑ ↔	↑ ↔
Arterial HCO_3	↔	↓	↓
Evaluation of lung function			
Vital capacity	↔	↔	↔
Maximum air flow rates	↑	↑	↑
Functional residual capacity	↔	↔	↔
Ventilatory response to inhaled CO_2	↔	↑	↑
Ventilatory response to hypoxia	↔	↔	↔
Pulmonary vascular resistance	↑	↑	↑
Oxygen transport			
Hemoglobin	↔	↑	↑
Erythropoietin	↑	↔	↔
P_{50}	↓	↑	↑
2-3 DPG	↔	↑	↑
Cardiac output	↑	↔	↔ ↓
Central nervous system			
Headaches, nausea, insomnia	↑	↔	↔
Perception, judgment	↓	↔	↔
Spinal fluid pH	↑	↔	↔
Spinal fluid HCO_3^-	↔	↓	↓

*These values apply to native sea-level inhabitants. See text for a discussion of discrepancies with native highlanders.

tilation results in decreased Pco_2 in the spinal fluid, which has a relatively fixed bicarbonate concentration. This results in an increase in spinal fluid pH, which tends to modify or suppress ventilation. As the bicarbonate is excreted from the blood, bicarbonate is gradually lost from the spinal fluid, and a new appropriate level is achieved with a lower bicarbonate level.[9] In face of this decreased buffer capacity, changes in CO_2 result in greater changes in hydrogen ion concentration and thus an increased sensitivity to carbon dioxide. At this point, control of respiration is slightly altered. Whereas ventilatory responses to inhaled carbon dioxide were initially normal, as the spinal fluid bicarbonate is excreted, small amounts of additional carbon dioxide result in greater increases in hydrogen ion concentration in the spinal fluid that bathes the respiratory centers centrally, and result in a greater increase in ventilation per unit change in carbon dioxide. The ventilatory response to hypoxia remains unchanged throughout the period at higher altitude. At extreme altitudes, resulting in arterial Po_2 less than 20 mm. Hg, there is profound depression of the central nervous system with suppressed ventilatory drive.

Although these effects on spontaneous ventilation are of considerable interest,

Table 1-4. Relationship of Pulmonary Artery Pressure to Altitude*

Location	*Altitude (feet)*	*Inspired* P_{O_2} *(mm. Hg)*	*Mean Pulmonary Artery Pressure (mm. Hg)*
Boston, MA	8	148	13
Halifax, N. S.	60	148	14
Denver, CO	5,250	121	16
Mexico City	7,400	111	16
La Paz, Bolivia	12,150	92	23
Morococha, Peru	14,900	83	28

*These figures are for natives of these locations.
(Adapted from Cudkowicz, L.: Mean pulmonary artery pressure and alveolar oxygen tension in man at different altitudes. Respiration, *27*:417, 1970[15])

additional effects on lung function occur. The vital capacity is unchanged; however, maximum air-flow rates (as measured by maximum mid-flow rates, peak-flow rates, and forced expiratory volumes at 1 second) are increased as a result of decreased density of the gases.[10,11] Numerous complex evaluations of respiratory function have been undertaken; it has been documented clearly that the diffusing capacity for carbon monoxide is increased,[8] and regional distribution of blood flow in the lungs is altered, with an improvement in blood flow to the apical regions.[12,13] Overall matching of ventilation in relation to perfusion, however, does not appear to be improved.[14] Pulmonary arterial pressure and pulmonary vascular resistance are increased in proportion to the degree of hypoxia (Table 1-4). As a result, increases in right ventricular pressures over prolonged periods of time produce right ventricular hypertrophy. Predictable electrocardiographic changes can be demonstrated, indicating right-axis deviation and right ventricular strain.[16,17]

Effects of Altitude on Oxygen Transport. Teleologically, one might anticipate that all the physiological responses to high altitude would be directed at improved oxygen delivery to the tissues. It is not surprising, then, that most aspects of the oxygen transport system are altered in the direction of improved oxygen delivery. As indicated previously, alveolar ventilation is increased by approximately the amount required to deliver the same molecular amount of oxygen to the alveolar spaces as takes place at sea level.

The oxygen-carrying capacity of the blood is predominantly determined by hemoglobin concentration. When a person travels to a higher altitude, the hemoglobin level initially is unchanged, but within hours it begins to rise. This early rise in hemoglobin is not due to increased red-cell mass, but is a result of hemoconcentration, which is not sustained over prolonged periods at higher altitude.[18,19] The hemoglobin concentration is eventually elevated, however, as a result of increased erythropoiesis and a true increase in red-cell mass. The mean increase in hemoglobin concentration is 1.5 to 2.0 g./100 ml. at 10,000 feet, and 3.0 to 4.5 g./100 ml. at 15,000 feet. Erythropoietin levels are elevated within the first hours at high altitude, but the true increase in red-cell mass resulting from increased production takes several weeks.[20] As the red-cell mass and hemoglobin concentration rise, the erythropoietin level decreases.

The ability of hemoglobin to transport oxygen is also dependent on hemoglobin affinity for oxygen. Initially, hemoglobin affinity for oxygen is increased because of the shift of the oxyhemoglobin dissociation curve to the left, which occurs with alkalosis. Since the alkalosis is transient, the curve would be expected to subsequently shift to its previous position. (See Chap. 4 for a detailed discussion of oxygen affinity for hemoglobin.) It is noteworthy, however, that soon after the development of the hypoxic state, there is an increase in production of 2-3 diphosphoglycerate (2-3 DPG). This increase in 2-3 DPG results in a shift of the oxyhemoglobin dissociation curve to the right. Although there is conflicting data regarding this shift in oxyhemoglobin affinity as a part of the early acclimatization to altitude, most studies have demonstrated at least a slight shift in this direction. The practical significance of this shift has not been established. It might be expected to permit increased unloading of oxygen at the tissue level (at the same tissue Po_2), but, certainly, at very high altitudes it might also interfere with oxygen uptake by the hemoglobin in the lungs.

Cardiac output is characteristically increased initially with the hypoxic state but has been demonstrated to decrease in the adaptive phases. Whether this eventual decrease is a result of the increased effectiveness of other components of the oxygen transport system, a mechanism for conserving energy, or a result of myocardial hypoxia, has not been established.

In spite of these adaptive responses to altitude, there is no significant change in resting oxygen consumption, or in the ability to perform vigorous exercise at moderate altitudes. Tolerance of higher work loads is limited by several factors, including tachycardia, hyperventilation, and easy fatigability.[21]

Effects of Altitude on the Nervous System. At very low levels of altitude, no changes can be demonstrated in the central nervous system function. At altitudes varying from 5,000 to 8,000 feet, there may be slight alterations in perception, impairment of judgment, and decreased efficiency of learning.[22] Certainly, these symptoms have been well documented at altitudes over 10,000 feet. Headaches, nausea, listlessness, insomnia, and alterations in breathing pattern (Cheyne-Stokes respiration) are all attributed to the effects of altitude. These effects have traditionally been ascribed to the hypoxia; however, there is some evidence that the symptoms can be modified not only by oxygen, but by pretreatment with drugs that prevent the marked respiratory alkalosis. (Carbonic anhydrase inhibitors such as acetazolamide increase excretion of bicarbonate by the kidney, thus reducing the serum bicarbonate.)[23] Fortunately, these symptoms generally improve spontaneously after 48 to 96 hours at higher altitude. Ascending too rapidly to altitudes over 17,000 feet may be associated with loss of consciousness as a result of the sudden, severe hypoxia.

A recent study of climbers on Mt. McKinley in Alaska demonstrated retinal hemorrhages in 36 per cent of thirty-nine subjects who climbed more than 14,000 feet. The severity of retinal hemorrhage was correlated with the severity of headaches. Subjects with a previous history of vascular headache experience a more severe altitude headache, and a more rapid ascent predisposed the climbers to more severe hemorrhages and headaches.[24]

Miscellaneous Effects of Severe Hypoxia. The acute hypoxia, when severe enough, may be expected to result in interference with function of organ systems in a more profound fashion than indicated above. These manifestations of severe hypoxia are more commonly seen as a result of hypoxia secondary to cardiorespiratory disease. Central nervous system manifestations may present a spectrum of symptoms, including impaired judgment, loss of memory, disorientation, hallucinations, tremor, stupor, coma, and death. The cardiovascular manifestations may include severe hypertension, hypotension, tachycardia, a wide variety of arrhythmias, heart failure (predominantly right ventricular failure due to pulmonary hypertension, but occasionally also left ventricular failure), and alterations in regional blood flow.

Renal manifestations of mild hypoxia are not striking; however, very severe degrees of hypoxia have been associated with a decrease in renal blood flow, with secondary effects including changes in concentrating and excreting capacity, as well as acute renal failure. Severe hypoxia is characteristically associated with development of anaerobic metabolism and metabolic acidosis.

Recent studies have dealt more

thoroughly with the effects of altitude on a variety of cellular functions and on endocrine function.[23,25]

Altitude Acclimatization as Seen in the High-Dwelling Native. It is noteworthy that man's capacity to adapt to such austere environments as elevations of 15,000 feet permits not only productive function, but perpetuation of the race. As indicated previously, the South American Indians' capacity to reproduce is in contrast with the infertility of sea-level dwellers who have moved to those altitudes. In addition, numerous other responses of the body appear to be modified in those who dwell at high altitudes.

Hurtado's studies demonstrated very large lung volumes in natives of the high-altitude plateau in the Andes. The principle of these findings has since been confirmed by animal studies that demonstrated an increase in lung volume and alveolar surface area in experimental animals raised in low-barometric-pressure atmospheres.[26] These changes may account for the much higher capacity for diffusing carbon monoxide documented in natives of high altitude when compared with sojourners to these altitudes.[8]

The "highlanders" have a "blunted" respiratory drive in response to hypoxia. As a consequence, they uniformly have a decreased minute ventilation at higher altitude, as compared with sea-level inhabitants ("lowlanders") of the same race, who have temporarily ascended to the same levels.[27] Additional degrees of hypoxia increase the ventilatory drive only minimally in these high-altitude natives. This modified response may be genetic, or it may have developed as a very early response to the environment, since natives of high altitudes sustain the blunted ventilatory response to hypoxia even after prolonged periods at sea level, and sea-level dwellers appear to acquire this response gradually, after prolonged periods at high altitude.[28] This effect may be due to a decrease in sensitivity of the peripheral chemoreceptors to the hypoxic stimulus, or to a decrease in sensitivity of central respiratory control mechanisms to inputs from the peripheral chemoreceptors.[29] The precise advantages of this blunted response to hypoxia are not entirely certain; however, it seems clear that at high levels of exercise, highlanders sustain a low work of breathing because of the lower ventilation.

Tissue adaptation may also take place, and, although convincing evidence in humans is not available, an increase in numbers of systemic capillaries may develop. If appropriate techniques were available, it would not be surprising to find cellular oxygen utilization accomplished more efficiently[8]; however, this remains to be demonstrated in humans.

Mountain Sickness and High-Altitude Pulmonary Edema. Early descriptions of explorations at high altitudes indicated that certain individuals develop severe illness not entirely explicable on the basis of predictable responses to altitude.[30] These are generally sojourners who demonstrate what appear to be excessive adaptive responses to the altitude. Characteristic findings are plethora, weakness and lethargy, somnolence, and, frequently, evidence of heart failure.[31,32] There is a wide variation in ability to adapt to high altitudes, and some persons, for reasons incompletely explained, may develop much greater increases in pulmonary vascular resistance, modified alveolar gas exchange with more profound hypoxia, and greater elevations in hemoglobin with increases in blood viscosity and, ultimately, poor peripheral perfusion. This condition has been referred to as chronic mountain sickness. A similar syndrome, Brisket disease, has been described in cattle.[33] This syndrome, known as chronic mountain sickness, has been treated effectively only by removal from the high-altitude environment, although long-term therapy with supplemental oxygen may be an alternative.

High-altitude pulmonary edema represents an entirely different problem.[34] It is most frequently seen in dwellers of lowlands who ascend to high altitude, but occurs in natives returning to high altitude after several weeks at sea level. It occurs within 36 hours of ascending to high altitude. It is frequently referred to by the uninitiated as "nocturnal asthma," or "altitude-induced asthma"; however, the major factor responsible for this condition is an increase of fluid in the lungs, characterized by all the symptomatology, physical signs, and roentgenographic features of acute pulmonary edema. No criteria have been established to predict who will develop high-altitude pulmonary edema. It may occur in individuals who have previously been to high altitude without developing it, and it may occur in persons without other manifestations of cardiorespiratory disease, and even in otherwise well-conditioned athletes. The precise altitude at which it will occur is also not certain. It has been suspected at levels as low as 8,000 feet, but generally does not occur at altitudes under 12,000 feet. Infection, exertion, age, or sex do not appear to be predisposing factors. In a large military airlift in India, a mean of 5.7 individuals out of each 1,000 flown to an altitude of 11,500 feet developed the syndrome.[35] Manifestations consist of tachypnea, dyspnea, weakness, and nausea, gradually progressing to full-blown pulmonary edema with cough and copious bronchial secretions. When contracted, it may progress to death.

The mechanisms of production of high-altitude-induced pulmonary edema are not at all clear. It is clear, from the limited number of available hemodynamic studies, that the pulmonary artery pressure is severely elevated, with a normal pulmonary venous pressure. This might be considered evidence against an increase in pulmonary capillary pressure. Pulmonary capillary pressure may, however, be elevated as a result of patchy pulmonary arteriolar constriction, with high capillary pressures in some vessels. On the other hand, there may be increased permeability of lung capillaries, thus producing increased fluid accumulation in the lung.[36]

Conventional therapy for pulmonary edema is ineffective, and the only known and absolutely reliable method of control for this condition is administration of oxygen or return to lower altitudes.[36]

Travel at Decreased Barometric Pressures. Early in aviation history, all flights were conducted in nonpressurized planes and, therefore, at decreased barometric pressures. The hazards were appropriate to the altitude, and high-altitude flights required inhalation of supplemental oxygen. More modern aircraft used for commercial passenger service, flying at high altitudes (30,000 to 40,000 feet), are pressurized to reasonable levels. In general, in-flight cabin pressures are equivalent to 5,000 to 8,000 feet, though many flights are conducted with cabin pressures near sea-level pressure. Normal persons at rest have no recognizable symptoms at these levels. Not infrequently, however, travelers with cardiorespiratory disease and reduced peripheral oxygen delivery develop symptoms while in flight, including weakness, dizziness, and, occasionally, loss of consciousness. They are generally improved by use of the available oxygen, and such problems may be readily avoided by supplying oxygen to persons at risk. Persons with disease who have severely reduced arterial Po_2 levels should probably be provided with oxygen throughout flight. Aside from hypoxia, persons with pulmonary disease rarely have adverse effects from flying. The presence of a large pneumothorax should be considered a contraindication to flying, because decompression results in expansion of the pneumothorax. Patients with sickle cell anemia may develop increased sickling and vascular occlusion at high altitudes.

More dramatic problems with atmospheric gases were experienced in the space exploration program. Although fringes of the earth's atmosphere extend approximately 350 miles (550 to 600 km.) above the earth (Table 1-5), the available oxygen diminishes markedly (Fig. 1-3). Space flights in the outer layers of the atmosphere or interplanetary flights are at barometric pressures that effectively provide no oxygen. After considerable experimentation, most United States manned flights were carried out with cabins pressurized to about one-third atmosphere (barometric pressure 250 mm. Hg). Most recent flights have had approximately 67 per cent oxygen (Po_2 150 mm. Hg), and the balance of the pressure was made up by nitrogen. Under these conditions, the major additional requirement has been for

Table 1-5. Characteristics and Composition of the Atmosphere

Region	*Altitude*	*Temperature*
Troposphere	Sea level to 19 km. at equator, 9 km. at poles (average, 10 km.)	Decreases with altitude about 6° C./km. rise
Stratosphere	10 to 20 km.	Constant at −60° C.
Mesosphere	20 to 80 km.	Rises to 0° C. at 30 to 50 km. due to absorption of ultraviolet- and x-radiation
Thermosphere	Greater than 80 km.	Rises to 900° C. at 200 km.
Ionosphere	Greater than 60 km.	Constant at 1,000° C. above 300 km. Temperature rise due to absorption of ultraviolet- and x-radiation, which is strongest at about 150 km.
Exosphere	Greater than 550 km.	Outer fringe of the atmosphere

(Adapted from Altman, P. L., and Dittmer, D. S.: Biological Handbooks. Environmental Biology. Federation of the American Society of Experimental Biologists, 1966[38])

efficient removal of carbon dioxide. When the cabin pressures are carefully controlled in these ranges, the predominant biological concern relates to problems of weightlessness, nutrition, and isolation. These are under active study.[37]

Effects of Latitude on Barometric Pressure. Numerous factors in addition to altitude affect barometric pressures, including atmospheric turbulence, temperature, and latitude. At sea level, barometric pressures have been recorded ranging from 664 to 805 mm. Hg, in various latitudes and under widely varying temperature conditions. Although the barometric pressure can be predicted with some confidence from the geometric altitude (as indicated in Fig. 1-3), the actual barometric pressure and thus the available inspired oxygen can be accurately assessed only by measurement of the barometric pressure in that location at a specific time. Thus, it is of interest that studies performed at the geographic South Pole[10] revealed barometric pressures substantially lower than would be anticipated for the geometric altitude of 9,280 feet. This decrease in barometric pressure is presumably due to the latitude (90° south) and is equivalent to the geometric altitude of about 11,000 feet in near-equatorial regions.[38]

Environments with Increased Barometric Pressure

It is only under water, where the pressure increases approximately 1 atmosphere with each 33-foot descent, that man encounters a natural environment in which the pressure is elevated significantly above 760 mm. Hg.

Underwater Diving. Direct body contact with increased barometric pressure is most commonly encountered during breath-hold diving.[39] Numerous important changes take place in the body during the breath-holding period. Continuous oxygen utilization by the body results in a progressive pickup of oxygen, eventually reducing available oxygen to critical levels. Similarly, the continuous production of carbon dioxide by the body results in progressively elevated blood and alveolar levels of carbon dioxide.

Under normal circumstances, the breath hold is terminated when the buildup of carbon dioxide in the blood acts as an almost irresistible drive to breathe. Since hypoxia is a mild stimulus to ventilation, it is a relatively mild stimulus to stop holding the breath. Breath holding beyond safe intervals is a major hazard in this form of diving, since oxygen is excessively depleted from the alveoli, and serious hypoxia develops. A common and hazardous error is made by swimmers who hyperventilate prior to the dive to increase the time of breath holding. This depletes the body carbon-dioxide stores, but the oxygen stores cannot be significantly hypersaturated. Under these circumstances, when a dive is undertaken, the accumulation of carbon dioxide, which generally forces the termination of breath holding, is considerably delayed. Particularly if exercise is continuing, the available oxygen may be utilized to a dangerously low level before the dive is terminated, and arrhythmias, seizures, or death may occur as a result of hypoxia. This is thought to account for many "swimming pool deaths."

A descent of approximately 33 feet in seawater results in an increase of pressure equivalent to 1 atmosphere. Only a few individuals can dive while holding their breath to depths where the pressure exceeds 5 atmospheres; most commonly such diving is confined to pressures of 2 or 3 atmospheres.

The external pressure exerted on the thorax during a dive results in a marked increase in intrathoracic pressure. This would impair venous return were it not for a concomitant increase in pressure surrounding all other portions of the body, thus compressing blood vessels throughout the body.

Increased intrathoracic pressure results in compression of the air-filled lung. Thus, a lung that was fully inflated as the dive began may be compressed to a very low volume during the dive. For example, if the dive were begun with the lungs inflated to total lung capacity, at a depth of 33 feet the volume would be reduced 50 per cent.

It becomes apparent that the individual with a large total lung capacity would be capable of dives to greater depths. Several studies suggest that persons particularly suited to diving, such as the diving women of Japan and Korea, have higher than normal ratios of total lung capacity to residual volume. Furthermore, divers who begin their dive with low lung volumes may be severely limited when the "lung squeeze" produces volumes near residual volume.

In addition to the net volume changes in the lung during "breath-hold diving," the compression of the chest cage results in increased gas pressures in the lung, with resultant increased alveolar Po_2 and Pco_2. Increased Po_2 merely improves availability of oxygen; however, increased carbon dioxide would be expected to stimulate respiration. The ability to dive in spite of this rise in Pco_2 can be cultivated. Submarine escape-training-tank instructors who spent many hours underwater, with prolonged breath holding and frequent periods of increased alveolar (and blood) Pco_2, eventually demonstrated sustained elevations in alveolar Pco_2 with appropriate changes in blood electrolytes.[39,40] These chronically elevated CO_2 levels returned to normal during a 3-month layoff period. A significant hazard to the diver develops as a result of the increased Po_2 produced by compression, in that the Po_2 is relatively high when at depth, but as the diver surfaces and the lung expands, the Po_2 decreases. If the lung has been depleted of oxygen by body utilization, the alveolar oxygen may reach critically low levels. The Pco_2, fortunately, decreases as the lung expands when the diver surfaces.

To overcome some of the dangers of breath-hold diving, modern equipment provides for respiration with continuous increased airway pressure, permitting much longer and deeper exposures. Under these circumstances, many of the problems cited below in the discussion of hyperbaric environments become relevant.

Preparation of artificial spaces under water has frequently resulted in the requirement of increased pressure, for example, when compressed air is used to exclude water during construction work in underwater caissons and tunnels. Although conventional submersion in submarines and similar vessels does not normally expose occupants to an elevation of atmospheric pressure, recent use of very deep-sea vessels has required pressurization.[39,41] Much of our knowledge of the body's responses to high-pressure environments is the result of high-pressure chambers used for experimental simulation of depth.

Early studies of diving under pressurized conditions encountered several important problems: (a) difficulty with adequate extraction of carbon dioxide from the respired gases in a closed environment; (b) high partial pressures of oxygen resulting in oxygen toxicity; (c) inert gas narcosis; and (d) decompression sickness.

Carbon Dioxide Removal. Under normal conditions, adequate alveolar ventilation meets the demands of both carbon dioxide removal and oxygen uptake. The virtual absence of carbon dioxide from the earth's atmosphere conveniently permits alveolar ventilation to be adjusted to the lowest level that will provide optimal oxygenation. Within a closed environment, however, higher levels of oxygen may be present, owing either to compression of atmospheric gases or to supplementation of oxygen, so that the available oxygen is markedly increased. On the other hand, if carbon dioxide removal is not complete, it will gradually accumulate in the environment. Such accumulation of even relatively small amounts of carbon dioxide (e.g., 0.2% at 5 atmospheres of pressure) would result in an increase in inspired P_{CO_2} of 8 mm. Hg, with the appropriately increased stimulation to ventilation. The effectiveness of atmospheric carbon dioxide removal systems would, of course, be even more critical at depths of 30 atmospheres or greater.

Oxygen Toxicity. At depths where the pressure is 2 to 3 atmospheres, the partial pressure of oxygen rises to from 300 to 500 mm. Hg. This is probably relatively safe even for prolonged periods. At greater depths, however, the partial pressure of oxygen begins to rise excessively. Grand mal epilepsy was first recognized as a central nervous system manifestation of oxygen poisoning in the late nineteenth century. Since that time, it has been well recognized that prolonged exposure to high partial pressures of oxygen, regardless of concentration, may result in numerous other manifestations of oxygen toxicity.[42,43] These include central-nervous-system excitation, seizures, and coma; production of interstitial edema, with endothelial damage and alterations in epithelial cells within the alveolar linings of the lung; and abnormalities of the red-cell membranes, resulting in hemolysis. The precise level of oxygen required to produce these effects is different in various animal species, and varies in different groups of individuals. It appears likely that partial pressures under 300 mm. Hg are not associated with detectable damage, but that increasing levels beyond this will be more likely to cause toxicity. (See Chap. 5 for a discussion of pulmonary effects of oxygen toxicity.)

Inert Gas Narcosis. The major respired gas, as indicated by volume, is nitrogen. Under normal circumstances, nitrogen does not cause any known chemical reaction in the body and is not produced or utilized by the body. The high concentration of nitrogen in the atmosphere makes it an important concern in high-pressure environments. Early experiences of divers at depths of from 5 to 10 atmospheres indicated problems arising from the high partial pressures of nitrogen. Its effects on the sensorium and performance are roughly comparable to those of alcohol and are indistinguishable from those of subanesthetic concentrations of nitrous oxide. Although marked individual susceptibility occurs, central nervous system manifestations become apparent at 4 or 5 atmospheres. Measurable effects on the electroencephalograph and impairment of function may be noted at considerably lower pressures. At pressures in excess of 10 atmospheres, virtually no one can continue to function effectively. Recent studies have established beyond doubt that other inert gases have variable effects. Substitution of helium for nitrogen in respired gases appears to avoid the narcotic effects, permitting descent to pressures of 45 atmospheres.[44]

Decompression Sickness. As a person ascends from a prolonged dive, he may develop illness characterized by muscle aches, headache, visual disturbances, and more profound alterations in cerebral function. These manifestations may be a result of the formation of bubbles in blood or tissues previously supersaturated with dissolved gas that was taken up during exposure to the high pressure. The likelihood of these bubbles forming and thus producing abnormalities of function as a result of accumulation in tissues, and interference with blood flow, is dependent on several factors. These include the solubility of the gas, the period of compression, and the rate of decompression. Because the illness associated with decompression was most commonly documented in caisson workers, it was frequently referred to as *caisson workers' disease*. The only effective method of dealing with this problem is recompression, which forces the gases back into solution, followed by more gradual decompression.[39,41] It is noteworthy that, at sea level, approximately 1 liter of nitrogen is dissolved in body fluids; however, at 2 atmospheres of pressure, approximately 2 liters are dissolved, and at 10 atmospheres, approximately 10 L. Therefore, the volume of nitrogen released is directly proportional to the partial pressure of the gas at the time of equilibration; this is the hazard of decompression illness.

In addition to the hazards posed by excessive quantities of gases dissolved at high pressure, the lungs (and other gas-filled organs) are at risk during decompression. So-called barotrauma most commonly results from a large pressure difference across the intrathoracic organs and may result in pneumothorax, pneumomediastinum, and mediastinal and interstitial emphysema in the lungs. Barotrauma in the sinuses (particularly seen in persons with obstructed sinuses during decompression) may result in mucosal damage, with pain and bleeding. The eardrums are occasionally injured by the same mechanism.[45]

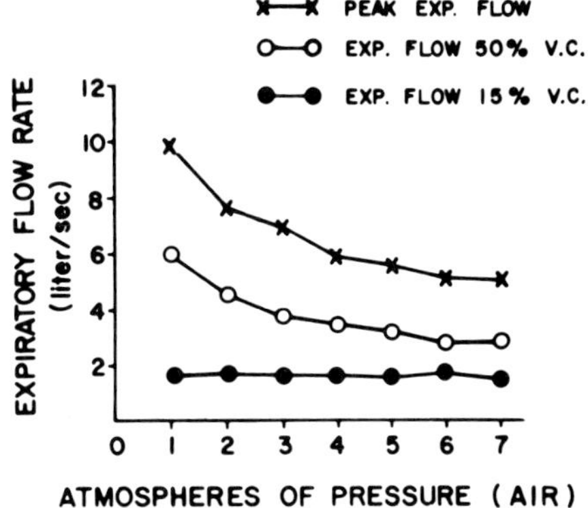

Fig. 1-5. Effect of increased atmospheric pressure on maximum exhaled flow rates. Expiratory flow rates are plotted at ambient pressures of 1 through 7 atmospheres of air. Note that the peak expiratory flow rate of 10 l. per second at sea level is reduced to approximately 5 l. per second at 7 atmospheres of pressure. The expiratory flow rates at 50 per cent of the vital capacity are similarly reduced from 6.1 per second to 2.8 l. per second at 7 atmospheres of pressure. Since the peak flow rate is substantially limited by turbulence, it is not surprising that the increase in density of the gases, as the result of increasing atmospheric pressure, provides increased resistance to flow. Substitution of the low-density gas, helium for nitrogen, in respired gases results in flow rates that are maintained at a much higher level at these atmospheric pressures. The observation that the flow rate at 15 per cent vital capacity is relatively unchanged by increasing atmospheric pressure supports the concept that flow is predominantly limited at this lung volume by laminar resistance rather than turbulent resistance. (Adapted from Overfield, E. M., Saltzman, H. A., Kylstra, J. A., and Salzano, J. V.: Respiratory gas exchange in normal men breathing 0.9% oxygen in helium at 31.3 atmospheres absolute. J. Appl. Physiol., 27:471, 1969,[46] and Wood, L. D. H., and Bryan, A. C.: Effect of increased ambient pressure on flow-volume curve of the lung. J. Appl. Physiol., 27:4, 1969[49])

Effect of Increased Atmospheric Pressure on Lung Function. The resistance to air flow in the bronchial tubes is determined by the caliber of the tubes, turbulence, and viscosity. Thus, it is clear that increased density of the gases affects the resistance to air flow, and therefore may modify the maximum flow rate that can be achieved. As illustrated in Figure 1-5, the peak expiratory air flow and the maximum expiratory flow at 50 per cent of vital capacity decrease progressively when the atmospheric pressure is increased from 1 to 7 atmospheres. The greatest change takes place in the range of 1 to 4 atmospheres. These limitations of air flow, when the density of a gas is increased due to a high barometric pressure, are entirely predictable and also occur with changes in density of gas as a result of a high molecular weight. Similarly, the density may be decreased by substitution of low-molecular-weight gases (for example, helium).[46-49]

Thus, it is perhaps fortuitous that the inert gas helium can be utilized in high-pressure environments, with several distinct advantages: (a) it is less soluble than nitrogen, so that body stores of the gas are diminished, and decompression can take place more rapidly; (b) it has a lower molecular weight, and therefore the rate of diffusion and elimination is increased; and (c) the density is markedly decreased, as compared with nitrogen, thus resulting in improved air flow within the bronchial tubes. Consequently, by substituting helium for nitrogen, ventilatory resistance is minimized, even at very high atmospheric pressures. Studies performed at 33.1 atmospheres of barometric pressure, with gases containing 99.1 per cent helium and 0.9 per cent oxygen, indicate that the density of the respiratory gases is 4.4 times the density of air at 1 atmosphere, and that the impairment of respiratory flow is comparable to that seen at a pressure of 4.4 atmospheres with normal atmospheric gases. Although a slight decrease in respiratory rate and an increase in tidal volume may occur under these circumstances, in order to overcome the increase in resistance to breathing, no clear evidence of significantly increased work of breathing is apparent in resting subjects. It is noteworthy that several individuals have had an increase in arterial carbon dioxide during exercise at these depths, and this may represent an adaptation by the body to the increased work of breathing. Certainly, normal subjects develop diminished ventilatory response to carbon dioxide when the airways' resistance is increased, and patients with sustained elevations of airway resistance frequently develop increased arterial carbon dioxide levels. Normal subjects studied at pressures of 4 atmospheres have been shown to have decreased ventilatory response to carbon dioxide.[50]

As a result of these observations, it has become conventional to develop gas combinations that seem optimally suited to the body's requirements. Generally, the oxygen partial pressure is maintained at approximately 200 mm. Hg, carefully avoiding the problems of oxygen toxicity. Methods of elimination of carbon dioxide are incorporated, with continuous monitoring of the respired atmosphere for traces of the carbon dioxide. The balance of the gas in the atmosphere is made up of helium. Recent studies, predominantly carried out in pressure chambers as part of the United States Navy Sea Lab Operation, have demonstrated the ability of man to function at a barometric pressure of 45 atmospheres (1,500 feet below seal level).[45] Healthy men, under these conditions, show no important changes in minute ventilation, tidal volume, oxygen consumption, carbon dioxide production, or alveolar gas exchange. They are able to function normally, including performance of exercise, at least for short periods, under these atmospheric conditions.

It is anticipated that the intrigue of underwater exploration will necessitate the development of increasingly efficient and safe environments for hyperbaric conditions. Many of the above generalizations regarding body responses may be modified after experience has been extended beyond the few selected and highly trained experimental subjects that have been studied up to now. Offshore oil explorations may be expected to stimulate great advances in the technology of underwater hyperbaric physiology. In any event, these exploratory data would support the concept that man is capable of enormous modification of his environment, to provide a unique and life-sustaining microenvironment under high barometric pressures.

Breathing Liquid Atmospheres

Some lines of evidence in history suggest that all mammalian origins occurred within aqueous environments. Certainly, the variety of animals capable of respiration in fluid environments today is ample evidence that with an appropriate fluid, and adequate exchanging surfaces, fresh- or seawater may serve as a perfectly acceptable source of respiratory gases. Small wonder that the prospect of a liquid medium has attracted mass interest. In 1962, in a talk entitled "Of Mice as Fish,"[51] Kylstra described the survival of mice in a saline environment specially prepared by oxygenation with hyperbaric oxygen.

The desirability of breathing liquids has several applications to humans. The possibilities of improved versatility during underwater exploration, submarine escape, and improved respiration in diseases where surface tension of the lung lining is severely altered, have encouraged the search for an optimal liquid.[52-55] Obvious problems can be recognized. The viscosity of fluids is greater than that of air; therefore, maximum ventilation rates would be altered. For example, the viscosity of saline solution is approximately 40 times that of air, and therefore a person with a maximum ventilatory rate of 200 liters per minute in air would be expected to have a maximum ventilatory rate of only 5 liters per minute in saline solution. It is not surprising, then, that resting animals breathing liquid have very low minute ventilations.[52] Ventilation with air is characterized by gas exchange in which diffusion of gases takes place along pressure gradients, but the gradients are largely maintained by ventilation and perfusion of the lungs. Thus, environmental gas is drawn into the tracheobronchial tree and alveolar spaces by convection. Then, to a small degree, diffusion within the alveolar space, and, to a much larger degree, diffusion across the alveolar membranes, results in transfer of gas into the blood. Under normal circumstances, the exchange of gas, then, is limited by convective forces. In the liquid environment, on the other hand, particularly with the low alveolar ventilation as a result of increased viscosity while breathing liquid, the gas exchange takes place predominantly by diffusion.

The technical complexities of providing ventilation with saline solution that has been hyperbarically oxygenated make this totally impractical. As a result, the search has been undertaken for a more suitable liquid. Such a liquid should have a high solubility for both oxygen and carbon dioxide, but at the same time should permit very rapid diffusion. Since the minute ventilation would be expected to be reduced as a result of the viscosity of the fluid, a very high solubility for oxygen would result in a high oxygen content in the inspired liquid and, consequently, an adequate arterial Po_2. The reduced alveolar ventilation would result in marked accumulation of carbon dioxide. Increases in arterial Pco_2, however, are limited biologically. Therefore, an appropriate combination of high solubility for carbon dioxide and rapid diffusion of carbon dioxide appear necessary for optimal transfer and removal of gases from the lungs.

At present, particular emphasis has been focused on fluorocarbon liquids. Several varieties have been developed that appear to be almost biologically inert, are immiscible with aqueous media, have very high solubility for oxygen and carbon dioxide, and permit survival following the period of breathing the liquids. Dogs and rodents have demonstrated that these liquids support life for 1 to 3 hours of breathing the liquid.[52] The solutions are oxygenated by bubbling oxygen through the liquid, and the animal is liquid ventilated by immersion or by a respirator. The solutions contain up to 31 volumes per cent of oxygen at 37° C. (more oxygen than is carried by equal volumes of blood), but in general, over a period of time, carbon dioxide accumulates, with marked increases in blood carbon dioxide and respiratory acidosis. These changes are attributable to hypoventilation, but in view of the difficulties with viscosity of the fluids, it is unlikely that they can be overcome by increasing ventilation. It is more likely that increased diffusion rates and altered solubility of carbon dioxide will be necessary as solutions are developed further. These liquids generally have very low surface tension and thus are very effective in wetting all surfaces that they contact. Initially, following a period during which these fluorocarbons were inhaled, the animal tended to have an altered respiratory pattern, and significant arterial hypoxemia. This persisted for days to weeks, but eventually the lungs appeared to be restored to normal. During the early phase after breathing fluorocarbon liquids, there was a considerable increase in numbers of alveolar macrophages and occasional evidence of disruption of alveolar walls, which may have been related to the mechanical trauma of artificial ventilation. The histological abnormalities also improved to normal within 3 weeks. In in-vitro and in-vivo experiments, there has been no evidence of alteration of the surface linings of the lungs; in fact, the elastic properties of the lungs and the surface tension characteristics of lung extracts appear to remain normal.[55] The application to humans of breathing liquids remains to be explored.

If a liquid can be developed that is capable of transporting large quantities of respiratory gases, it might also be used as a blood substitute to transport oxygen and carbon dioxide.[53] Fluorocarbon emulsions have been demonstrated to support life by transporting oxygen and carbon dioxide in the circulatory system of animals.

Table 1-6. Atmospheric Gases

Nitrogen	78.08%
Oxygen	20.95%
Argon	0.93%
Carbon dioxide	0.033%
Neon	18 ppm
Helium	5 ppm
Methane	2.0 ppm
Krypton	1.0 ppm
Hydrogen	0.5 ppm
Nitrous oxide	0.5 ppm
Xenon	0.09 ppm
Sulfur dioxide	0.1 ppm
Nitrogen dioxide	0–0.02 ppm
NH_3	Trace
Ozone	0.07 ppm (winter) 0.02 ppm (summer)

(Adapted from Altman, P. L., and Dittmer, D. S.: Biological Handbooks. Environmental Biology. p. 269. Federation of the American Society of Experimental Biologists, 1966[38])

Atmospheric Components With Adverse Effects

In general, the gases in the atmosphere are present in predictable concentations, as illustrated in Table 1-6. As reviewed previously, the concentration of oxygen appears to be very stable indeed, in spite of the extensive utilization by combustion of fossil fuels. The concentration of carbon dioxide, on the other hand, has demonstrated measurable changes since the beginning of the nineteenth century; it is thought to have increased from 0.029 per cent in 1900 to the present level of 0.033 per cent as a result of fuel combustion. The other gases appear to be present in relatively stable concentrations in the environment in general.

Many of the gases listed in Table 1-6, and others, may be present in much higher concentrations as a result of special circumstances. In recent years, the presence of significantly increased concentrations of gases or particles in the atmosphere, above generally accepted levels of normal, has come to be known as "air pollution." In present use, this is a sociopolitical term, and not one that can always be associated with scientific evidence of adverse effects.

Altered composition of atmospheric contents generally may be considered in the context of either gases or aerosols (particulate). Many changes in atmospheric composition have no demonstrable adverse effects; furthermore, those adverse effects that are recognized may be related to nonhuman biological changes in plants and vegetables, effects on inanimate objects such as buildings and other structures, or biological effects involving human and animal life. For example, sulfur dioxide at a concentration of 0.5 parts per million for 4 hours results in demonstrable injury to numerous vegetables, including alfalfa, lettuce, rhubarb, and spinach. Concentrations in excess of 1.5 parts per million produce similar injury in periods of an hour or more. In contrast, citrus fruits are resistant to sulfur dioxide. Many of these biological effects have been reviewed, and new information is acquired rapidly as a result of the renewed societal interest in this area.[56-60]

In addition to direct effects on structure and function of plants and animals and corrosive and destructive processes involving inanimate objects, an indirect, major effect of pollution is change in visibility. This may have important effects on daily sunshine and on aircraft operations, but to many persons, it is more impressive because of its esthetic effects.

Gaseous Pollution. *Carbon Monoxide.* This is the most common air pollutant when measured in tonnage and exceeds the amount of all other contaminants added together. Some estimates indicate that the annual world emission is about 250 million tons, and the estimated annual emission of carbon monoxide in the United States is more than 100 million tons. Although the major emission is from the combustion of fuels (in gasoline-powered engines), industrial processes and miscellaneous sources such as forest fires contribute 25 to 30 per cent. Many factors affect the carbon monoxide production of a gasoline engine. The average emission rates listed in Table 1-7 represent random vehicles in city driving, at an average speed of 25 miles per hour. Emission rates, however, vary widely with the size of the engine, the speed of operation, the environmental temperature, and, to a certain extent, the fuel. Furthermore, recent advances have permitted the modification of the emission by altering combustion temperature, the air-to-fuel ratio, and other factors. The level of carbon monoxide in the regional environment, thus, is totally dependent on the sources. In a city, high concentrations of carbon monoxide would be anticipated in areas of high traffic density. Atmospheric conditions may influence the rate of dispersion of pollutants. Temperature inversions, in which cold air immediately on the earth's surface is sealed in by a layer of warm air above, limit the escape of gases into the surrounding atmosphere.

Carbon monoxide accumulation would be expected to be a greater problem in areas where wind is minimal, in poorly ventilated buildings, and in heated or enclosed parking lots in northern climates. Values under 30 parts per million are generally conceded to be safe biologically, even for prolonged periods of time; 50 parts per million may be associated with certain biological hazards. The odorless and colorless nature of the gas permits it to accumulate undetected.

Table 1-7. Emission of Pollutants from Motor-Vehicle Gasoline Engines*

Carbon monoxide	2,400 lb./1,000 gal.
Nitrogen oxide	185 lb./1,000 gal.
Hydrocarbons	132 lb./1,000 gal.
Particulates	11 lb./1,000 gal.
Sulfur dioxide	9 lb./1,000 gal.
Organic acids	7 lb./1,000 gal.
Aldehydes	4 lb./1,000 gal.

*Average emission rates from vehicles, in two large cities, driving at speeds of about 25 miles per hour. (Adapted from Altman, P. L., and Dittmer, D. S.: Biological Handbooks. Environmental Biology. Federation of the American Society of Experimental Biologists, 1966[56])

Urban populations may be exposed to average carbon monoxide levels of 9 to 15 parts per million at street level, with peak levels of 30 to 60 parts per million.[61] In enclosed parkades, we have observed levels of 50 to 150 parts per million commonly, with occasional peak traffic levels as high as 400 parts per million. High-rise buildings with no air conditioning demonstrate higher levels at street level than in upper floors, and buildings with air-conditioning intakes in the upper floors have lower carbon monoxide levels than those with intakes at street level. Buildings heated with oil burners have higher carbon monoxide levels than those with gas or electric heat. It is noteworthy that a common cause of carbon monoxide poisoning in northern climates is the poorly ventilated tent or camper heated by a low-heat gas or oil heater.

Fortunately, there has not been a demonstrable accumulation of carbon monoxide in the atmosphere at large. This indicates that the massive quantities of carbon monoxide being dumped into the atmosphere are in some way also being removed. It has not been established by what method carbon monoxide removal occurs, but some recent experiments suggest that soil bacteria are capable of removing carbon monoxide from the air above the soil and thus act as a carbon-monoxide sink. If this mechanism is in effect and is capable of recycling, it is unlikely that carbon monoxide will be a major hazard in terms of general atmospheric pollution.

The most predictable and common cause of carbon monoxide inhalation is cigarette smoking. Smoking a single cigarette measurably modifies the level of carbon monoxide in the alveolar gas and in the circulating blood. Thus, the average city dweller may have an increase of 1 to 2 per cent in carbon monoxide in his blood as a result of the general atmospheric pollution, but the two- to three-pack-per-day cigarette smoker may have levels as high as 10 per cent in his blood. The biological effect is of equal importance regardless of the source.

Several studies have emphasized the increased risk of carbon monoxide toxicity in the cigarette smoker who is also exposed to otherwise mild elevations in environmental carbon monoxide levels.[62-64] When restricted to poorly ventilated areas, even the nonsmoker is at risk from the carbon monoxide generated by the smoker. In one study of subjects in a cigarette-smoke-filled room, carboxyhemoglobin levels of nonsmokers increased from 1.6 to 2.6 per cent, whereas the levels of smokers increased from 5.9 to 9.6 per cent.[65] It has been estimated that cigarette smoke contains up to 5 per cent carbon monoxide. Samples of taxicabs with smoking drivers have documented levels as high as 90 parts per million. In general, both pipe and cigar smokers have lower levels of inhaled carbon monoxide.

Endogenous sources of carbon monoxide as a by-product of porphyrin metabolism produce negligible levels when compared with exogenous exposures. The average healthy adult produces about 0.4 ml. of carbon monoxide per hour, and this value increases in diseases with an increased rate of red-blood-cell breakdown.

Adverse effects of carbon monoxide are under vigorous investigation. Its interference with oxygen transport in the blood is well understood. Other potential effects of less severe exposure may include accelerated development of atherosclerosis and decreased fetal growth rate.

The best-understood adverse effect of carbon monoxide is its interference with oxygen transport in the body. Oxygen binds reversibly with hemoglobin in order to provide adequate transport of oxygen in the blood. Carbon monoxide has a much greater affinity (210 times) for hemoglobin than does oxygen. As a consequence, small amounts of carbon monoxide, when in equilibrium with the blood, result in relatively high concentrations of carboxyhemoglobin.

The relationship of inhaled carbon monoxide to carboxyhemoglobin is predictable. It is described over a wide range of inhaled concentrations by the equation:

$$\text{Carboxyhemoglobin (\%)} = 0.35 \times \text{carbon monoxide}^{0.8} \text{ (ppm)}.$$

For concentrations of less than 100 parts per million, this simpler equation may be used[66]:

$$\text{Carboxyhemoglobin (\%)} = 0.16 \times \text{carbon monoxide (ppm)}.$$

This equation applies only to equilibrium conditions, when the carbon monoxide levels are stable, and the gas has been inhaled long enough. At low levels of carbon monoxide and at resting levels of alveolar ventilation, it may require 4 to 8 hours to reach equilibrium. The rate of equilibration is increased when minute ventilation is increased.[67] Table 1-8 compares the levels of carboxyhemoglobin that occur at various levels of inhaled carbon monoxide. Note that the increased ventilation associated with exercise results in higher levels of carboxyhemoglobin after 2 hours, reflecting more complete equilibration of respired gases with the blood. Even this exercise value, however, does not represent complete equilibration. The time necessary for equilibration has been worked out for a wide range of inspired carbon monoxide levels.[67,68]

Table 1-8. Effects of Exposure to Carbon Monoxide for 2 Hours

CO Concentration Inhaled (ppm)	*COHb in Blood of Sedentary Subject* %	*COHb in Blood with Light Exercise* %
20	1.25	2.5
40	2.0	4.0
70	3.8	7.6
100	5.0	10.0
200	10.0	20.0

(Adapted from Bates, D. V.: A Citizen's Guide to Air Pollution. Montreal, McGill-Queen's University Press, 1972[58])

The adverse effects of carbon monoxide on the living organism are summarized below. There is some evidence in humans for most of the characteristics, and substantial evidence in various animal models. Impairment of oxygen delivery is of questionable significance in normal individuals below levels of 5 per cent. Minor alterations in sensory function, however, as indicated by impaired judgment of duration of a tone,[69] and a deficit in "careful-driving" skills have been reported[70] at levels below 5 per cent carboxyhemoglobin. In the range between 5 and 10 per cent carboxyhemoglobin, more definite alterations in perception and mental agility are demonstrable,[71] and in the range of 10 to 20 per cent carboxyhemoglobin, headaches, nausea, and decreased mental acuity occur. As carboxyhemoglobin levels increase beyond this, approaching 50 per cent, coma eventually develops, and carboxyhemoglobin levels above 50 per cent are commonly associated with permanent cerebral damage or death.

The oxygen transport system is affected in several ways. The binding of carbon monoxide to hemoglobin displaces oxygen, thus leaving less hemoglobin available for oxygen transport. In addition, the remaining hemoglobin is altered in such a way that oxygen is bound with greater affinity, thus decreasing the release of oxygen at tissue levels. The net effect, of course, is to decrease the tissue partial pressure of oxygen in order to facilitate extraction of oxygen from the circulating blood. In chronic carbon monoxide exposure, the hypoxia results in an erythropoietic response, and measurable increases in the red-cell mass occur.[72]

Not only does carbon monoxide bind to hemoglobin, but it binds to other porphyrin groups in the body, including myoglobin and the cytochrome oxidase system. These latter groups have a much lower affinity for carbon monoxide than does hemoglobin, and in general are considered of less importance in relation to carbon monoxide toxicity.

In early studies, it was thought that carbon monoxide exposure resulted in injury to lung tissues. Recently, it has been demonstrated that reduced arterial Po_2 may occur due to modifications in gas exchange in the lungs as a result of the altered oxyhemoglobin dissociation curve.[73] As a result, patients with ventilation and perfusion imbalance who have arterial hypoxemia develop much more profound hypoxemia when their hemoglobin is partly bound to carbon monoxide. No

Adverse Effects of Carbon Monoxide

Normal Persons

1. Decreased oxygen delivery
   a. Less oxygen bound to hemoglobin
   b. Increased affinity of remaining hemoglobin for oxygen with impaired release at the tissue level
   c. Increased red-cell mass
2. Interference with oxygen binding to myoglobin and cytochrome oxidase system
3. Possible increase in atherosclerosis
4. Reduced birth weight and increased neonatal mortality

Persons With Cardiac Disease

1. Anaerobic myocardial metabolism
2. Increased mortality from myocardial infarction
3. Angina pectoris and intermittent claudication at lower levels of exercise

demonstrable change in the alveolar membrane is apparent in experimental exposure to carbon monoxide in moderate concentrations.

Experimental studies[74] and some evidence in humans[75] have shown an increase in atherosclerotic lesions in the vascular system after exposure to carbon monoxide. The authors of the animal studies have postulated that prolonged exposure to low levels of carbon monoxide result in increased permeability of vascular endothelium. This increased permeability may result in increased deposition of lipids in the vascular wall, with the development of earlier atherosclerosis. In humans, it was demonstrated that the increased incidence of coronary artery disease was related more directly to carboxyhemoglobin levels in the smokers than to the actual smoking history. Whether the findings of these early exploratory studies will be borne out by additional, more vigorous analysis is uncertain.

The demonstration that the infants of women who smoked during pregnancy had a higher rate of neonatal death and lower birth weights raised the possibility that carbon monoxide was the offending agent. Studies performed on animals with moderate carbon monoxide exposure have demonstrated substantial decreases in birth weight and increases in neonatal mortality. This relationship also requires much further study before it can be established.[76] As might be anticipated, persons with preexisting disease that limits oxygen delivery to specific tissues may demonstrate adverse effects of carbon monoxide at levels lower than those that produce measurable changes in normal subjects. Thus, it was demonstrated that anaerobic myocardial metabolism increased in patients with coronary disease at carboxyhemoglobin concentrations as low as 6 per cent.[77] It is anticipated that other manifestations of disease may be more prominent in such persons. Angina pectoris has been difficult to assess but may be increased when the carboxyhemoglobin concentration is increased to less than 3 per cent.[78] Few detailed studies of patients with hypoxemia related to pulmonary disease are available, but it would be surprising if these persons were not more susceptible to the effects of carboxyhemoglobin, as are persons who are hypoxic at high altitude and as a result of anemia.

Epidemiological studies suggest that the fatality rate due to myocardial infarction is increased in persons from high-pollution areas. It is likely that a high level of carbon monoxide adversely affects the prognosis of patients suffering myocardial infarctions.[79]

Acute carbon monoxide poisoning may result in demonstrable evidence of tissue hypoxia, ranging from mild alterations in cerebral function to clear-cut evidence of cellular damage in the central nervous system, heart muscle, skeletal muscle, liver, peripheral nerves, and skin. Biochemical evidence of anaerobic metabolism, as reflected by metabolic acidosis and lactic acid accumulation, is present in severe acute toxicity.

The management of acute carbon monoxide poisoning follows entirely from its known effects on oxygen transport. First the subject must be removed from the environment. Obviously, the urgency of the situation is dictated by the degree of impairment. Mild degrees of intoxication are quickly improved by removal from the environment and the addition of supplemental oxygen. More severe degrees of intoxication require immediate institution of high inhaled oxygen therapy. When available in the ambulance or hospital, hyperbaric oxygenation should be immediately instituted. When this is not available, 100 per cent oxygen should be administered. Traditional physiological thinking and early experiments suggested that, since the carbon monoxide was present in small concentrations, it would not affect alveolar or arterial Po_2 and, therefore, would not interfere with the normal respiratory control mechanisms (which act partially through the effect of partial pressure of oxygen on the peripheral chemoreceptors). It is now commonly recognized, however, that sufficient reduction in arterial Po_2 is present to increase the respiratory drive in the majority of patients. This hypoxemia may be the result of central nervous system depression, causing prolonged immobilization and ventilation-perfusion imbalance in the lungs. This is particularly likely because most victims of carbon monoxide poisoning have developed severe central nervous system depression quite gradually. Thus, the use of supplemental oxygen overcomes the low arterial Po_2, increases dissolved oxygen in the blood, and increases the rate of displacement of carbon monoxide from the hemoglobin.

The washout of carbon monoxide, like the initial accumulation of carbon monoxide in the blood, is dependent on the minute ventilation.[67,80] Inhalation of carbon dioxide may be utilized in order to drive ventilation and thus further increase the rate of washout. If adequate ventilation is maintained, however, spontaneously or by an artificial respirator, in the presence of 100 per cent oxygen the carbon monoxide levels of most subjects quickly reduce to a safer range.[67,68] Normal men, breathing ordinary air will have an average half-time of carbon monoxide elimination of about 250 minutes; if oxygen is substituted, this is reduced to 40 minutes, and if 5 to 7 per cent carbon dioxide is added, the half-time is further reduced.

Sulfur Dioxide. Sulfur dioxide, which is normally virtually absent from the atmosphere, is a product of burning fuels containing sulfur. The most common source is the burning of coal and oil. Consequently, this, too, is predominantly a problem of urban "progress." Both sulfur dioxide and sulfur trioxide are released, and when dissolved in water, they form sulfurous- and sulfuric acid. Sulfur dioxide is commonly oxidized in the air, in association with particles, to form sulfur trioxide. It is not surprising then, that sulfur dioxide ultimately has major effects on inanimate substances, such as increased rate of corrosion of metals; substantial deterioration and discoloration of limestone, marble, and slate; and damage to textile fibers, including cotton, rayon, and nylon. Sulfur dioxide can be detected by most persons by taste, rather than odor, at concentrations in the range of 0.3 to 1.0 parts per million. For most persons, the odor threshold appears to be about 0.5 parts per million. At levels of 10 to 25 parts per million, substantial irritation of mucous membranes is experienced.[57] Recent processes for eliminating and reclaiming sulfur from fuel oils have been very effective in reducing the emission of sulfur dioxide when combustion of these fuels occurs. Studies of oil refinery workers in Persia exposed for 1 to 19 years with levels commonly as high as 25 parts per million and, on occasion, as high as 100 parts per million, failed to demonstrate evidence of chronic systemic effects. On the other hand, paper pulp workers in Norway exposed to SO_2 levels of 2 to 36 parts per million showed increased frequency of cough, expectoration, and dyspnea on exertion, and reduced maximum expiratory flow rates. It is now accepted that the adverse effects of sulfur dioxide on the respiratory tract are potentiated by environmental factors such as humidity, and are additive in the presence of other preexisting diseases.[57] In relation to the latter factor, most epidemiological studies that demonstrate increased morbidity and mortality in relation to sulfur dioxide pollution indicate that the cigarette smoker is much more susceptible to sulfur dioxide than the nonsmoker. Furthermore, during times of peak air pollution in London, New York, and Chicago, excessive mortality rates were correlated with a rise in sulfur-dioxide smog levels. In a recent air pollution peak in New York City, an increase of from 0.2 to 0.4 parts per million was associated with an increase in morbidity and mortality. The population at greatest risk appears to be elderly persons with chronic bronchitis or emphysema. Substantial evidence also suggests that patients with true bronchial asthma have increased morbidity and mortality at times of increased sulfur dioxide levels. The latter group has, on occasion, been shown to be susceptible to acute attacks, particularly when exposed to levels of sulfur dioxide above the odor-detection threshold.[81] Recently, excessive acute respiratory disease, including laryngotracheobronchitis, has been reported in children and adults with increased levels of sulfur dioxide.[82]

The pulmonary effects of sulfur dioxide inhalation have been well defined during acute, high-level exposures.[83-85] Increased airway resistance in the bronchial tubes is reflected in decreased respiratory air-flow rates. Although 10 to 15 parts per million are generally required to produce perceptible mucosal irritation, the mechanism of the bronchoconstriction has not been established; it is possible that irritation of airway mucous membranes results in reflex increase in bronchial muscle tone. Mucociliary activity is demonstrably impaired by 10 to 20 parts per million sulfur dioxide, but it should be recalled that this is far in excess of the 0.5 part per million commonly present during peak pollution periods.

No conclusive evidence is available to support actual histological pulmonary damage from the low levels of sulfur dioxide commonly present as an urban pollutant, and no completely satisfactory data are available to substantiate long-term tissue injury.

Oxides of Nitrogen. Combustion occurring under pressure and with heat is likely to result in the fixation of nitrogen and oxygen, which are normal constituents of air. Initially, most commonly, nitrous oxide is produced, but this quickly becomes oxidized in the atmosphere to become the more irritant nitrogen dioxide. When dissolved, this of course produces the highly corrosive H_2NO_3. The major source of nitrogen dioxide in the environment is fuel combustion, particularly coal and natural gas, and a close runner-up is the production of NO_2 by combustion of gasoline in motor vehicles. In general, the oxides of nitrogen do not achieve high concentrations; the average monthly urban concentrations range from 0.04 to 0.14 part per million, with peak concentrations rarely exceeding 0.5 part per million. Thus, it is uncommon to achieve concentrations that can be demonstrated to cause direct irritation to the tracheobronchial tree. The commonly cited measured concentration in cities with populations of more than 500,000 persons is 0.06 part per million. There is some evidence that this may be associated with an increase in respiratory symptoms, though this is not entirely certain.[57-59] Animal experiments have demonstrated histological abnormalities suggesting early emphysema and injury to terminal bronchioles, after prolonged exposure to nitrogen dioxide.

Hydrocarbons. Twenty-six aromatic hydrocarbons have been identified in the air in several urban areas of the United States. These are produced primarily by automobiles, and the principal compound is methane, which may average 3 parts per million in urban air. Other alkanes and alkenes are produced, and much of the smell of diesel and gasoline exhaust is thought to be the result of the presence of aldehydes. Fortunately, the biological effects of these substances seem to be predominantly related to changes in vegetation, and ethylene appears to have the most direct effect on certain forms of plant life. Small amounts of polycyclic hydrocarbons have been identified, including benzopyrene, which is of particular interest because of its experimentally demonstrated capacity to induce cancer. Concentrations are usually very low, and the measurements are not readily performed.[57-59]

Ozone. See below under photochemical smog.

Particulate Pollution. Soil, dust, and naturally air-borne particles will not be considered in this section. Their role as a health hazard is almost totally unexplored. We refer here to solid or liquid matter suspended in air (called *aerosols*).[86] These are comprised of a wide variety of substances with one common feature: a submicron size. Large particulate matter originating as dust from windswept fields tends to be readily deposited due to its size (in the range of 1 to 10 microns). Smaller particles (less than 1 micron), however, tend to remain suspended for prolonged periods. Thus, these may be suspended in air for periods of several months under suitable meteorologic conditions. Because of their widely diversified nature, such particulates have varying consequences. The sources of particulate emission are multiple, but major urban sources include combustion from space heaters, incineration processes (either commercial or individual), motor-vehicle exhaust, and a variety of sources such as brake linings of vehicles, construction work, road repairs, and so forth. These widely divergent sources of particles contain many common materials, such as carbon and silicon, but also a wide range of metals, such as cadmium, chromium, copper, iron, lead (particularly from leaded gasolines), manganese, nickel, and many others. In addition, asbestos and beryllium play some role. The pulmonary effects of these specific pollutants will be discussed in Chapter 12.

It is of considerable concern that particulate pollution in the urban areas now occurs in the presence of gaseous pollution. Although it has not been clearly established, the possibility that irritant gases may be adsorbed to particles and thus deposited in the lungs, with high local concentrations in the lung tissue, is a very real concern.[57-59]

The most important single particulate emitted from the automobile appears to be lead. At present, it has been estimated that approximately 180,000 tons of lead are emitted into the atmosphere in the United States annually as a result of motor-vehicle exhaust. Although little definite evidence of lead toxicity (from this source) has been demonstrated in humans, current studies suggest that the lead has been incorporated into vegetation, which is ultimately consumed by humans, where it may accumulate and the well-recognized deleterious effects of lead become manifest. Current efforts to severely limit the use of leaded gasolines may be early enough to avert some of these consequences.

The adverse effects of particulate pollution may be categorized as follows[57]:

Effects on Health. At the present state of our knowledge, the aerosols are recognized more as potential health hazards than as definite health hazards. The absorption of noxious gases, and the body reactions to deposition of very small particles deep in the tracheobronchial tree all represent areas of concern.

Effects on Visibility. Air-borne particles in smog reduce visibility by scattering and absorbing light. Such particulate pollution occasionally requires restriction of aircraft operations. The effects on visibility may be a result of "dust" smog or photochemical smog. These circumstances might be anticipated only in densely populated metropolitan areas; however, the beautiful city of Calgary, Alberta, with a population of less than half a million persons, located in the foothills of the Canadian Rocky Mountains, has frequent periods of distinct haze, occurring during days in which there is a temperature inversion.

Effects on Materials. Substantial evidence has been accumulated showing that the corrosiveness of sulfur dioxide and nitrogen dioxide are increased when adsorbed to particulate material.

Undesirable Odor Sources. These refer particularly to motor exhausts, street-paving asphalts, and trash burning.

Effects on Direct Sunlight. At concentrations ranging from 100 to 150 micrograms per cubic meter, where large smoke-turbidity factors persist, particles reduce direct sunlight up to one-third in summer and two-thirds in winter in the middle and high latitudes. The color of sunsets is changed by particulates.

Effects on Climate. The scattering and adsorption of sunlight by airborne particulates reduces the amount of sunlight reaching the ground. Total sunlight is reduced 50 per cent for each doubling of the concentration above 100 micrograms per cubic meter, and this reduction is most pronounced for ultraviolet radiation.

Photochemical Smog. This most commonly occurs in the environment as a result of secondary effects on pollutants exhausted from gasoline engines. In this circumstance, quantities of oxides of nitrogen and hydrocarbons discharged into the air in the presence of intense sunlight and under still-air conditions may result in a series of reactions by which secondary products are formed. The major effect is the production of ozone, which apparently is formed at an accelerated rate in the presence of hydrocarbons or carbon monoxide. Thus, the production of the ozone is frequently delayed substantially after the initial emission of the pollutants necessary for its formation. Although high concentrations of ozone have not been found in most cities, Los Angeles, for example, has measured 0.5 part per million for short periods. The precise noxious effects of ozone and the critical levels that produce them have not been established, but experimental emphysema has been demonstrated to occur in the presence of modest levels of ozone, and ozone is an intensely irritating gas. Men exercising in an environment of 0.7 part per million of ozone experience irritation of the windpipe. Levels of 0.37 and 0.75 part per million during a 2-hour period produced evidence of airway obstruction in normal men.[87] The levels of ozone have not been well established in most urban areas, and therefore its significance as a health hazard is not clear.

Automobile Exhaust. The major emission products of automobile exhaust, as listed in Table 1-7, are carbon monoxide, oxides of nitrogen, hydrocarbons, particulates, sulfur dioxide, organic acid, and aldehydes. The emission rate is dependent on operating temperature of the combustion engine, speed of travel, and, to a certain extent, the type of fuel burned (for example, the emission rate of lead is entirely dependent on the lead content of the gasoline). Furthermore, the precise emission products are modified by recently instituted pollution-control systems that markedly reduce certain constituents.

The health effects of automobile exhaust are also determined by location. For example, carbon monoxide may accumulate in high concentrations within a motor vehicle that has an unsatisfactory exhaust system. General atmospheric pollution, however, involving carbon monoxide, oxides of nitrogen, hydrocarbons, and the products of photochemical action, predominantly ozone, has adverse effects only when these substances accumulate in sufficiently high concentrations. These factors depend on wind conditions, temperature inversions, and traffic density.

The adverse effects of carbon monoxide have been discussed under Gaseous Pollution. The oxides of nitrogen may have direct deleterious effects on the airways, as discussed previously, and, in conjunction with hydrocarbons and photochemical factors (with the production of ozone), may have direct noxious effects on the lungs. The ozone concentration may, of course, increase in the atmosphere considerably later than the peak concentrations of the pollutants, because it is produced by the action of sunlight. Among the most troublesome effects of automobile-exhaust pollution is the emission of lead by combustion of leaded gasolines. Lead is probably the pollutant with the most long-range adverse effects; however, definite documentation of human illness resulting from it has not been accumulated in substantive form. Strict legislative control has been developed for this pollutant.

Each of the major products of emission and its health hazard have been discussed above. General studies of the overall health effects of motor-vehicle exhaust have failed to demonstrate any additional effects on lung function,[88] or on safety of operation of motor vehicles.[89]

Smoking. The effects of inhaled tobacco smoke vary tremendously with the nature of the smoking device (cigarette, pipe, or cigar), the presence of a filter, the length of the tube or tobacco through which the smoke is inhaled, and the method of the smoker. Smoke produced by an average cigarette weighs about 500 mg. Five to 10 per cent of this is moist particulate matter; 12 to 15 per cent, carbon dioxide; 3 to 6 per cent, carbon monoxide; and the remainder mainly nitrogen, oxygen, and water. More than 1,200 components have been identified in tobacco smoke, predominantly residing in the particulate matter. These include nicotine and the so-called tobacco tar.[90]

Effects on the human body are also determined by the temperature of the inhaled smoke, the amount of inhalation, the depth of inhalation into the lungs, and the duration of smoking history. As a consequence, cigarette smokers in general have more severe respiratory effects than do smokers of cigars and pipes, and the number of cigarettes smoked relates directly to the health consequences. Table 1-9 indicates approximate carbon monoxide

Table 1-9. Carbon Monoxide Levels in Relation to Smoking*

Category	*CO Measured in Expired Air (ppm)*	*Carboxyhemoglobin (%)*
Nonsmoker	3.2	1.2
Smoker		
Pipe and/or cigar only	5.4	1.7
Cigarette:		
Light (less than ½ pack/day)		
Inhaler	17.1	3.8
Noninhaler	19.0	2.3
Moderate (½ to 2 packs/day)		
Inhaler	27.5	5.9
Noninhaler	14.4	3.6
Heavy (more than 2 packs/day)		
Inhaler	32.4	6.8
Noninhaler	25.2	5.6

*The carboxyhemoglobin level tends to remain fairly stable in a habitual smoker. A random blood sample is generally indicative of the approximate level through the day.[91]
(Adapted from Castleden, C., and Cole, P.: Variations in carboxyhemoglobin levels in smokers. Br. Med. J., 4:736, 1974[91])

levels for various smoking habits. So-called tumorigenic agents in tobacco are largely contained in the particulate matter, tar. The well-established carcinogenicity of tobacco tar in a variety of animal species makes this a likely offender in the production of lung cancer. Selected carcinogenic polynuclear aromatic hydrocarbons are borne in the particulate component of the smoke. The introduction of tobacco sheets and filters has led to a significant reduction in the tar and polynuclear aromatic hydrocarbons in the inhaled tobacco smoke.

The lifespan of cigarette smokers is reduced in proportion to their cigarette consumption.[92-94] In early studies, a relative death rate of 1.68 was found in cigarette smokers, compared with 1.0 in nonsmokers. Furthermore, there was a direct relationship between the amount of cigarette consumption and death rates. Thus, the one-half- to one-pack-per-day smoker had a relative death rate of 1.70 and the two-pack-per-day smoker had a rate of 2.23. Of course, these overall mortality statistics only hint at the disability and morbidity. The disability varies from minutes, in those who suffer sudden death after acute myocardial infarction, to several years of severe impairment in persons with chronic obstructive pulmonary disease. Specific health consequences of smoking continue to be elucidated. Epidemiological data provide strong circumstantial evidence for the adverse effects of smoking[95]; however, the specific mechanisms of tissue injury are not always clear.[96] The health hazard to the nonsmoker in an environment of smokers appears to be small.[97]

Smoking and Cardiovascular Diseases. The death rate from coronary heart disease and stroke is higher in smokers than in nonsmokers (Table 1-10). This higher death rate due to arteriosclerotic vascular disease has been confirmed in many studies. Furthermore, there is some evidence that the risk of sudden death is increased in individuals who are smoking at the time of a myocardial infarction and that this risk is decreased soon after the cessation of smoking cigarettes.[98] The precise mechanism of development of atherosclerosis has not been established, but as indicated in the discussion of carbon monoxide, this gas has been implicated in experimental development of ath-

Table 1-10. Mortality Ratios for Coronary Heart Disease and Stroke by Amount of Cigarette Smoking, Sex, and Age

Sex and Age	*Never Smoked Cigarettes Regularly*	*Smoked Cigarettes Regularly*			
		Number Smoked Daily			
		1–9	*10–19*	*20–39*	*40 +*
		Coronary Heart Disease			
Males					
40–49 years	1.00	1.60	2.59	3.76	5.51
50–59 years	1.00	1.59	2.13	2.40	2.79
60–69 years	1.00	1.48	1.82	1.91	1.79
70–79 years	1.00	1.14	1.41	1.49	1.47
Females					
40–49 years	1.00	1.31	2.08	3.62	3.31
50–59 years	1.00	1.15	2.37	2.68	3.73
60–69 years	1.00	1.04	1.79	2.08	2.02
70–79 years	1.00	.76	.98	1.27	—
		Stroke			
Males					
40–49 years	1.00	2.79	1.14	2.21	1.64
50–59 years	1.00	1.95	1.48	2.03	2.40
60–69 years	1.00	1.30	1.44	1.62	1.72
70–79 years	1.00	.95	.92	1.22	.68
Females					
40–49 years	1.00	1.50	2.60	2.90	5.70
50–59 years	1.00	1.26	2.70	2.67	3.52
60–69 years	1.00	1.26	2.15	1.83	—
70–79 years	1.00	.83	.57	1.28	—

erosclerosis. The potential role of nicotine has also been explored, and the effects of smoking on thrombus formation and blood flow have been considered.[95] Aggregation of platelets, increased levels of catecholamine, increased free fatty acids, and probable mobilization of polymorphonuclear leukocytes have all been demonstrated in various studies of the intravascular circulation.

Smoking and Chronic Obstructive Bronchopulmonary Disease. Studies of populations of working men in Italy, the Netherlands, England, the United States, Sweden, and Australia, all demonstrate a higher incidence of chronic obstructive lung disease in cigarette smokers as compared with nonsmokers. The precise mechanism whereby cigarette smoke produces chronic obstructive lung disease has not been entirely elucidated. Acute inhalation of cigarette smoke produces an increase in central airway resistance and a decrease in lung compliance, but it does not appear to affect the small airways of the lung.[99-101] Cigarette smoke lowers the effectiveness of pulmonary surfactant, thereby increasing the surface-tension properties of the lung lining. It exerts a powerful ciliostatic effect on the bronchial lining under some circumstances,[95] but may actually result in increased mucociliary transport under other circumstances.[102] The metabolism and function of the pulmonary alveolar macrophages and their role in clearing the lungs are impaired by cigarette smoke.[103] Each of these factors might play a role in diminishing clearance of noxious agents from the peripheral lung units, thus predisposing to disease. On the other hand, entirely separate lines of evidence indicate that in some persons, other host factors become important. Persons with hereditary alpha$_1$ globulin deficiency (alpha$_1$ antitrypsin deficiency) may lack the inhibitor that prevents proteolytic lung destruction, and they may consequently develop emphysema. This suggests that persons who inhale tobacco smoke may, in some way, increase the concentration of proteolytic enzymes near critical lung tissues and thereby develop destructive changes in the lungs. Alveolar macrophages, circulating leukocytes, and bronchial leukocytes, as a result of inflammatory reaction, all are potential sources.[104,105] It is possible that many persons have a genetic predisposition to lung injury. The pathogenesis of bronchitis and emphysema will be discussed in further detail in Chapter 13.

Smoking and Cancer. The death rate from squamous-cell carcinoma of the lung has been shown to range from 6 to 51 times as high in smokers as in nonsmokers.[92,94,106] There is strong evidence for a cumulative effect, because the cancer death rate rises steadily and markedly as the amount of smoking per day increases. Thus, the rate per 100,000 man-years is 3.4 in nonsmokers, 61 in those smoking less than a pack per day, 143 in the one- to two-packs-per-day group, and 217 for the two-or-more-packs-per-day group.[93]

Numerous changes in bronchial epithelium, including hyperplasia, stratification, atypical metaplasia, and carcinoma in situ, are more common in patients who smoke. Direct evidence regarding the specific carcinogenic component and the precise early cytologic change that constitutes neoplasia has not been established. Animal studies,[92,95] however, have provided ample evidence that certain components of cigarette smoke are potential tumorigenic factors. (See also a detailed discussion of Bronchogenic Carcinoma in Chap. 14.)

Effects of Smoking on Pregnancy. Although the total health effects of cigarette smoking on pregnancy have not been determined, maternal smoking during pregnancy is associated with decreased infant birth weight and increased incidence of prematurity (as defined by weight alone). It may also be associated with an increased incidence of spontaneous abortion, stillbirth, and neonatal death. The precise mechanism again, has not been established; however, carbon monoxide concentrations may be important, as discussed previously in relation to carbon monoxide hazard.

Thus, the specific noxious agents in cigarette smoke, their precise site of action, and, in many instances, the actual health hazard and disability have not been established. The enormous impact of this habit on mortality, health-care economy, and human suffering warrants the tremendous research effort currently being expended. It is anticipated that solutions to the theoretical concerns cited will soon be forthcoming. Therapeutically oriented persons experience great distress when they recognize that, in the face of such convincing circumstantial evidence, the simplest solution to the cigarette health hazard is proving unsatisfactory to society. Most smokers will not quit! Furthermore, the number of cigarette smokers among teenagers appears to be at least stable or on the increase despite vigorous anti-smoking campaigns. Legislation regarding warning of cigarette health hazards, restriction of cigarette advertising, and enormous tax expenditures in the areas of health-care research have not provided the incentive needed by the masses to deal with this habit. The solution to the smoking problem lies in the understanding of human motivation.

The health benefits of quitting smoking include lower risk of bronchitis.[107] Not all studies have demonstrated improvement in obstructive lung disease, and it still remains to be shown whether the small-airways disease prevalent in cigarette smokers is uniformly reversible or whether patients with established chronic bronchitis indeed have significant improvement in life expectancy or disability. Furthermore, the death rate from coronary artery disease is substantially diminished in ex-smokers.[92] This probably does not represent a decrease in atherosclerosis, but other factors responsible for myocardial infarction and sudden death appear to be improved. There is evidence suggesting that cessation of smoking decreases the risk of cancer of the lung several years after the smoker quits.[94] The emotional and metabolic effects of quitting smoking have also been studied in some depth but will not be discussed here.[108,109]

Pitfalls of Air Pollution Epidemiology. Current epidemiological approaches to the analysis of air pollution have resulted in several problems: (a) the expending of meaningless effort in the measurement of pollutants that have no adverse effects; (b) the organization of agencies or bureaus that are incapable of taking serious action; (c) the selection of only certain industries or types of emissions as the targets for control efforts, when numerous emissions are contributing; (d) the introduction, without prior evaluation, of control efforts that, in themselves, present certain hazards; and (e) preoccupation with air pollution concentrations thousands of times greater than those that actually occur.[110,111]

The retrospective study, the failure to identify multiple variables that may be responsible for effects, genetic population differences, and insensitive techniques for determining early abnormalities all prevent our effective utilization of large-scale studies to identify health hazards in large populations. Consequently, the purist argues that cigarette tar extracts painted on bald epithelium of rodents may, in spite of their carcinogenic effect, have no bearing on human disease. Similarly, the purist may argue that increased mortality due to myocardial infarction, or chronic obstructive bronchopulmonary disease, relates to other genetic or physiological characteristics of the persons involved rather than the pollutants in cigarette smoke. It is not new to biomedical science that folklore, intuition, and circumstantial evidence provide useful clues regarding health benefits. Biblical prohibition of the eating of pork may well have spared the Israelis from generations of diseased muscles due to trichinosis. While the ultimate in experimental design is being developed and the final mechanisms of histological damage are elucidated, careful avoidance of health hazards, which are identified by strong circumstantial evidence, may prolong active life.

REFERENCES

1. Altman, P. L., and Dittmer, D. S.: Biological Handbooks. Respiration and Circulation. p. 14. Federation of the American Society of Experimental Biologists, 1971.
2. Van Valen, L.: The history and stability of atmospheric oxygen. Science, *171*:439, 1971.
3. Altman, P. L., and Dittmer, D. S.: Biological Handbooks. Respiration and Circulation. p. 383. Federation of the American Society of Experimental Biologists, 1971.
4. Saltzman, H. A., and Salzano, J. V.: Effects of carbohydrate metabolism upon respiratory gas exchange in normal men. J. Appl. Physiol., *30*:228, 1971.
5. Naimark, A., Wasserman, K., and McIlroy, M. B.: Continuous measurement of ventilatory exchange ratio during exercise. J. Appl. Physiol., *19*:644, 1964.
6. Baker, P. T.: Human adaptation to high altitude. Science, *163*:1149, 1969.
7. Altman, P. L., and Dittmer, D. S.: Biological Handbooks. Environmental Biology. p. 350. Federation of the American Society of Experimental Biologists, 1966.
8. Lenfant, C., and Sullivan, K.: Adaptation to high altitude. N. Engl. J. Med., *284*:1298, 1971.
9. Mitchell, R. A.: Control of respiration. *In* Frohlich, E. D. (ed.): Pathophysiology: Altered Regulatory Mechanisms in Disease. 2 ed. Philadelphia, J. B. Lippincott, 1976.
10. Guenter, C. A., Joern, A. T., Shurley, J. T., and Pierce, C. M.: Cardiorespiratory and metabolic effects in men on the South Polar Plateau. Arch. Intern. Med., *125*:630, 1970.
11. Cruz, J. C.: Mechanics of breathing in high altitude and sea level subjects. Respir. Physiol., *17*:146, 1973.
12. Dawson, A.: Regional pulmonary blood flow in sitting and supine man during and after acute hypoxia. J. Clin. Invest., *48*:301, 1969.
13. Bisgard, G., *et al.*: Distribution of regional lung function during mild exercise in residents of 3100 m. Respir. Physiol., 22:369, 1974.
14. Haab, P., Held, D. R., Ernst, H., and Farhi, L. E.: Ventilation-perfusion relationships during high altitude adaptation. J. Appl. Physiol., *26*:77, 1969.
15. Cudkowicz, L.: Mean pulmonary artery pressure and alveolar oxygen tension in man at different altitudes. Respiration, *27*:417, 1970.

16. Blount, S. G., Jr., and Vogel, J. H. K.: Altitude and the pulmonary circulation. Adv. Intern. Med., *13*:11, 1967.
17. Vogel, J. H. K. (ed.): Hypoxia, High Altitude and the Heart. Advances in Cardiology. vol. 5. New York, S. Karger, 1970.
18. Krzywicki, H. J., *et al.*: Water metabolism in humans during acute high altitude exposure (4,300 m) J. Appl. Physiol., *30*:806, 1971.
19. Myhre, L. G., Dill, D. B., Hall, F. G., and Brown, D. K.: Blood volume changes during three-week residence at high altitude. Clin. Chem., *16*:7, 1970.
20. Whitcomb, W. H., *et al.*: Effect of the South Polar Plateau on plasma and urine erythropoietin levels. Arch. Intern. Med., *125*:638, 1970.
21. Vogel, J. A., Hansen, J. E., and Harris, C. W.: Cardiovascular responses in man during exhaustive work at sea level and high altitude. J. Appl. Physiol., *23*:531, 1967.
22. Kelman, G. R., and Crow, T. J.: Impairment of mental performance at a simulated altitude of 8,000 feet. Aerosp. Med., *40*:981, 1969.
23. Frayser, R., Drummond, R., Gray, G. W., and Houston, C. S.: Hormonal and electrolyte response to exposure to 17,500 feet. J. Appl. Physiol., *38*:636, 1975.
24. Schumacher, G., and Petajan, J.: High altitude stress and retinal hemorrhage. Arch. Environ. Health, *30*:217, 1975.
25. Hart, J. S. (ed.): Proceedings of the international symposium on altitude and cold. Fed. Proc., *28*:919, 1969.
26. Bartlett, D., Jr., and Remmers, J. E.: Effects of high altitude exposure on the lungs of young rats. Respir. Physiol., *13*:116, 1971.
27. Lahiri, S., *et al.*: Irreversible blunted respiratory sensitivity to hypoxia in high altitude natives. Respir. Physiol., *6*:360, 1969.
28. Weil, J., *et al.*: Acquired attenuation of chemoreceptor function in chronically hypoxic man at high altitude. J. Clin. Invest., *50*:186, 1971.
29. Lahiri, S., and Edelman, N. H.: Peripheral chemoreflexes in the regulation of breathing of high altitude natives. Respir. Physiol., *6*:375, 1969.
30. Mosso, A.: Life of Man on the High Alps. London, T. Fisher Unwin, 1898.
31. Monge, M. C.: High altitude disease. Arch. Intern. Med., *59*:32, 1937.
32. ———: Life in the Andes and chronic mountain sickness. Science, *95*:79, 1942.
33. Hecht, H. H., *et al.*: Brisket disease. III. Clinical features and hemodynamic observations in high altitude dependent right heart failure of cattle. Am. J. Med., *32*:171, 1962.
34. Houston, C. S.: Acute pulmonary edema of high altitude. N. Engl. J. Med., *263*:478, 1960.
35. Menon, N. D.: High altitude pulmonary edema. N. Engl. J. Med., *273*:66, 1965.
36. Kleiner, John P., and Nelson, W. P.: High altitude pulmonary edema. A rare disease? J.A.M.A., *234*:491, 1975.
37. Bullard, R. W.: Physiological problems of space travel. Annu. Rev. Physiol. *34*:205, 1972.
38. Altman, P. L., and Dittmer, D. S.: Biological Handbooks. Environmental Biology. p. 269. Federation of the American Society of Experimental Biologists, 1966.
39. Sanford, J. P.: Medical aspects of recreational skin and scuba diving. Annu. Rev. Med., *25*:401, 1974.
40. Lanphier, E. H.: Man in High Pressure. Handbook of Physiology: Adaptations to the Environment. American Physiological Society, 1964.
41. Lambertson, C. J. (ed.): Proceedings of the Third Symposium on Underwater Physiology. Baltimore, Williams & Wilkins, 1967.
42. Wada, J., and Iwa, T.: Proceedings of the Fourth International Congress on Hyperbaric Medicine. Baltimore, Williams & Wilkins, 1970.
43. Clark, J. M., and Lambertson, C. J.: Pulmonary oxygen toxicity: a review. Pharmacol. Rev., *23*:37, 1971.
44. Morrison, J. B., and Florio, J. T.: Respiratory function during simulated saturation dive to 1,500 feet. J. Appl. Physiol., *30*:724, 1971.
45. Johnson, D. G., and Burger, W. D.: Injury and disease of scuba and skin divers. Postgrad. Med., *49*:134, 1971.
46. Overfield, E. M., Saltzman, H. A., Kylstra, J. A., and Salzano, J. V.: Respiratory gas exchange in normal men breathing 0.9% oxygen in helium at 31.3 atmospheres absolute. J. Appl. Physiol., *27*:471, 1969.
47. Salzano, J., Rausch, D. C., and Saltzman, H. A.: Cardiorespiratory responses to exercise at a simulated seawater depth of 1,000 feet. J. Appl. Physiol., *28*:34, 1970.
48. Lord, G. P., Bond, G. F., and Schaefer, K. E.: Breathing under high ambient pressure. J. Appl. Physiol., *21*:1833, 1966.
49. Wood, L. D. H., and Bryan, A. C.: Effect of increased ambient pressure on flow-volume curve of the lung. J. Appl. Physiol., *27*:4, 1969.

50. Doell, D., Zutter, M., and Anthonisen, N. R.: Ventilatory responses to hypercapnia and hypoxia AT 1 and 4 ATA. Respir. Physiol., *18*:338, 1973.
51. Kylstra, J. A., Tissing, M. O., and Van Der Moen, A.: Of mice as fish. Trans. Am. Soc. Artif. Intern. Organs, *8*:378, 1962.
52. Symposium on inert organic liquids for biological oxygen transport. Fed. Proc., *29*:1696, 1970.
53. Symposium on artificial blood. Fed. Proc., *34*:1428, 1975.
54. Modell, J. H., Hood, C. I., Kuck, E. J., and Ruiz, B. C.: Oxygenation by ventilation with fluorocarbon liquid (FX-80). Anesthesiology, *34*:312, 1971.
55. Modell, J. H., Gollan, F., Giammona, S. T., and Parker, D.: Effect of Fluorocarbon liquid on surface tension properties of pulmonary surfactant. Chest, *57*:263, 1970.
56. Altman, P. L., and Dittmer, D. S.: Biological Handbooks. Environmental Biology, pages 270-315. Federation of the American Society of Experimental Biologists, 1966.
57. Stokinger, H. E.: Toxicity of airborne chemicals: air quality standards—a national and international view. Annu. Rev. Pharmacol., *12*:407, 1972.
58. Bates, D. V.: A Citizen's Guide to Air Pollution. Montreal, McGill-Queen's University Press, 1972.
59. Ayres, S. M., Evans, R. G., and Buehler, M. E.: Air pollution: a major public health problem. CRC Crit. Rev. Clin. Lab. Sci., *1*, 1972.
60. Larsen, R. I.: Air pollution from motor vehicles. Ann. N.Y. Acad. Sci., *136*:277, 1967.
61. Godin, G., Wright, G., and Shephard, R. J.: Urban exposure to carbon monoxide. Arch. Environ. Health, *25*:305, 1972.
62. Gothe, C. J., *et al.*: Carbon monoxide hazard in city traffic. Arch. Environ. Health, *19*:310, 1969.
63. Lawther, P. J., and Commins, B. T.: Cigarette smoking and exposure to carbon monoxide. Ann. N.Y. Acad. Sci., *174*:135, 1970.
64. Goldsmith, J. R.: Contribution of motor vehicle exhaust, industry, and cigarette smoking to community carbon monoxide exposures. Ann. N.Y. Acad. Sci., *174*:122, 1970.
65. Russell, M. A. H., Cole, P. V., and Brown, E.: Absorption by non-smokers of carbon monoxide from room air polluted by tobacco smoke. Lancet, *1*:576, 1973.
66. Goldsmith, J. R., and Landaw, S. A.: Carbon monoxide and human health. Science, *162*:1352, 1968.
67. Roughton, F. J. W., and Root, W. S.: The fate of carbon monoxide in the body during recovery from mild carbon monoxide poisoning in man. Am. J. Physiol., *145*:239, 1945.
68. Roughton, F. J. W.: Kinetics of gas transport in the blood. Br. Med. Bull., *19*:80, 1963.
69. Beard, R. L., and Wertheim, G. A.: Behavioral impairment associated with small doses of carbon monoxide. Am. J. Public Health, *57*:7012, 1967.
70. Wright, G., Randell, P., and Shephard, R. J.: Carbon monoxide and driving skills. Arch. Environ. Health, *27*:349, 1973.
71. McFarland, R. A.: Low level exposure to carbon monoxide and driving performance. Arch. Environ. Health, *27*:355, 1973.
72. Sagone, A. L., Jr., Lawrence, T., and Balcerzak, S. P.: Effect of smoking on tissue oxygen supply. Blood, *41*:845, 1973.
73. Brody, J. S., and Coburn, R. F.: Effects of elevated carboxyhemoglobin on gas exchange in the lung. Ann. N.Y. Acad. Sci., *174*:255, 1970.
74. Astrup, P.: Some physiological and pathological effects of moderate carbon monoxide exposure. Br. Med. J., *4*:447, 1972.
75. Wald, N., Howard, S., Smith, P. G., and Kjeldsen, K.: Association between atherosclerotic diseases and carboxyhemoglobin levels in tobacco smokers. Br. Med. J., *1*:761, 1973.
76. Astrup, P., Olsen, H. M., Trolle, D., and Kjeldsen, K.: Effect of moderate carbon monoxide exposure on fetal development. Lancet, *2*:1220, 1972.
77. Ayres, S. M., Giannelli, S., Jr., and Mueller, H.: Myocardial and systemic responses to carboxyhemoglobin. Ann. N.Y. Acad. Sci., *174*:268, 1970.
78. Aronow, W. S., and Isbell, M. W.: Carbon monoxide effect on exercise-induced angina pectoris. Ann. Intern. Med., *79*:392, 1973.
79. Cohen, S. I., Deane, M., and Goldsmith, J. R.: Carbon monoxide and survival from myocardial infarction. Arch. Environ. Health, *19*:510, 1969.
80. Norman, J. W., and Ledingham, I. M. A.: Carbon monoxide poisoning: investiga-

tion and treatment. Prog. Brain Res., *24*:101, 1967.

81. Zweiman, B., *et al.*: Effects of air pollution on asthma: a review. J. Allergy Clin. Immunol., *50*:305, 1972.
82. French, J. G., *et al.*: The effect of sulfur dioxide and suspended sulfates on acute respiratory disease. Arch. Environ. Health, *27*:129, 1973.
83. Frank, N. R., and Speicer, F. E.: Effects of acute controlled exposure to sulfur dioxide on respiratory mechanisms in healthy male adults. J. Appl. Physiol., *17*:252, 1962.
84. Nadel, J. A., and Salem, H.: Mechanisms of broncho-constriction during inhalation of sulfur dioxide and cigarette smoke. Arch. Environ. Health, *16*:651, 1968.
85. Amdus, M. O.: Toxicologic appraisal of particulate matter, oxides of sulfur, and sulfuric acid. J. Air Pollut. Control Assoc., *19*:639, 1969.
86. First, M. W.: Aerosols in nature. Arch. Intern. Med., *131*:24, 1973.
87. Hazucha, M., *et al.*: Pulmonary function in man after short term exposure to ozone. Arch. Environ. Health, *27*:183, 1973.
88. Speizer, F. E., and Ferris, B. G.: Exposure to automobile exhaust. Arch. Environ. Health, *26*:319, 1973.
89. Ury, H. K., Perkins, N. M., and Goldsmith, J. R.: Motor vehicle accidents and vehicular pollution. Arch. Environ. Health, *25*:314, 1972.
90. Wynder, E. L., and Hoffman, D.: Experimental tobacco carcinogenesis. Science, *162*:862, 1968.
91. Castleden, C., and Cole, P.: Variations in carboxyhemoglobin levels in smokers. Br. Med. J., *4*:736, 1974.
92. Smoking and health: a report of the American Thoracic Society Committee on Therapy. Am. Rev. Respir. Dis., *96*:613, 1967.
93. Hammond, E. C.: The effects of smoking. Sci. Am., *207*:39, 1962.
94. Doll, R., and Hill, A. B.: Mortality in relation to smoking: ten years' observation of British doctors. Bri. Med. J., *1*:1399, 1964.
95. The health consequences of smoking. U.S. Department of Health, Education and Welfare, Public Health Service. Annual reports, 1967, 1969, 1975.
96. Kilburn, K.: Effects of tobacco smoke on biological systems. Scand. J. Respir. Dis. [Suppl.], *91*:64, 1974.
97. Huber, G.: Smoking and nonsmokers—What is the issue? N. Engl. J. Med., *292*:858, 1975.
98. Doyle, J. T., *et al.*: The relationship of cigarette smoking to coronary heart disease. J.A.M.A., *190*:886, 1964.
99. Nadel, J. A., and Comroe, J. H., Jr.: Acute effects of inhalation of cigarette smoke on airway conductance. J. Appl. Physiol., *16*:713, 1961.
100. Furnass, F. N., and Halebsky, N. (eds.): Cardiovascular effects of nicotine and smoking. Ann. N.Y. Acad. Sci., *90*:1, 1960.
101. Da Silva, A. M. T., and Hamosh, P.: Effect of smoking a single cigarette on the "small airways." J. Appl. Physiol., *34*:361, 1973.
102. Camner, P., Philipson, K., and Arvidsson, T.: Cigarette smoking in man. Arch. Environ. Health, *23*:421, 1971.
103. Green, G. M.: Pulmonary clearance of infectious agents. Annu. Rev. Med., *19*:315, 1968.
104. Mittman, C., Lieberman, J., Marasso, F., and Miranda, A.: Smoking and chronic obstructive lung disease in $alpha_1$ antitrypsin deficiency. Chest, *60*:214, 1971.
105. Guenter, C. A., Welch, M. H., and Hammarsten, J. F.: $Alpha_1$ antitrypsin deficiency and pulmonary emphysema. Annu. Rev. Med., *22*:283, 1971.
106. Doll, R., and Hill, A. B.: Lung cancer and other causes of death in relation to smoking: a second report on the mortality of British doctors. Br. Med. J., *2*:1071, 1956.
107. Anderson, D. O., and Ferris, B. G., Jr.: Role of tobacco smoking in the causation of chronic respiratory disease. N. Engl. J. Med., *267*:787, 1962.
108. Glauser, S. C., *et al.*: Metabolic changes associated with the cessation of cigarette smoking. Arch. Environ. Health, *20*:377, 1970.
109. Krumholz, R. A., Chevalier, R. B., and Ross, J. C.: Changes in cardiopulmonary functions related to abstinence from smoking. Ann. Intern. Med., *62*:197, 1965.
110. Goldsmith, J. R.: Air pollution epidemiology: a wicked problem, an informational maze, and a professional responsibility. Arch. Environ. Health, *18*:516, 1969.
111. Braun, D. C., Jurgiel, J. A., and Gross, P.: Establishing environmental criteria: medical perspectives. Arch. Environ. Health, *27*:121, 1973.

2 The Respiratory Airways

James C. Hogg, M.D., Ph.D.

In this chapter, two basic approaches will be taken in an attempt to present the normal structure and function of the airways and to discuss the changes that occur in them with disease. The first approach will be to present theoretical concepts concerning aerodynamics and mechanics that are useful to the understanding of airways function. These basic principles are fundamental to the analysis of many physiological measurements and commonly used clinical techniques. The second section will deal with airway anatomy, the morphological changes that occur with disease, and the relationship of disordered morphology to function.

THEORETICAL ASPECTS OF AIRWAYS FUNCTION

Ideally, to understand airflow in the lung, one should be able to describe the characteristics of flow through an irregularly branched system of distensible tubes, where the geometry of the system changes considerably during inflation and deflation of the lung. Unfortunately, the mathematical approach to such a system is poorly developed, and an adequate description of the recent attempts at such an analysis is beyond the scope of this presentation. A more simplified approach to fluid mechanics, however, can still provide us with information necessary for a minimum understanding of airflow in the lung. The basic concepts describing the relationships of flow to pressure, resistance, and dimensions of the conduit are presented.

POISEUILLE'S LAW

An empirical law governing the flow of a viscous liquid through a fine tube was reported by Poiseuille in 1842. He found that the volume of liquid passing through a tube per unit of time was proportional (a) to the difference in pressure at the two ends of the tube, (b) to the fourth power of the radius of the tube, and (c) to the reciprocal of the length. Hagenbach later defined the coefficient of viscosity (μ) and worked out the formula now referred to as Hagen-Poiseuille's law:

$$\dot{V} = \Delta P \frac{\pi}{8} \times \frac{r^4}{l} \times \frac{1}{\mu} \quad \text{(Equation 1)}$$

($\dot{V}$ = flow, r = radius, l = length of tube, μ is the viscosity of the liquid, and ΔP is the difference in pressure at the inlet and outlet of the tube).

Although this relationship is often applied to flow through the airways, it has definite limitations because it is valid only for laminar flow. Furthermore, the geometric factor r^4/l does not take branch points and bends into account, or allow for the fact that changes in driving pressure (ΔP) also change the transmural pressure of the airways, thereby increasing their diameter and altering the geometric relationship.

One important factor in considering the flow through a parent tube and its two daughter branches is that the pressure drop along the two daughters will be greater than that along the parent until the cross-sectional area of daughters exceeds that of the parent by a factor of $1/\sqrt{2}$.

CONTINUITY EQUATION

Under conditions of steady flow through a tube of changing dimension (Fig. 2-1), the law of conservation of matter is expressed by the equation:

$$A_1V_1W_1 = A_2V_2W_2 \quad \text{(Equation 2)}$$

(A is the area in cm.^{2}, V is the velocity in cm./sec., and W is the specific weight of the substance in grams/cm.^{3}).

Since the units are in grams/sec., the equation states that the weight rate of flow is the same in both diameter tubes. When the flowing gas is not compressed, the W term is dropped, and the volume rate of flow is constant.

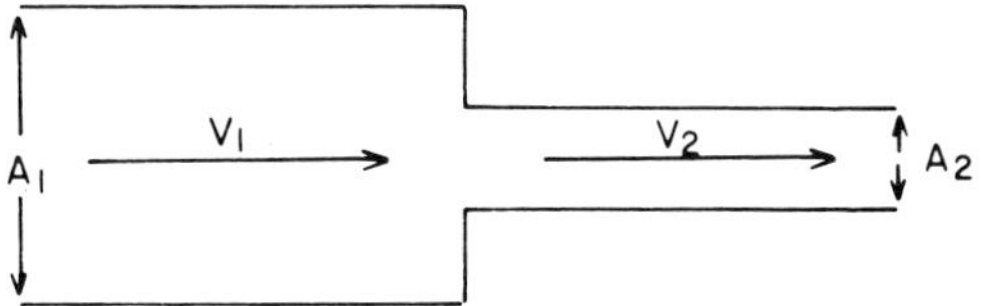

Fig. 2-1. When flow is constant and incompressible, the rate of flow through the tube of large diameter is exactly equal to the rate of flow through the tube of small diameter. (See text, Equation 2.)

MOMENTUM EQUATION

Newton's first law states that the momentum of a body is constant unless it is acted on by an external force, and his second law states that the external force acting on a body is equal to the time rate of change of its momentum. Therefore, it follows that if a liquid loses velocity as it flows through a tube, there will be a loss of momentum. The force (F) acting on the liquid to change its momentum will be:

$$F = m\frac{V_1 - V_2}{t} \text{ or } F = m\frac{dv}{dt} \quad \text{(Equation 3)}$$

(where m is the mass of the liquid, V_2 and V_1 are the initial and final velocities, and t is the time during which the velocity changed.)

The work done to accomplish this change in momentum will be the force (F) times the distance through which it acts.

ENERGY EQUATION

The energy of a body is defined as the capacity for doing work, where work is the product of force and displacement. The total force resulting from the movement of the liquid that is available to do work can be found by integrating the momentum equation and is equal to ½ mv.^{2} A liquid also has potential energy in proportion to its height above some arbitrary datum and has hydrostatic energy in proportion to its depth below the same point. By the law of conservation of energy, as a liquid flows through the tube, the loss in energy will equal the work done on the liquid plus the heat produced, when the heat equivalent of work has a definite value (1 BTU = 778 ft. lbs.). Under conditions of constant temperature, there is no heat lost by the fluid, so that the loss in energy is equal to the work done. If flow occurs through a pipe of varying diameter, it is obvious that as the velocity of the fluid increases, there will be a rise in kinetic energy and a fall in hydrostatic energy, because the total energy is constant. The fall in hydrostatic pressure that accompanies an increase in kinetic energy when a continuous flow passes through a narrowing in a tube is referred to as the *Bernoulli effect*.

INTERNAL FRICTION

When liquid or air flows through a pipe, the thin layer of liquid that adheres to the pipe wall has zero velocity. The velocity of concentric rings of fluid toward the center of the pipe gradually increases. The distance between the ring with zero velocity and that with the greatest velocity is referred to as the boundary layer, and it is in this boundary layer that all the viscous forces are concentrated. Figure 2-2 shows that if a column of fluid enters a pipe with uniform velocity, the effect of friction is initially limited to the layer of liquid closest to the pipe wall. As a parabolic or laminar flow profile is established, the boundary layer can be seen to grow, so that the frictional forces become distributed throughout the liquid.

A force is required to overcome the internal friction or viscosity between layers. The dynamic viscosity between the layers of the fluid may be assessed as follows:

$$\text{dynamic viscosity} = \frac{\text{shear stress}}{\text{rate of shear stress}} \quad \text{(Equation 4)}$$

(Shear stress equals the force divided by the area of contact between the layers; the rate of shear strain is the velocity of the layer divided by its thickness.

The unit of dynamic viscosity is the poise, and its symbol is μ. Therefore,

$$\mu = \frac{\frac{\text{dynes}}{\text{cm.}^2}}{\frac{\text{cm./sec.}}{\text{cm.}}} = \frac{\text{dynes./sec.}}{\text{cm.}^2} \quad \text{(Equation 5)}$$

$$\text{and since a dyne} = \frac{1\ \text{gram/cm.}}{\text{sec.}^2},$$

$$1\ \text{poise} = \frac{\text{gram}}{\text{cm./sec.}}$$

Kinematic viscosity is the ratio of dynamic viscosity to density, and its unit is the stoke.

$$\text{Kinematic viscosity} = \frac{\frac{\text{gram}}{\text{cm./sec.}}}{\frac{\text{grams}}{\text{cm.}^3}} = \frac{\text{cm.}^2}{\text{sec.}} \text{ or } \textit{stoke} \quad \text{(Equation 6)}$$

The viscosity of viscous fluids such as glycerine is about 15 poise, whereas that of water is about 0.01 poise, and air, 0.0001 poise. Once motion of a liquid begins, the forces acting to slow it down are frictional, and one might think that those which were the most viscous would slow at the fastest rate. This is not so in practice, as one can demonstrate by the fact that stirred air slows much faster than stirred water, after the stirring force is removed. Dividing the viscosity by the density takes into account the momentum of the stirred air, and we find that the kinematic viscosity of air is 0.162 stoke, whereas that of water is 0.01 stoke.

REYNOLD'S NUMBER

When the flow through a tube is laminar, the interaction between concentric layers of fluid is dependent on friction alone, so that only viscous forces are exerted between layers. When flow becomes turbulent, however, there is an actual transfer of fluid mass between concentric layers, so that inertial forces interact between layers. The exact nature of turbulent flow has not been completely determined, but flow can be described in terms of the ratio between inertial and viscous forces in the liquid. This ratio is known as the Reynold's number.

The Reynold's number for flow in a tube

$$= \frac{\text{inertial forces}}{\text{viscous forces}} \quad \text{(Equation 7)}$$

$$= \frac{2\rho v}{\pi r \mu}, \text{ where } \rho = \text{the density of the fluid in } \frac{\text{grams}}{\text{cm.}^3}$$

$v =$ the velocity of the fluid $\frac{\text{cm.}^3}{\text{sec.}}$

$r =$ the radius of the tube (cm.)

$\mu =$ the viscosity of the fluid in poises or $\frac{\text{gram}}{\text{cm./sec.}}$

If all units are inserted into the equation as indicated below, all the units cancel, and the Reynold's number is dimensionless:

$$\frac{\frac{\text{gram}}{\text{cm.}^3}\ \frac{\text{cm.}^3}{\text{sec.}}}{\text{cm.}\ \frac{\text{gram}}{\text{cm./sec.}}}$$

For incompressible flow in pipes, flow is found to be laminar when the Reynold's number is less than 2000, transitional between 2000 and 3000, and turbulent when the Reynold's number is above 3000.

ENTRANCE LENGTH PHENOMENA

If the velocity of a fluid entering a tube is uniform (Fig. 2-2), a boundary layer is set up in the tube. The concentric laminae near the tube wall decelerate, and the concentric laminae at the center of the tube accelerate to satisfy the conservation of momentum. The boundary layer grows during the period, so that viscous forces become more widely dispersed. During the development of a laminar profile, liquid mass exchanges between laminae, so that energy is re-

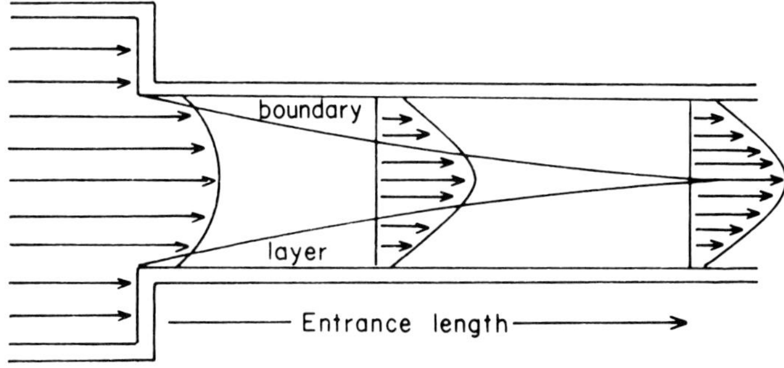

Fig. 2-2. During the development of laminar flow, the inertial forces developed by fluid exchange between layers fall to a minimum, and the boundary layer, where viscous forces are concentrated, expands throughout the liquid.

quired to overcome both inertial force and viscous forces. The length of the tube required for a laminar profile of flow to develop is called the *entrance length*. It follows that the pressure drop along the entrance length is greater than the pressure drop along an equal length of tube when laminar flow is fully established, because in the former, energy is required to overcome both inertial and viscous forces, whereas in the latter, only viscous forces must be overcome. In the normal human lung, entrance length phenomena are observed primarily in the central airways, whereas in the peripheral airways, fully developed laminar flow prevails. This fact has been utilized recently to determine sites of airways resistance. In the normal subject, the cross-sectional area of the central airways is small in relation to that of the peripheral airways (see Fig. 2-8D), so that the velocity is greater in the central airways than in the periphery. Under these circumstances, one would expect the flow profiles to be turbulent in large airways and laminar in the small airways.

Reviewing Equation 7, it is clear that decreasing gas density or increasing viscosity results in a decrease in the Reynold's number, and the pressure required to drive flow through the central airways decreases. Breathing a helium-oxygen mixture, which is less dense and more viscous than air decreases the resistance by this mechanism (primarily in the central airways), so that normal persons achieve increased flow rates under these circumstances. If the major site of resistance is in the peripheral airways, where flow is laminar, however, breathing a helium-oxygen mixture does not have this effect.

A number of authors[1,2] have recently taken advantage of this property of helium to localize the site of airways obstruction. For example, asthmatics who have primary disease in the central airways increase their maximum flow rates with helium-oxygen mixtures; whereas chronic bronchitics who have primarily peripheral airways obstruction do not.

THE APPLICATION OF THEORY TO THE LUNG

GENERAL PRINCIPLES

The Swiss physiologist, Rohrer, was the first to apply Newtonian mechanics to the lung. By making two assumptions, he wrote an equation of motion for the lung that related its elastic, viscous, and inertial properties to the applied force. Although his analysis was not appreciated during his lifetime, it was so thorough that in a modern review of lung mechanics, Mead[3] stated that a bibliography combining Rohrer's name with those of his pupil Neergaard and a few contemporaries would encompass most of the ideas and techniques in this field. Therefore, prior to reviewing the measurements of mechanical properties of lungs, this analysis and its underlying assumptions will be discussed.

The assumptions that have to be made in order to write an equation of motion for the respiratory system are that the system behaves as a rectilinear system of one degree of freedom, in which the elements are nonlinear. This means that when a force is applied, the lung should move in only one dimension. To make this clear, let us consider a point in three-dimensional space.

Such a point has three degrees of freedom, because it is free to move in any one of three dimensions. If the point were a block of wood fastened to a stick held in the hand, the block would be free to move in three dimensions and therefore would have three degrees of freedom. If the block is placed in a groove on a flat surface, however, any force applied by the hand can only move the block up and down the groove, so that it moves in a single dimension and therefore has only one degree of freedom. It follows that in one-dimensional systems, the single degree of movement can be characterized by a linear change; in two-dimensional systems, by an area change; and in three-dimensional systems, by a volume change. Lung motion can be described by volume change, and the lung can be considered to be a system with one degree of freedom if the motion at each position in the lung bears a fixed relationship to the total motion of the lung. The evidence that suggests that this is so in the lung relates to the fact that the distribution of air along the various pathways within the lung is normally independent of breathing frequency, and this fact suggests that the motion of each unit always has a fixed relationship to the motion of the whole lung.[4] Because the lung behaves as a system of one degree of freedom, it follows that its motion can be described by a single variable, lung volume. When a force is applied to the lung, it must overcome elastic, viscous, and inertial forces that are developed by the lung. It can be shown that the elastic forces are proportional to the volume change, the viscous forces to the rate of volume change ($\dot{V}$) or flow, and the inertial force to the rate of change in flow ($\ddot{V}$), which is the acceleration. The equation of motion can then be written:

$$F \text{ (applied)} = K1V + K2\dot{V} + K3\ddot{V} \quad \text{(Equation 8)}$$

(K1, K2, and K3 are constants; the applied force (F) is the transpulmonary pressure; and V, $\dot{V}$, and $\ddot{V}$ are volume, flow, and volume acceleration, respectively.) This equation can be written more simply:

$$P_L = P_{CL} + P_{RL} + P_{IL} \quad \text{(Equation 9)}$$

(P_L is the instantaneous value for the pressure drop from the airway opening to the outer pleural surface; P_{CL} is the component of P_L required to overcome elastic forces; P_{RL} is the component of P_L required to overcome flow-resistive forces; and P_{IL} is the component of P_L required to overcome inertial forces.)

This simply states that the sum of elastic, flow-resistive, and inertial forces equals the total force developed by the lung to oppose the force applied to it and that these forces are proportional to the volume, flow, and volume acceleration that occur when the force is applied.

The phase relationship of these forces can be examined by determining these parameters during breathing. These relationships are shown in Figure 2-3. A full inspiration from RV (residual volume) to TLC (total lung capacity) and back to FRC (functional residual capacity) is shown in the volume tracing for orientation. By comparing the tracings during a sinusoidal pattern of respiration that approximates tidal breathing, it can be seen that the flow tracing is 90° out of phase with volume and that volume acceleration lags behind flow by another 90°, so that it is 180° out of phase with volume. When the frequency of breathing is increased at a constant tidal volume, both flow and volume acceleration increase.

Figure 2-3B shows the relationship between P_{CL} and P_{IL} as breathing frequency is increased. It is clear from Figure 2-3A that the pressures required to overcome elasticity remain the same at a higher frequency because tidal volume is constant. The pressures required to overcome inertia, however, increase with increased breathing frequency, because volume acceleration increases. This means that at some frequency, inertial and elastic forces will be equal, and because they are 180° out of phase, they cancel. This is known as the resonant frequency of the lung, and at this frequency the applied force has to overcome only the resistive properties of the lung. This relationship can therefore be used to measure airways resistance of normal lungs, and equipment has been devised to take advantage of it.

This resonant frequency method is useful in assessing lung mechanics, because the lung has a high degree of viscous

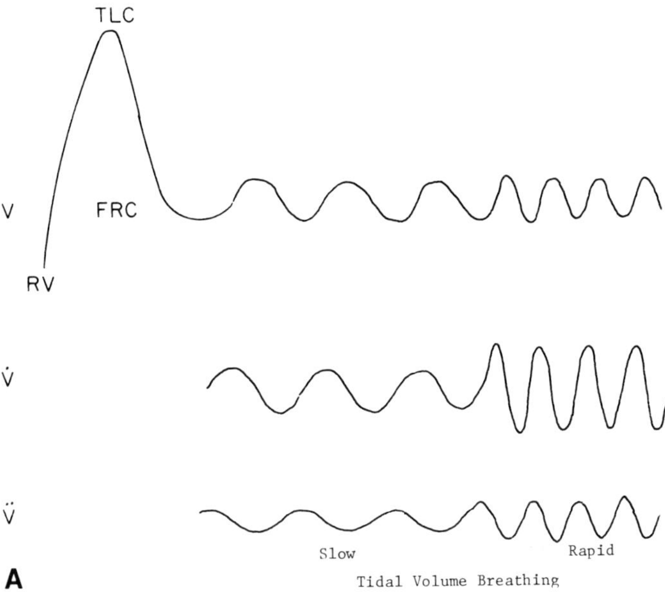

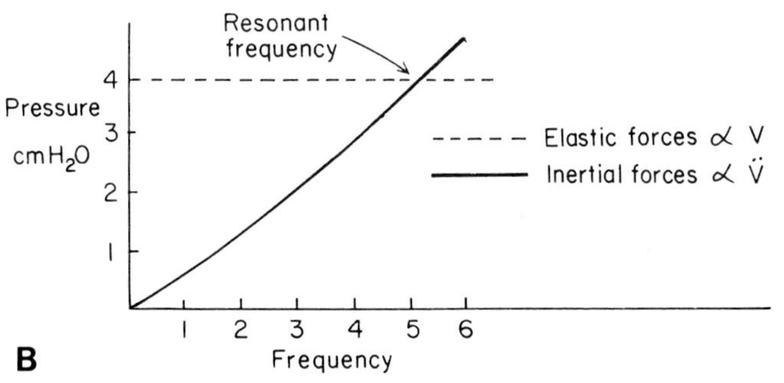

Fig. 2-3. (*A*) These graphs show that volume (V) is 90° out of phase with the flow ($\dot{V}$) and 180° out of phase with volume acceleration ($\ddot{V}$), when the breathing pattern is a sine wave. When frequency is increased at a constant tidal volume, the inertial forces increase. When the inertial forces equal the elastic forces, they cancel, because they are 180° out of phase. (*B*) The elastic forces remain constant in spite of an increased rate of breathing; they are proportional to lung volume. The inertial forces are proportional to the rate of acceleration; therefore, they are increased at rapid breathing frequencies. Since these forces are 180° out of phase, they cancel.

damping, and therefore it approaches the resonant frequency in a stable fashion. The stability of a mechanical system as it approaches resonance is a function of damping. Figure 2-4 shows the magnitude of the response to a particular applied force as the frequency with which the force is applied is increased. With an underdamped system, the magnitude of the response increases dramatically near the resonant frequency, because as the elastic and inertial forces cancel, the applied force has only the resistive forces to overcome. Thus, a singer's note can shatter a wineglass under appropriate conditions. Damping decreases the amplitude of this response in the manner indicated, and with an overdamped system, the amplitude of the response decreases as soon as the frequency is increased. In a critically damped system, the amplitude of the response to an applied force remains constant as the resonant frequency is approached. This fact is often alluded to by manufacturers of measuring instruments such as pressure transducers, who describe the frequency response of their instruments as being flat to so many cycles/second. It follows that in order to measure the flow and volume changes that occur in the lung, the frequency response of the measuring devices must be such that they remain flat well beyond the cycling frequencies at which the measurements are made.

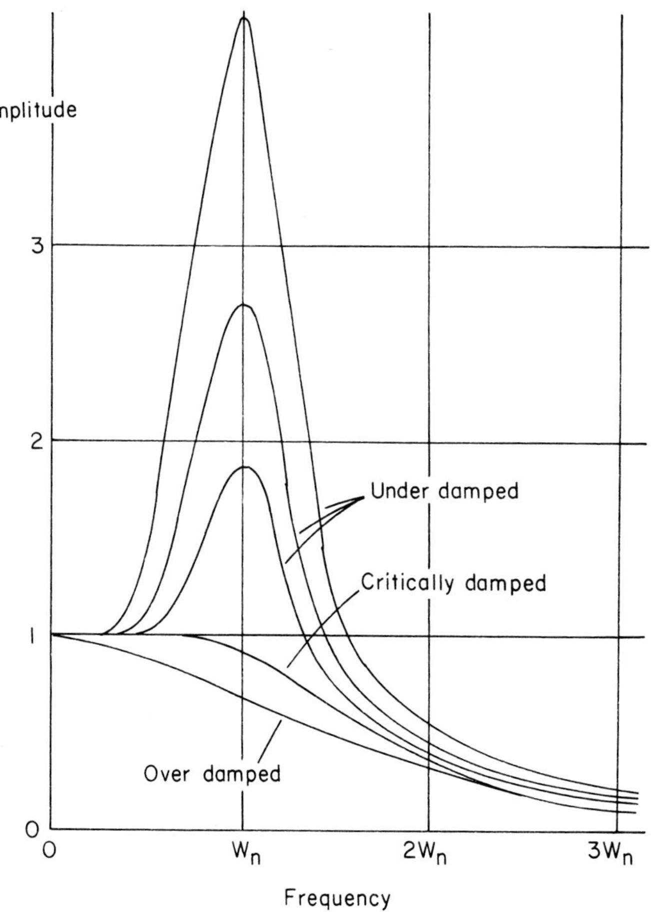

Fig. 2-4. The amplitude of a response to a constant input in relation to frequency and damping. The maximum response occurs at the resonant frequency (W_n), but increasing the damping decreases this response. If the system is over-damped, the response decreases as soon as the frequency is increased, but when critical damping is achieved, the response is the same at all frequencies up to the resonant frequency.

MEASUREMENT OF TOTAL PULMONARY RESISTANCE

Pulmonary resistance measurements, then, require an analysis of the flow-resistive forces reflected in the pressure gradient from the alveolus to the mouth, and an analysis of elastic and inertial forces reflected in total transpulmonary pressure (mouth pressure minus pleural pressure). At zero flow, the flow-resistive and inertial forces are zero, and the only force is elastic, which is easily measured (Equation 9).

Total lung resistance can be assessed during flow by construction of a pressure-volume diagram during respiration,[3] and with minor changes in technique and instrumentation this can be readily applied clinically[5,6] to differentiate elastic from flow-resistive components. These techniques are discussed in relation to clinical applications in Chapter 3.

The study by Dubois and associates[7] of the oscillatory mechanics of the lungs and chest wall led to the ingenious method of measuring the resistance of the respiratory system by using an oscillating system. They found that the lung and chest wall constituted a highly damped system, with a resonant frequency of from 4 to 6 cycles per second. As we have seen, inertial and elastic forces cancel at the resonant frequency, so that the pressure required to drive the lung at this frequency has to overcome only the flow-resistive components (Fig. 2-3). In the initial studies with this method, a pump was used to drive flow in a sine-wave frequency. Mead and his associates modified the technique by using a loudspeaker in an enclosed box to produce the oscillations, and this method is now in common use in many laboratories to measure airways resistance.

The introduction of a satisfactory body plethysmograph[8,9] allowed alveolar pressure to be estimated for the first time. This permitted a direct analysis of flow resistance, because the mouth-to-alveolus pressure gradient could be assessed. The clinical applications of this method are discussed in Chapter 3.

THE EFFECT OF LUNG INFLATION AND LUNG SIZE ON PULMONARY RESISTANCE

As we have seen, resistance refers to the relationship between the pressure drop from the alveoli to the atmosphere divided by the instantaneous airflow. With increasing rates of airflow, the relationship between pressure and flow becomes curvilinear. Fry and his associates[10,11] have shown that there is a specific pressure flow curve for each lung volume and introduced the term *isovolume pressure flow curve* to describe them. At high lung volumes, much higher expiratory flow rates can be achieved than at low lung volumes, because the airways are larger. The relationship between resistance and lung volume has been thought to be hyperbolic,[12] so that the smallest values for resistance occurred at the highest lung volumes. Macklem and Mead[13] have shown that the minimal value for resistance actually occurred at about 70 per cent VC (vital capacity). These authors found it difficult to explain the increase in the resistance that occurred in both central and peripheral airways at higher lung volumes to changes in airway length. They suggested that the pressure-to-area relationship of the airways might change as the airways lengthened, so that the airways might narrow somewhat at high lung volumes.

Briscoe and Dubois[14] have studied the effect of lung size on airway conductance and have shown that there is a linear relationship. Although their number of cases studied is small, their results indicate that for adults of similar age but different size, the linear dimensions of the lungs and airways change nearly equally.

THE EFFECT OF LUNG GROWTH ON PULMONARY RESISTANCE

In comparing lungs of persons of different ages, it is helpful to use the inverse of resistance (i.e., pulmonary conductance), because conductance is positively correlated with increases in volume. In examining the relationship between airways conductance and lung volume in the data of Briscoe and Dubois,[14] and Cook and associates,[15] Mead[3] drew attention to the fact that between the ages of 9 and 15, lung volume increases at a greater rate than conductance, whereas between 15 years and adulthood, conductance increases at a much faster rate than volume. Mead suggested that this might mean that initially the size and number of alveoli increase out of proportion to the size of the airways, whereas later on in life, the airways more than catch up. It has been shown that the number of conducting airways is complete at birth,[16] whereas the number of alveoli increase rapidly after birth and approach the adult number at between 5 and 8 years of age.

In the normal adult lung, the bulk of the resistance is in the central airways, and the resistance beyond the twelfth generation of airways is very small. (See the section on lung anatomy for a further description and see Fig. 2-9.) This relative distribution of airways resistance is different in early life, because the growth of the conducting airways lags behind during the period of rapid alveolar multiplication, from birth to age 5. Indeed, a series of experiments in our laboratory indicated that significant changes in airway resistance occur at the lung periphery about the same time that the number of alveoli reach the adult value.[17,18] Figure 2-5 shows the data from these experiments. A catheter was carefully placed in the same position in the airways of lungs of persons of various ages so that airways conductance could be measured. In the adult lung, the conductance of the peripheral airways was much greater than that of central airways, and this relationship held true down to about 6 or 7 years of age. In the younger children, however, the peripheral airways conductance fell off markedly.

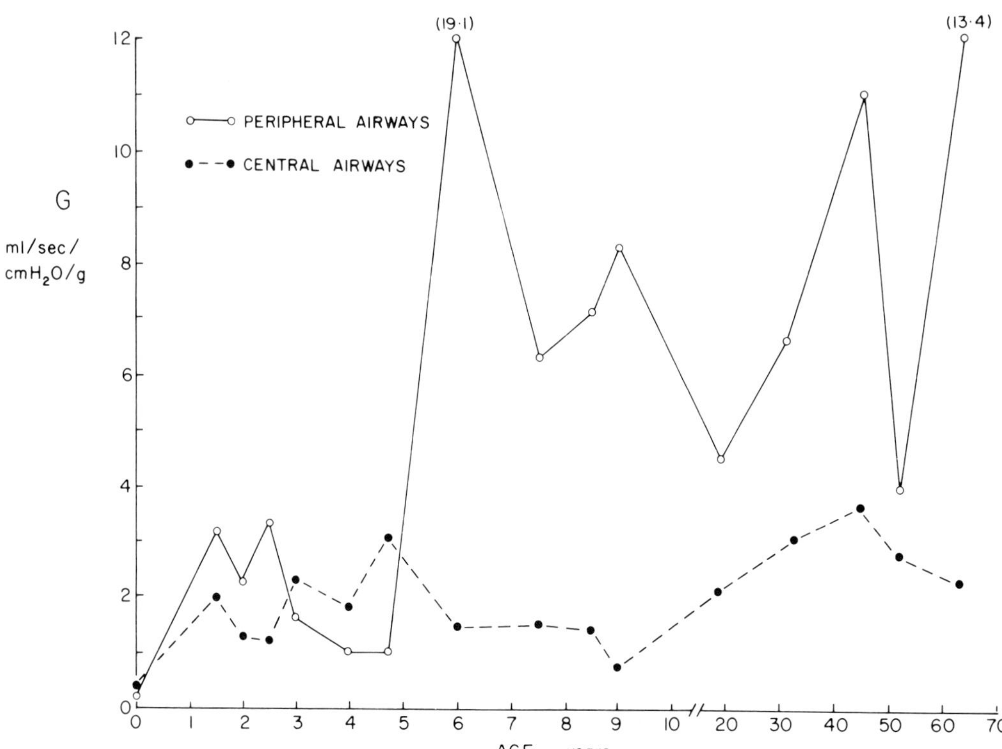

Fig. 2-5. Airways conductance of lungs from subjects of varying ages. The central and peripheral airways are plotted separately. Although the central airways conductance remains uniform at all ages, the peripheral airways conductance increases markedly at about age 5. This is thought to be due to the fact that the peripheral airways increase their radii relatively slowly during the first few years of life, but later, these increase very strikingly.

This observed increase in peripheral airways conductance after about age 5 could be explained if the total number of conducting airways in the periphery of the lung increased, or if their size increased at a more rapid rate than the central airways. We know that the number of conducting airways is fixed by the third month of intrauterine life[16]; therefore, it is likely that the peripheral airways increase in size at a more rapid rate than the central airways, beginning at about age 5. When the number of alveoli is nearly complete at age 5, further lung growth, due to an increase in alveolar dimensions, is probably associated with an increase in small airways diameter.

To understand why a tiny change in airways caliber causes such an increase in conductance requires a return to our previous consideration of flow through tubes. If a single tube branches and if the total cross-sectional area of the two daughter branches is exactly equal to that of the parent, the pressure drop along the daughters is greater than that along the parent. If the daughters increase their cross-sectional area in relation to the parent, the pressure drop along the daughters decreases, and when the ratio of cross-sectional area of parent to daughters becomes greater than $1/\sqrt{2}$, the pressure drop along the daughters is less than that along the parent. Weibel[19] has shown that in adult lungs, the total cross-sectional area increases with each generation at a rate that is much greater than $1/\sqrt{2}$ (Fig. 2-8D). Our data suggest, however, that the same may not be true in children under 5 years of age. Indeed, Charles Bryan and his colleagues* have shown that the ratio is less than $1/\sqrt{2}$ in this age group. The disproportionately high peripheral airways resistance in children is an important concept as it relates to their lung pathology, a point to which we will return later.

CHANGES IN AIRWAY RESISTANCE WITH THE RESPIRATORY CYCLE

In 1892, Einthoven[20] predicted that airway resistance would be greater during expiration because of dynamic widening of the airways during inspiration and narrowing during expiration. He reasoned that if the pressure outside the airways is equal to the pleural pressure, then when no air flow occurs, the pressure across the wall of the airways is equal to the difference between atmospheric pressure and pleural pressure.

During the respiratory cycle, there is a gradient of pressure across the airway wall, as well as a gradient from trachea to alveoli, to produce air flow. During inspiration, the pressure at the outer wall becomes more negative, and a gradient in pressure is introduced at the inner wall, varying from atmospheric pressure near the airway-opening to a value less than atmospheric pressure in the alveoli. The distending pressure difference across the airway wall is, therefore, greater in the large airways than in the small airways. During expiration, the pressure at the outer wall of the airway increases toward atmospheric and the gradient of pressure on the inner wall of the airways is reversed, with pressure falling from greater than atmospheric near the alveoli to atmospheric pressure at the airway-opening. Therefore, when the airways near the airway opening are compared with those near the alveoli, the large airways have a greater distending force exerted on them during inspiration and a lesser distending force exerted on them during expiration than do the small airways. Much later, Dayman[21] measured a variation in airway resistance during the breathing cycle in normal subjects and

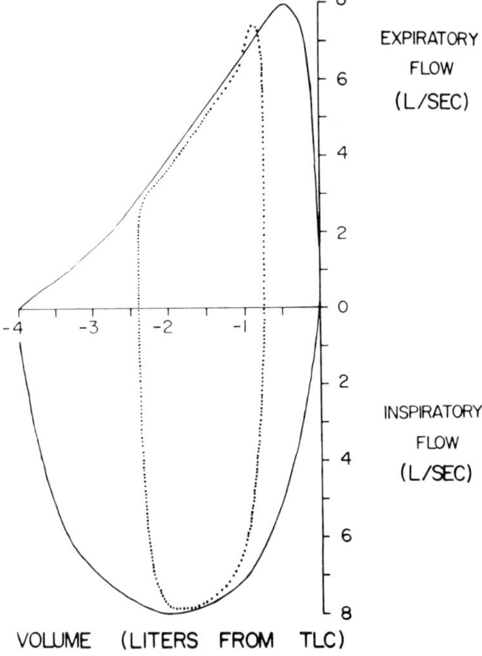

Fig. 2-6. Inspiratory and expiratory flow volume curves. The solid line represents a maximal effort, from TLC to RV. The dotted line represents a submaximal effort.

independently proposed the same mechanism that Einthoven did. Dekker and associates[22] measured intrabronchial pressure directly during voluntary wheezing in normal subjects and showed that the major obstruction during expiration was in the large bronchi. Fry and Hyatt[11] have shown that when flow is plotted against volume during inspiration, flow increases with each increase in effort throughout the inspiration (Fig. 2-6). During forced expiration, however, the maximum flows over the lower two-thirds of the vital capacity are extremely reproducible, uninfluenced by external resistances and independent of effort once maximum flows are reached. To further clarify this, they showed that when transpulmonary pressure is plotted against different flow rates at a particular lung volume in the range of the vital capacity, expiratory flow could not be increased beyond a certain maximum value by increasing driving pressure. This suggested that flow was being limited during expiration

*Personal communication.

by dynamic compression of the intrathoracic airways and led Fry[10] to develop the concept of flow-limiting segments of the airways. The analysis of these segments has proved extremely complex because of the difficulty in characterizing events in the compressed airways.

Mead and associates[23] avoided the compressed segment entirely when they introduced the "equal pressure point" theory in their analysis of expiratory flow. During forced expiration, alveolar pressure drives flow. Because alveolar pressure is made up of the static recoil pressure of the lung and the pleural pressure, it follows that as the pressure drops from the alveolus to the atmosphere, there are points along the airway where the pressure outside the airway (pleural pressure) and the pressure inside the airway are equal. The driving pressure for the segment from the alveolus to the equal pressure points is, therefore, the static recoil pressure of the lung. The equal pressure point (EPP) divides the airways into an upstream segment (alveolus to EPP), where the transmural pressure is positive, and a downstream segment (EPP to mouth), where the transmural pressure is negative. Flow through the upstream segment can be characterized by the resistance of the small airways and the elastic recoil pressure, both of which can be measured. Because the upstream and downstream segments act as resistances in series, characterizing flow through one of them characterizes the flow through the entire system. Using this approach to interpret the isovolume pressure flow curve, Mead and co-workers theorized that the equal pressure point is at the airway opening when pleural pressure is atmospheric. As the pleural pressure becomes more positive than atmospheric pressure, the equal pressure point moves upstream (toward the alveoli) and shortens the upstream segment, decreasing its resistance, so that flow increases. When the equal pressure point becomes fixed, the resistance of the upstream segment is fixed, and this coincides with the flat parts of the isovolume pressure flow curve. The disadvantage of the theory is that it ignores the compressed downstream segment and therefore cannot be used to attempt to explain the mechanisms that actually limit flow.

A third attempt to explain flow limitation on forced expiration, based on the model of a starling resistor, has been put forward by Pride and associates.[24] A starling resistor is a collapsible tube whose resistance depends on the relationship between inlet pressure and surrounding pressure, as long as surrounding pressure is greater than the outlet pressure. Pride and co-workers have applied this to the lungs, where pleural pressure is the surrounding pressure, alveolar pressure is the driving pressure, and outlet pressure is atmospheric pressure. By their analysis, flow continues to increase at a particular volume until the transmural pressure at some point in the airways causes the airway to narrow. They refer to this pressure, which is just sufficient to limit flow, as PTm′ and suggest that it is the same as the transmural pressure required to close the airway under static conditions.

It is important to note that the compression of intrathoracic airways, which limits flow, presents a problem for each of these three theories and that they are not mutually exclusive, but rather focus on one or another part of a complex mechanism. It is of interest that the airway narrowing produced during forced expiration is of greater significance than flow limitation; airway narrowing markedly increases the velocity of the air flow, which is an important feature of the clearance of the airways by the cough mechanism.

SINGLE-BREATH ANALYSIS OF DISTRIBUTION OF VENTILATION

Considerable information can be obtained about the distribution of gases in the ventilated lung regions by analyzing a single respiratory cycle. If nitrogen is measured in the expirate after a single inspiration of pure oxygen, a rapid increase in the amount of nitrogen is observed as the dead space is washed out, followed by a gradually increasing alveolar plateau (Fig. 2-7B). Krogh and Lindhard[25] thought that this plateau was due to the fact that gas mixing

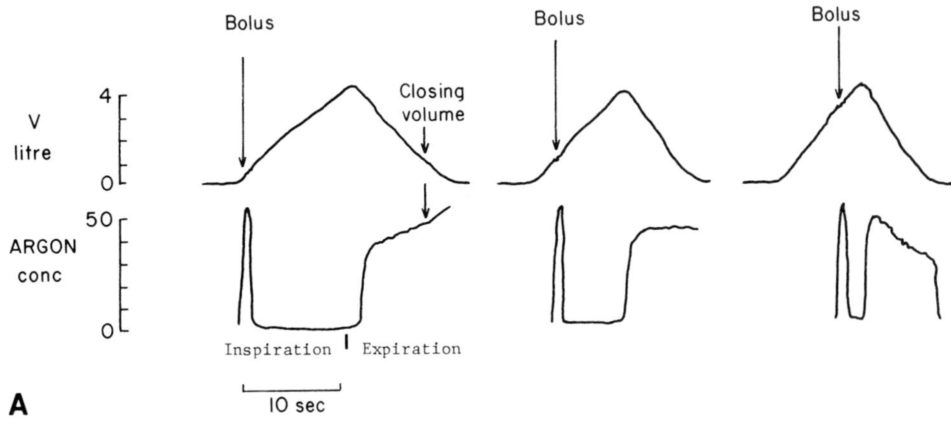

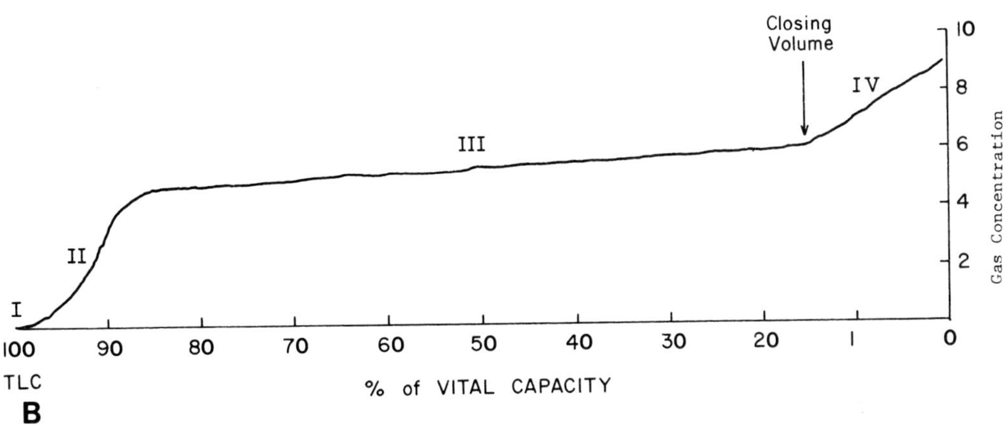

Fig. 2-7. (*A*) The continuous analysis of expired breaths following an inhalation of a bolus of argon. When the bolus is inhaled near residual volume, the argon trace slopes upward throughout expiration, with an inflection and a steeper upward slope as residual volume is approached. When the bolus is inhaled higher in inspiration, the argon trace is flat throughout expiration, and when it is inhaled near TLC, it slopes downward. (Data modified from Fowler, K.: Relative compliances of the well and poorly ventilated spaces in the normal human lung. J. Appl. Physiol., *19*:937, 1964) (*B*) This shows the tracer gas plotted against the vital capacity. The bolus is introduced at RV; the subject inhales to TLC; and the expired breath is analyzed at the mouth. Phase II represents the washout of mixed alveolar and dead-space gas. Phase III represents alveolar gas, which is upward-sloping because of the continuous addition of gas from poorly ventilated spaces. Phase IV represents the contribution from the poorly ventilated space following closure of the airways. The point of inflection of this trace is labeled *closing volume* and can also be seen on the argon trace of the RV bolus in Fowler's data (*A*). A similar curve is obtained for nitrogen, when a single breath of oxygen is inhaled from RV to TLC. (Modified from Dolfuss, R., Milic-Emili, J., and Bates, D.: Regional ventilation of the lung studied with boluses of xenon. Respir. Physiol., *22*:760, 1967)

was slow enough to leave a gradient in nitrogen within the lungs. Rauwerda,[26] however, calculated that diffusion in the lungs is rapid enough to make this gradient unlikely and concluded that Krogh and Lindhard's explanation of the alveolar plateau was incorrect. This led to the consideration that the plateau could be explained by regional inhomogeneity in the distribution of the inspired air.

The relative importance of compliance over resistance in the distribution of ventilation was first suggested by Fowler.[27] He estimated that the time constant (i.e., the product of resistance and compliance) of the lower airways and lung was about 0.15 second. He concluded, from theoretical considerations, that the threefold changes in the time constant produced by changes in resistance would have little effect on ventilation distribution. He therefore analyzed single expired breaths obtained after the introduction of argon and calculated the effective compliance of the well-ventilated and poorly ventilated spaces. When the expired air is analyzed for argon after a single inspiration of the argon mixture, a downward-sloping plateau is observed. This indicates that the flow from the space receiving the least amount of argon is greatest at low lung volumes. By introducing boluses of argon at RV, FRC, and near TLC in separate tests (Fig. 2-7A), he observed that the argon-concentration in the expired breath was upward sloping, flat, and downward sloping, respectively. He concluded that the poorly ventilated space received the highest flow near RV, whereas the well-ventilated space received the highest flow between FRC and TLC. Because of the location of the cardiac oscillations during these expired breaths, he speculated that the well-ventilated space was in the lower lung and the poorly ventilated space in the upper lung.

The introduction of radioactive gas methods made it possible to demonstrate the topographical difference in the distribution of ventilation between lung regions. Milic-Emili and associates[28] showed that at RV the upper lung regions expand to about 35 per cent of their total capacity, whereas the lower lung regions expand to only about 10 per cent. During the initial expansion of the lung above RV, the upper regions expand rapidly, with very little expansion in the lower zones. At lung volumes above 40 per cent of TLC, however, the expansion is greatest in the lower regions, and this relative distribution of regional expansion remains the same up to TLC. They assumed that there was no difference in the pressure volume characteristics of lung regions and attributed the differences in expansion that they observed to the pleural pressure gradient. It followed that because the pleural pressure is more negative at the lung top, the upper lung regions would expand more at RV, and because they were on the steep portion of the pressure-volume curve, they would expand most rapidly close to RV. The lower regions would be much less expanded, so that closure of the lower airways would explain the fact that these regions expand little during the initial phase of respiration. Above FRC, the upper lung regions approach the flatter, less compliant portion of the lung pressure volume curve and expand slowly, whereas the lower lung regions remain on the steep, more compliant portion of the curve and expand rapidly. Dolfuss and associates[29] used the bolus technique with radioactive xenon as the test gas. This allowed the distribution of gases in the inspired breath to be studied both by examination of the expired breath and by external counting of the xenon over the chest. They tied together the observations of Fowler and of Milic-Emili and associates by demonstrating a gradual progression from the poorly ventilated upper lung regions to the well-ventilated lower lung regions. The slope of the alveolar plateau (Phase III, Fig. 2-7B) was found to be consistent with small progressive increases in the contribution of alveolar gas from the upper lung regions, and the steep rise in the slope of Phase IV (Fig. 2-7B) was found to be consistent with lower airway closure, so that all of the remaining expired breath came from the upper regions.

In recent years, there has been a great deal of interest in the analysis of single expired breaths. By displaying volume on one axis and gas concentration on the other axis of an X-Y recorder (Fig. 2-7B), the volume at which Phase IV begins has been called *the closing volume*. Currently, a great deal of interest is being shown in the measurement of both closing volume and the slope of Phase III, and it is possible that they may provide good tests for minimal airways obstruction. This is discussed further in relation to the early detection of disease in Chapter 3.

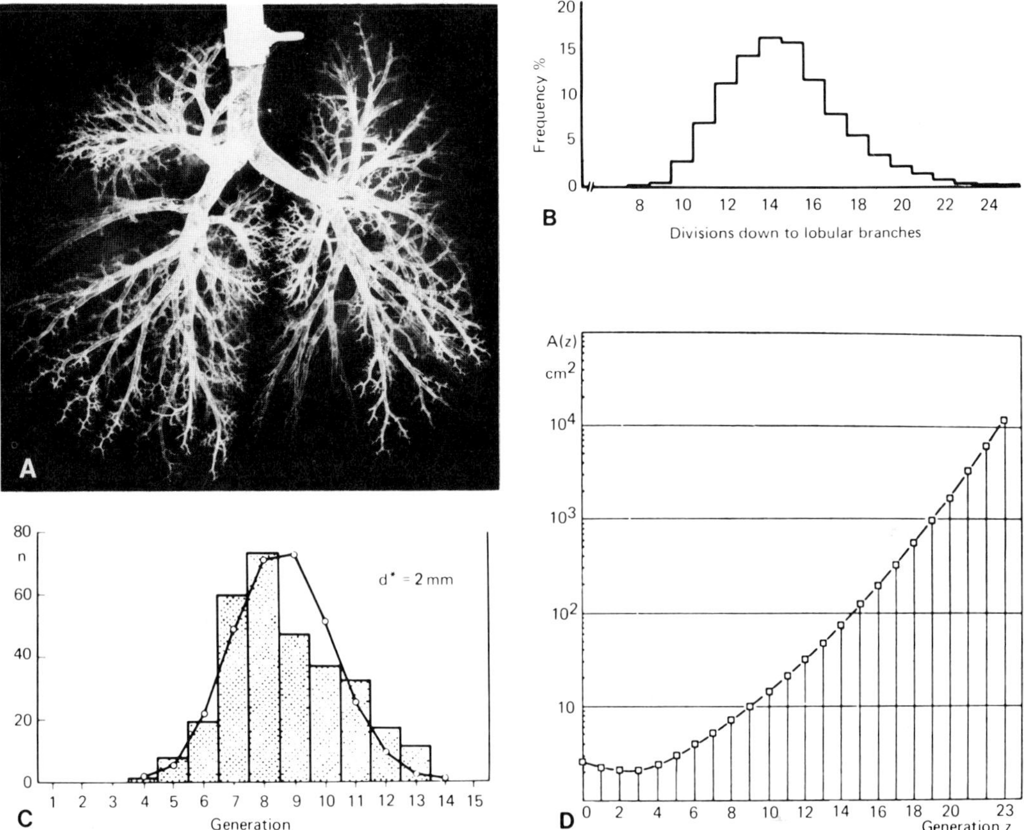

Fig. 2-8. (*A*) A normal human bronchogram. Note the differing size of bronchi and the varying number of branches. (*B*) The number of branches along the bronchial tree. Eight to twenty-four branches may occur, depending on the lung region. The most frequent number is fourteen. (*C*) The distribution of small airways may occur after a highly variable degree of bronchial branching. This graph demonstrates the number of divisions of bronchi that result in 2-mm. diameter airways. Although they are found after four to fourteen divisions, they most commonly occur after eight. (*D*) The cross-sectional area of the airways may decrease slightly at the time of the first or second division. Thereafter, it progressively increases to the most distal generation of bronchi. (*B* modified from Horsfield, K., and Cumming, G.: The morphology of the bronchial tree in man. J. Appl. Physiol., *24*:373, 1968. *C* and *D* reproduced with permission from Weibel, E.: Morphometry of the Human Lung. New York, Academic Press, 1963)

THE ANATOMY OF THE AIRWAYS AND THEIR RESPONSE TO INJURY

In this presentation, we will not provide a description of the segmental anatomy of the airways, because this has been adequately covered in numerous other texts. This omission will allow us to concentrate on the quantitative anatomy of the airways and the alterations that occur in the lung in response to injury.

ANATOMY OF THE CONDUCTING AIRWAYS

A great deal of pertinent information concerning the nature and branching of the airways can be gained by looking at a normal bronchogram. Careful examination of the tracheobronchial tree (Fig. 2-8A) shows that it is slightly asymmetrical, because the branches are not always equal in size. It also shows that it is possible to reach the

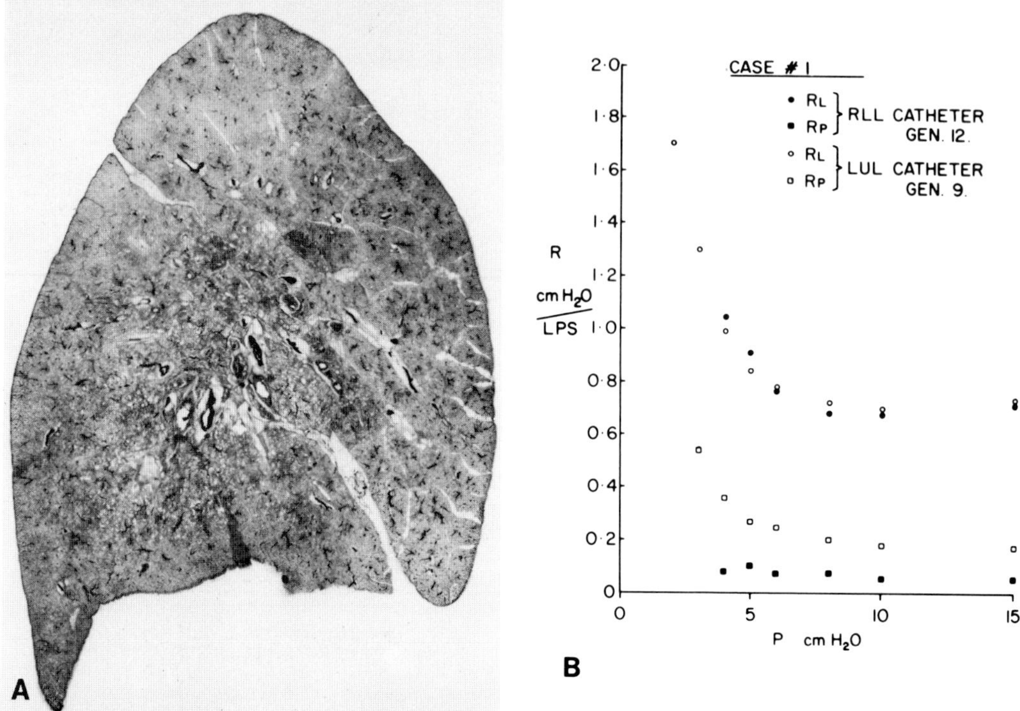

Fig. 2-9. (*A*) A normal, paper-mounted, whole lung section. (*B*) The distribution of airways resistance in an excised normal human lung. R_L is total airway resistance, and R_P is the resistance of the peripheral airways. Total resistance at a transpulmonary pressure of 4 mm. Hg is about 1 cm. of water per liter per second; about 10 per cent of this is located in airways distal to generation twelve. This compares favorably with values in life, which are about 2 cm. of water per liter per second, with the remainder being accounted for by the larynx, which was not present in these experiments. (*B* modified from Hogg, J., Macklem, P., and Thurlbeck, W.: Site and nature of airways obstruction in chronic obstructive lung disease. N. Engl. J. Med., *278*:1355, 1968)

alveolated structures from the trachea by traversing a different number of branch points, depending on the pathway followed. The exact number of branch points or generations traversed as different pathways are followed has been computed by Horsfield and Cumming,[30] who showed that the path from the trachea to the alveolated structures may traverse as few as eight or as many as twenty-four branch points (Fig. 2-8B). This means that airways of a particular size are found at a variety of positions along the length of the airway, because they narrow at different rates. For example, Weibel[19] (Fig. 2-8C) has shown that 2-mm. airways may be found anywhere from the fourth to the fourteenth bronchial divisions. The size of the total cross section of airways of different generations is also of interest, because this information is crucial in understanding the distribution of airways resistance. For many years, it was thought that the peripheral airways (i.e., 2 mm. and smaller) constituted the narrowest point in the tracheobronchial tree. This information was based on the work of the great Swiss physiologist, Rohrer, who measured the diameter of airways in excised uninflated lungs with calibrated bougies. Much more recently, Weibel[19] measured the diameter of these airways from casts of human lungs

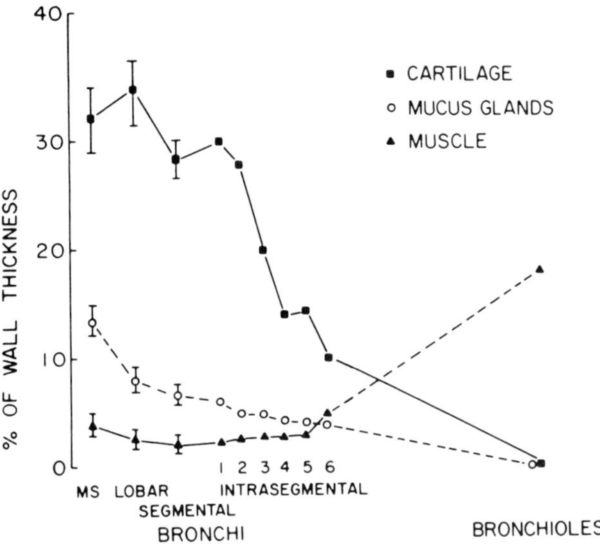

Fig. 2-10. The distribution of cartilage, mucous glands, and muscle, from main-stem bronchi to bronchioles, in the tracheobronchial tree. Note that bronchioles have no cartilage but are muscular.

and found that Rohrer had grossly underestimated both the number and the total cross-sectional area of these small airways. Weibel showed that as one progressed towards the peripheral generations of airways, the total cross-sectional area increased markedly (Fig. 2-8D). This information has important physiological implications, because it means that the peripheral airways should account for a very small proportion of the total airways resistance. This was shown to be the case by Macklem and Mead,[13] who introduced an ingenious method for measuring pressure in the small airways, so that peripheral airways resistance could be measured. Similar data[17] have also been obtained using this technique in human lungs (Fig. 2-9). An important corollary of this is that disease must be very severe in these airways before it can be detected by measuring total airways resistance. Returning to our discussion of lung growth, it is possible that the cross-sectional area of children's lungs, from trachea to alveoli, increases at a slower rate than the rate Weibel has shown for adult lungs, because peripheral airways may show little or no increase in dimension during the period from 1 to 5 years of age, when lung growth occurs primarily by an increase in the number of alveoli. If this is so, it would explain why the peripheral airways resistance in children's lungs is disproportionately high and perhaps why airways disease can be so devastating in the younger child.

MICROSCOPIC ANATOMY OF THE AIRWAYS

The airways are made up of cartilage, smooth muscle, mucous-producing glands, connective tissue, and epithelium. The relative amounts of cartilage, smooth muscle, and mucous gland that make up the walls of the airways are shown in Figure 2-10. Cartilage makes up about 30 per cent of the wall thickness in the main-stem and lobar bronchi and gradually decreases. By definition, the bronchioles are airways that do not contain cartilage in their walls. The bronchial mucous glands make up about 12 per cent of the wall thickness in the main-stem bronchi, and then these, too, gradually diminish as the more peripheral airways are reached. The bronchioles contain no mucous glands in their walls. Smooth muscle, on the other hand, represents only about 5 per cent of the airway thickness in the main-stem airway, but this increases along the airways. The wall thickness of the bronchioles, which are the most muscular airways, is composed of about 20 per cent muscle.

The Bronchial Epithelium

The epithelium in the airways is a pseudostratified columnar type. The cells of which it is primarily comprised are the goblet cell and the ciliated cell. Other cells such as the nonciliated bronchial epithelial cell (Clara cell) and the representatives of the APUD system have also been described, but their function is less certain.[31] The major functions of the epithelium are to protect the lung from injurious agents and to trap and clear particulate matter from the airways. The two major cell types responsible for these functions are the ciliated epithelial cell and the goblet cell. These cells are responsible for maintaining the mucociliary blanket that serves to protect the tracheobronchial tree by trapping and removing foreign material. The mucous layer is produced by both the goblet cells and the bronchial mucous glands. Reid has shown that the number of cells producing mucus in the glands is greater than the number of goblet cells, and it has been assumed that the glands are more important as a source of mucus than are the goblet cells. Study of the physical characteristics of the mucous layer shows that the superficial layer is more viscous than the deep layer. This is important with respect to the ciliary function, because the cilia are allowed to recover rapidly in the less viscous lower layer; whereas they attach to the highly viscous superficial layer during their power stroke to propel this layer toward the mouth. The cilia beat in unison to provide an effective escalator type of mechanism to clear the airway. The structure of cilia is similar in all biological species, in that they all have a characteristic 9 + 2 structure. This means that there are nine pairs of microtubular structures arranged in doublets around the periphery of each cilia, with one central pair of microtubules that are separated from each other (i.e., non-doublet). The structure and function of the microtubules in many cell types are presently under active investigation, but their specific function in the ciliated epithelial cell of the tracheobronchial tree is only beginning to be studied. The fact that the cilia maintain a constant length in both the power and recovery strokes, however, suggests that the microtubules move as a system of sliding filaments, with a powerful winding of the filaments during the slow power stroke, followed by a quick release and rapid unwinding during the higher-velocity recovery stroke.[32,33]

In addition to the mucous layer, the epithelium provides a further protective mechanism by the arrangements of the cell junctions. The junctional complexes of most epithelial cells have three components that succeed one another, proceeding from the luminal surface to the base of the cell. The zonula occludens provides membrane-to-membrane contact around the periphery of the cells at the luminal surface. This function represents a fusion of the outer leaflet of the membranes of adjacent cells. This fusion is not continuous but represents a series of fusions arranged in parallel. The number and extent of these fusions appear to determine the permeability of the junctional complexes and vary with epithelia in different organs. The second component of the junctional complex is the zonula adherens, where the membranes of the adjacent cells are separated by a space of about 200°, which is filled by protein filaments. The third component of the functional complex is the desmosome or macula adherens, where the adjacent cell membranes are separated but are joined by an intermediate line that may represent condensation of the material of the cell coat.

In addition to the junctional complex, the epithelial cells are joined at various other sites by the nexus or gap junction. This junction provides direct communication between cells without communication with the intercellular space, but its function is unknown. Whether or not these communications are important in controlling the uniformity of the ciliary beat remains to be investigated, but it is worth noting that these junctions are thought to be important in the electrical coupling of cells and in the passage of small molecules between cells. Of great interest is the fact that these junctions have been shown to decrease in number during the development of squamous-cell carcinoma of the cervix and to be related to the phenomenon of contact inhibition of cells growing in tissue culture. The investigation of the precise structural and functional relationships will provide intriguing questions for the investigator interested in the biology and pathology of the airway epithelium.

The Bronchial Glands

The secretory portions of the mucous glands are embedded in the submucosa. The ducts from these glands extend to the luminal surface of the airway, where they empty their contents onto the mucociliary blanket. Their secretion can be influenced by the autonomic nervous system, in that stimulation of the vagus or injection of acetylcholine can cause beads of secretion to appear where the duct opens onto the epithelial surface. Just what part the autonomic nervous system plays in the normal function of the glands is more difficult to determine.

Airway Cartilage

The trachea and the extrapulmonary bronchi consist of a framework of incomplete rings of hyaline cartilage united by fibrous tissue and nonstriated muscle. The trachea has from sixteen to twenty horseshoe-shaped cartilages that open posteriorly. Two or more of these cartilage plates often unite either partially or completely; they may calcify and sometimes contain bone in advanced age. The cartilages are enclosed by an elastic fibrous membrane, with a dense layer passing over the outer surface of the rings and a less dense layer over the inner surface. These layers fuse to form a tough membrane both between the rings and in the posterior part of the trachea and main-stem bronchi, where the rings are deficient.

The horseshoe-shaped rings of cartilage in the trachea and extrapulmonary bronchi are replaced by irregularly shaped cartilage plates in the intrapulmonary bronchi. Although their irregularity in shape suggests that they might not encircle the bronchus, Miller showed, by reconstruction, that these cartilages do encircle the lumen of the airway completely in many instances. The cartilage, like the mucous glands, decreases in amount with successive generations of airway, until it disappears completely in the bronchioles.

Smooth Muscle

Muscle is present only in the posterior part of the trachea and extrapulmonary bronchi, where it is located within the fibrous membrane. The longitudinal fibers are external and consist of a few scattered bundles, whereas the transverse fibers form the tracheal muscle, which extends between the ends of the cartilage and passes across in the intervals between them.

In the intrapulmonary airways, the muscle lies between the epithelium and cartilage in a layer that encircles the lumen. It is formed by two sets of fibers, one rotating around the airway in a clockwise fashion and the other in a counterclockwise fashion. The function of this muscle is not at all clear, but it is influenced by the autonomic nervous system. Stimulation of the parasympathetic nervous system causes contraction, and stimulation of the β-adrenergic system causes dilation. The contribution of the α-adrenergic system to bronchoconstriction is controversial.

Bronchial Circulation

The various elements of the airways that have been described all receive their blood supply from the systemic circulation. The tracheal blood supply is variable but usually arises from the inferior thyroid vessels and drains into the inferior thyroid venous plexus. The bronchial arteries supply the extrathoracic airways, and these usually arise from the descending thoracic aorta and form the upper posterior intercostal arteries. In the bronchi, they form a capillary plexus that supplies the muscle and submucosa of the airways. This plexus communicates with branches of the pulmonary artery and empties into the pulmonary veins. Other branches supply the interlobular tissue and the pleura, and these drain into the bronchial veins, which empty into the azygos vein on the right side and into the superior intercostal or superior hemiazygos vein on the left side.

THE PATHOLOGY OF TRACHEOBRONCHIAL INJURY

ACUTE TRACHEOBRONCHIAL INJURY

Tracheitis and Bronchitis

Acute tracheitis and bronchitis are very common afflictions of man. Indeed, most persons suffer these illnesses many times during their life. A wide variety of agents can produce laryngotracheobronchitis; these include noxious gases, particulate irritants, and a variety of living organisms.

The conducting airways of the lung have a limited way in which to respond, so that the appearance of the airways is similar with a wide variety of etiologic agents. The common denominator of all of the agents is that they induce an inflammatory response that follows a sequence, progressing from vasoconstriction, followed by vasodilatation, to transudation of fluid from capillaries into the airways lumen. As most irritants also increase the mucus production, the fluid has a characteristically sticky white appearance until the polymorphonuclear cells migrate from the capillaries into the mucous exudate and change it to the characteristically yellow-green sputum of purulent tracheobronchitis. The exfoliation of superficial bronchial epithelial cells is increased by this process. If the injury is severe, large ulcerations of the mucosa may develop, and bleeding may occur, giving the sputum a blood-tinged appearance.

The extent and degree of the injury depend on the distribution of the agent and its concentration at various levels of the tracheobronchial tree. The factors determining this are very complex. For example, nitrogen dioxide gas is extremely soluble in water and is therefore absorbed rapidly in the airways, so that it primarily damages the upper airways, trachea, and main bronchi. The tracheobronchial tree may also be contaminated by bacteria and viruses that are carried in water droplets. Distribution of these aerosols depends on the particles' or droplets' weight, size, velocity, settling time, and so forth. Large droplets tend to impact by inertial forces, so that they leave the flowing stream of air at bends and branch points in the nose and larynx. Smaller particles remain in the stream and penetrate deeper into the lung. Differences between the agents producing disease in the airways and those producing disease in the alveoli may relate to the physical characteristics of the agents, which determine how they are delivered to the lungs. The responses of the airways and parenchyma could differ, because the conducting airways are supplied by the bronchial circulation, where a higher capillary pressure might result in exudates that are sticky and remain localized, as in the so-called bronchopneumonic processes; whereas the lung parenchyma is supplied by the pulmonary circulation, where capillary injury might produce a transudate that would spread quickly through the alveolar spaces, as in the early stages of pneumococcal pneumonia. Direct evidence in support of these hypotheses, however, is difficult to come by.

Bronchiolitis

There probably is involvement of the bronchioles in most cases of airway injury. In adults, however, this has relatively little effect on airways resistance, and since it is usually not life-threatening, we seldom have the opportunity to observe the pathology of this condition. Quite the reverse is true in children, where the peripheral airways make up a significant proportion of total resistance, and disease in the bronchioles can be serious. Bronchiolitis has been defined as an acute illness, mainly affecting infants, in which the principal lesion is an inflammatory obstruction of the small airways.[34] It is usually preceded by several days of mild upper-respiratory infection, followed by an acute onset of respiratory distress when the lower-respiratory tract becomes involved. Physical examination at this time reveals a rapid respiratory rate; a

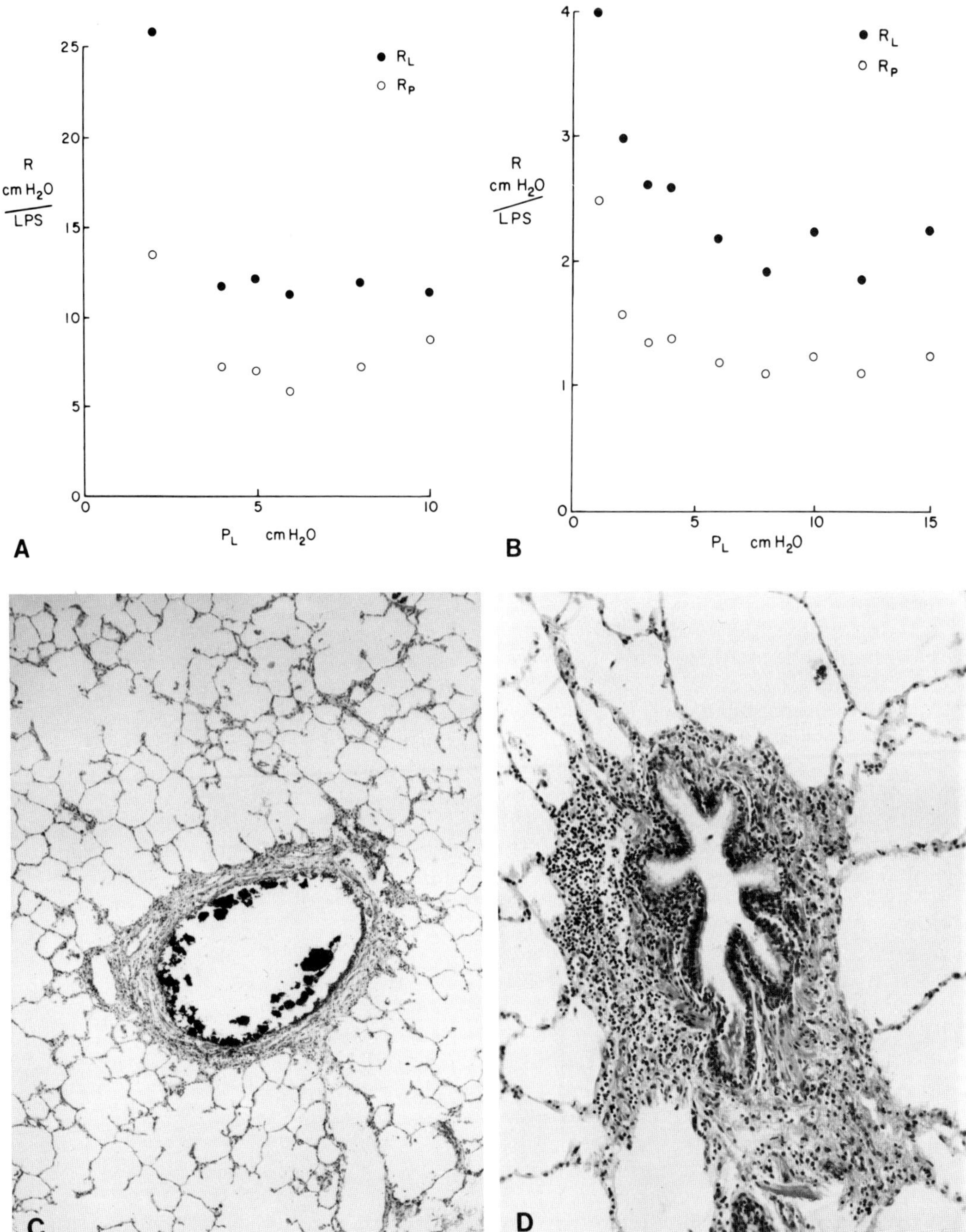

Fig. 2-11. The distribution of airways resistance in a 6-month-old child (*A*) and in a 63-year-old adult (*B*), both of whom have bronchiolitis. In both cases, the total airways resistance (R_L) is high, with a large portion of the resistance being accounted for by an increase in peripheral airways resistance (R_P). Compare this with the normal lung in Figure 2-9B. The morphological features of the child (*C*) and the adult (*D*). In both cases, note the thickening of the airway wall due to the inflammation of the wall. The surrounding parenchyma is normal in both cases.

hyperinflated chest, with marked activity of the accessory muscles of respiration; a dry, unproductive cough; and a low-grade fever.

In a study of forty-one cases, High[34] found that twenty-one cases occurred in children less than 6 months of age, ten cases in children between 6 months and a year, and eight of the remaining ten cases in children in the second year of life. Only two of the forty-one cases were in older children, and the oldest was 4 years of age.

Laboratory investigation reveals signs of overinflation on the chest reontgenogram, with little or no parenchymal change. Bacterial pathogens are often isolated from the throat and sputum of these patients and are thought to represent secondary invasion rather than a primary cause. The etiological agent in the disease is generally thought to be of viral origin.[35] Further information on this topic is included in the section on viral infections, Chapter 6.

The most consistent disorder of anatomy in bronchiolitis is a lymphocytic infiltration of the bronchiolar wall, with a proliferation of the basal cells and extrusion of the columnar cells toward the center of the lumen. This produces a marked thickening of the bronchiolar wall and a narrowing of the lumen, but actual plugging of the lumen with inflammatory mucus is a less obvious feature of the disease.[34] It is of interest that even though upper-respiratory infections with later involvement of the lower-respiratory tract are common in adults as well as in children, this sequence of events rarely has a serious effect on older children and adults. Studies done on human lungs obtained at autopsy have shown that bronchiolitis does occur in adults, but that it probably goes unrecognized, because it produces little effect on total airway resistance. Results from two postmortem studies shown in Figure 2-11A and B illustrate this point. Both cases had morphological evidence of bronchiolitis (Fig. 2-11C, D), and both had physiological evidence of increased central and peripheral airways resistance. The 6-month-old child, however, died from the disease, whereas the 63-year-old patient had only minor respiratory symptoms at the time of sudden death from a cerbrovascular accident. One possible reason for this could be the anatomy of the airways. In the child, the peripheral airways are disproportionately narrow, and collateral ventilation is poorly developed, so that airway closure with overinflation might easily occur. This could result in defective gas exchange and a life-threatening situation. On the other hand, in the adult, the peripheral airways total cross-sectional area is large, and collateral ventilation is well developed, so that the interference with gas exchange may be minimal.

CHRONIC BRONCHIAL INJURY

When the tracheobronchial tree is subjected to injurious agents over long periods of time, fundamental changes occur in the airways. The ciliated cells of the epithelium are replaced by either goblet cells or squamous cells, as a result of a metaplastic process. This change, which must be an attempt at protection, leads to difficulty by both increasing the production of and decreasing the clearance of the mucus. In the later stages of chronic bronchitis, the inflammatory process becomes less impressive, with the striking pathological features being enlargement of the bronchial mucous glands and some increase in the number of goblet cells. Study of postmortem lungs has shown that the greatest degree of obstruction with chronic disease occurs in the peripheral airways, and this seems to be due to mucus plugging the lumen of these small airways, chronic inflammation of their walls with fibrosis, and even obliteration of the small airways in some cases.

Chronic Bronchitis

This condition has been defined as persistent excess mucus in the tracheobronchial tree that is not caused by other specific conditions such as bronchiectasis.[36] It is recognized clinically by excessive sputum production, which is usually associated with cough. (For a complete clinical definition, see Chap. 13.) The morphological criteria for diagnosis involve a description of the mucous glands and the mucosal goblet cells. Because the mucous glands have been estimated to have 100 times the volume of the goblet cells, their size has been taken as a morphological criterion for the diagnosis of chronic bronchitis. Although the Reid index, or ratio of gland thickness to wall thickness, offered some promise in separating patients with bronchitis from those without bronchitis, it is now apparent that there is a considerable overlap in the values obtained for this ratio between these two groups. Thurlbeck and Angus[37] have recently shown that the distribution curve of the Reid index in the general autopsy population is bell-shaped, where those subjects with values less than 0.35 usually did not have symptoms of bronchitis during life, and those with values greater than 0.55 usually had clinical evidence of bronchitis. The bulk of the values for the patients in their study fell in the intermediate range, however, where there was a varying incidence of bronchitis. They suggested that since the clinical criterion of sputum production is open to considerable error, it may be more realistic to consider a continuum from normal to bronchitis, without an arbitrary separation of the two distinct groups (bronchitics and nonbronchitics), based on rigid morphological criteria.

The possibility that decreased bronchial clearance might result in excessive tracheobronchial mucus has not been adequately investigated. Although the use of radiopaque and radioactive materials shows promise for the study of clearance mechanisms in the lung, these mechanisms have not been satisfactorily characterized. The morphology of the bronchial cilia and the excessive mucus found in the airways at autopsy, however, suggest that abnormal clearance may be of great importance in this disease.[38] The physical properties of mucus in health and disease are of equal importance, but although descriptions of "viscid, sticky, highly viscous and thick" mucus abound in the literature, the study of the exact visco-elastic nature of the material has proved to be difficult.

Pulmonary Emphysema

Introduction. Emphysema has been defined as an increase, beyond normal size, of the air spaces that are distal to the terminal bronchioles, accompanied by destructive change.[36] The relative importance of overinflation and actual destruction of lung tissue in emphysema has been controversial. The published works supporting each side of the controversy are very extensive, and a discussion of them is not relevant here. Laennec[39] provided the first lucid account of the condition in 1819 and gave excellent gross descriptions of air-dried specimens of lungs from patients who had died of the disease. In his review of the morbid anatomy of emphysema, Strawbridge[40] stated, "Since the original microscopic description of chronic emphysema by Rainey in 1848 there has been virtually complete agreement that the basic lesion is destruction of the alveolar walls by the process of fenestration." The exact etiology of the fenestration (and whether the fenestrae represent enlarged pores of Kohn or new holes in the alveolar wall) is, of course, much more controversial.

Morphological Types of Emphysema. *Centrilobular Emphysema.* A renewal of interest in the morphology of emphysema was brought about by the description of centrilobular emphysema by Gough.[41] He and Leopold[42] showed that centrilobular emphysematous spaces are respiratory bronchioles, arising from more than one of the terminal bronchioles within a lobule, that have enlarged and become confluent. In the classic case, the alveolar ducts and sacs at the rim of the lobule are preserved, so that the cut surface of the lung appears to have punched-out holes that are separated by relatively normal-appearing alveolated structures. In many instances, however, the parenchyma at the rim of the lobule is not normal, and arbitrary decisions have to be made concerning the type of emphysema that is present. In general, the disease is more severe in the upper zones of the lung (Fig. 2-12).

Panlobular Emphysema. In this form, the entire acinus is involved. In the early stages, effacement of the alveoli produces a

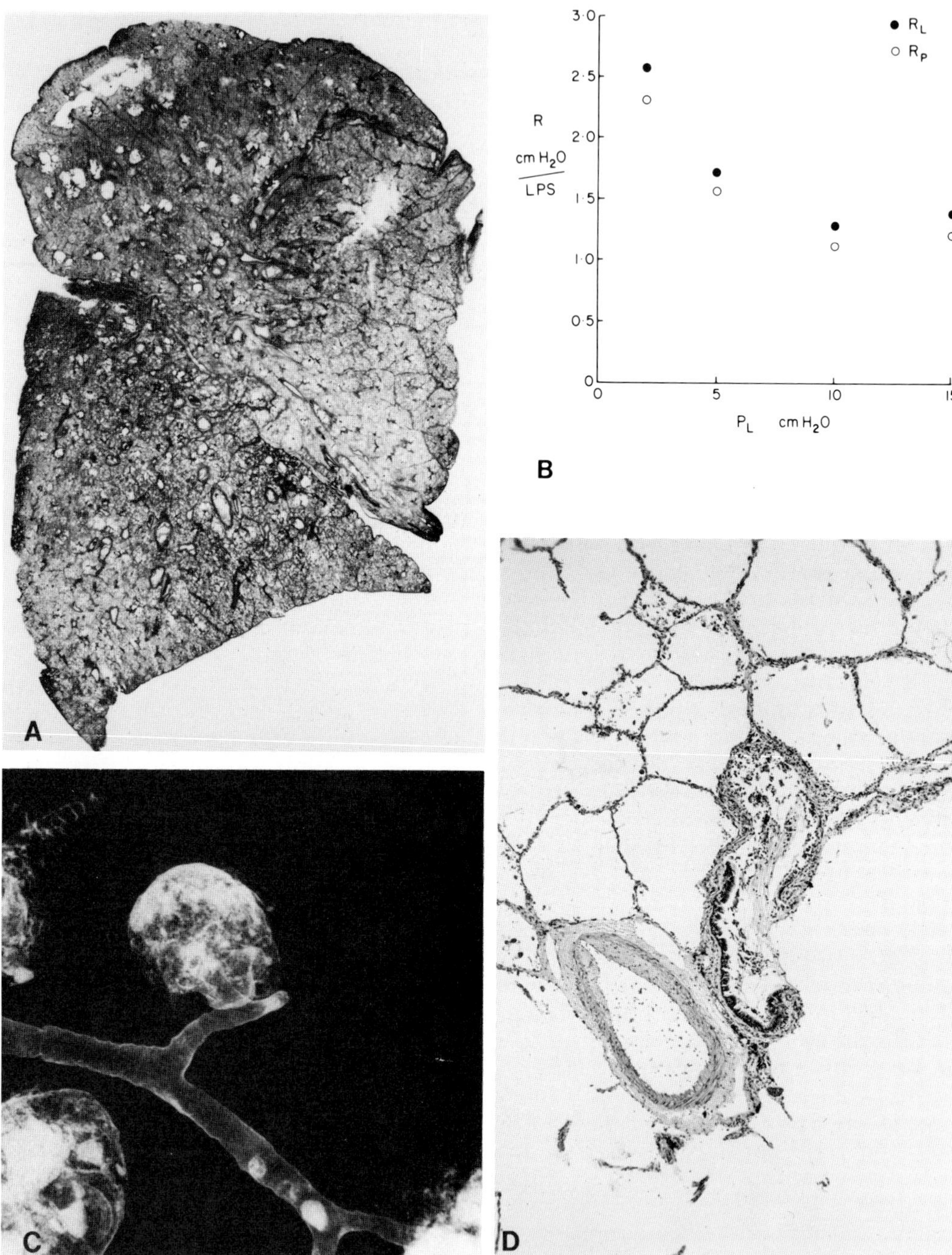

Fig. 2-12. (*A*) A paper-mounted, whole lung section with centrilobular emphysema. (*B*) The distribution of airways resistance in a case of centrilobular emphysema. In this case, the total airways resistance is increased (R_L), primarily because of the increase in peripheral airways resistance (R_P). (*C*) A bronchogram of the centrilobular emphysematous space. (*D*) Histological section of the airways near a centrilobular emphysematous space, showing narrowing and mucous plugging.

loss of the sharp distinction between alveoli and ducts, so that some scientists have referred to this as *alveolar duct emphysema*. As the disease progresses, however, there is a gradual destruction of the entire acinus. Panlobular emphysema is more or less random in its distribution within the lung, but there is a tendency for more frequent occurrence in the anterior basal segment and the tip of the lingula (Fig. 2-13).

Other Types of Emphysema. Heard and Izukawa[43] have described a form of emphysema that selectively involves the periphery of the lobule, and because of its relationship to the lobular septae, it was referred to as *paraseptal emphysema*. Since the lobular septae are often imcomplete, some prefer to call this *periacinar, linear,* or *superficial* emphysema.

Emphysema that shows no particular localization within the acinus is termed *irregular emphysema*, and as this is often seen in relation to scars, it is also referred to as *scar emphysema*.

***Incidence of Emphysema*.** If examples of scar emphysema are included, emphysema can be demonstrated in 80 to 90 per cent of random adult necropsies. Only about 50 per cent, however, show well-defined panlobular or centrilobular forms. The disease occurs from the third to the ninth decade, with the majority of cases occurring in the sixth, seventh, and eighth decades, and although all forms of emphysema are more common in men than women, panlobular emphysema is more common than centrilobular emphysema in women.[44]

Measurement of Emphysema. There have been many attempts to quantitate the extent and severity of emphysema in lungs obtained at autopsy. Thurlbeck[45] has recently reviewed the methods that have been used and pointed out that because most of them are subjective, it is difficult to compare observations obtained by one method to those obtained by another. The type of measurement selected depends on the exact correlation between structure and function that is being attempted. For example, a simple method would be preferred if one were interested in the incidence of emphysema in a large population, because many lungs would have to be studied; whereas a more exact method, providing specific information about the number and size of the airways, would be required in a study attempting to correlate airway resistance with the morphology of the lung.

The extent of emphysema is usually assessed on the cut surface of a whole lung fixed in inflation. Heard and Izukawa[43] divided the surface of the lung into six zones and assessed the extent separately in each zone. Sweet and colleagues[46] covered the lung with a grid 1 cm. square and assessed the amount of emphysema in each square. Dunnill[47] used a grid with holes in it and assessed the lung he could see through the holes, using the Delesse principle to quantitate the amount of emphysema in the lung. Pratt and co-workers,[48] on the other hand, planimetered the area of the lung and the area of the surface that was involved with emphysema. Thurlbeck[45] assessed the amount of emphysema in each of ten zones in the lung and graded the emphysema in each zone on a 0-to-3 scale, depending on its severity. This gave a possible score ranging from 0 emphysema to 30 units of emphysema in extremely severe cases. His attempt to grade both extent and severity of the disease has an advantage over the methods that only measure the extent of the condition. A recent attempt to correlate these measurements with a rough visual estimate based on photographs provides a useful alternative to these measurements.[49]

A quantitative assessment of disease in the airways is of great importance in emphysema, but the methods employed have not been completely satisfactory. The Reid index for quantitating bronchitis has been referred to earlier in this chapter, and other attempts to measure the volume of the mucous glands have been described.[50] It is difficult, however, to know if enlarged bronchial mucous glands actually indicate the presence of excessive tracheobronchial mucus, because the size of the glands might in fact be a poor indication of their ability to produce mucus. Quantitative as-

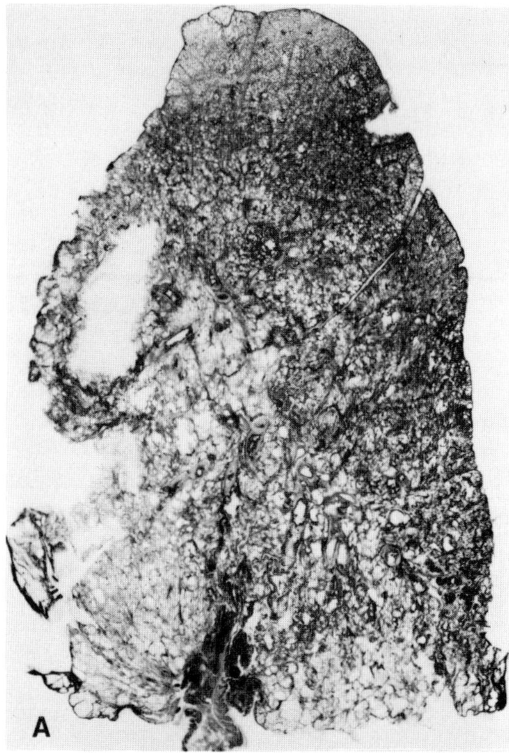

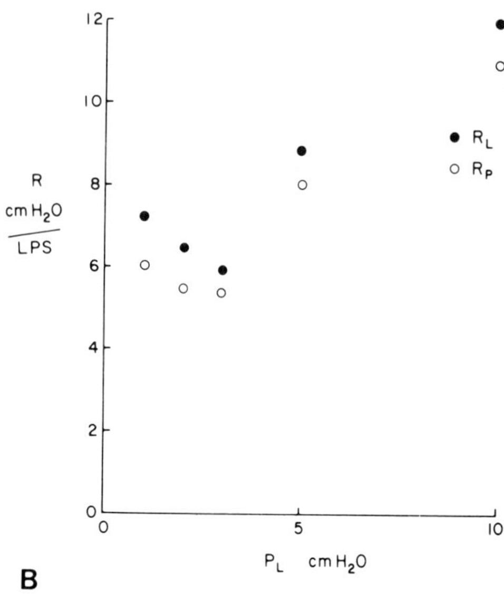

Fig. 2-13. (A) Paper-mounted, whole lung section with panlobular emphysema. *(B)* A case of panlobular emphysema, with a marked increase in total airways resistance (R_L) caused by the disease in the peripheral airways (R_P). *(Continued opposite)*

sessment of disease in the smaller airways tends to show that there is evidence of mucous plugging and inflammatory narrowing in these airways.[51]

Mechanical Properties of the Lung in Emphysema. *Lung Compliance.* In 1934, Christie[52] observed that patients with emphysema had a much smaller elastic recoil pressure at a given lung volume than normal persons. Since that time, it has been well documented that these patients have an increased static compliance and that this falls rapidly with breathing frequency.[53] The work of Otis and associates[4] has shown that the fall in compliance with increased breathing frequency is due to an inequality of the time constants of the various parallel pathways.

The fact that static lung compliance is increased means that in advanced cases, it is impossible to determine whether inequality in time constants is due to changes in the resistance of the airways or changes in the elastic property of the parenchyma. (In early disease, when the lung's elastic properties are normal and airways resistance is not increased, the presence of dependence of compliance on frequency has been taken as evidence of disease in the peripheral airways.[54])

Pulmonary Resistance in Emphysema. An increase in total pulmonary resistance is a characteristic finding in patients with clinical emphysema. Since this is not a result of elastic resistance, it represents increased flow resistance, but the site and nature of this increase have been centers of controversy. Laennec[39] attributed the airway obstruction to mucous plugging of the small bronchi and bronchioles and felt that the inspiratory muscles could overcome this obstruction but the expiratory muscles could not. Dayman[21] showed that the tendency for the pulmonary resistance to rise during expiration was increased in emphysema, and he attributed this to the fact that emphysema destroyed the peribronchiolar supporting structures, causing the bronchioles to act as a check valve. Butler and associates[55] proposed a third

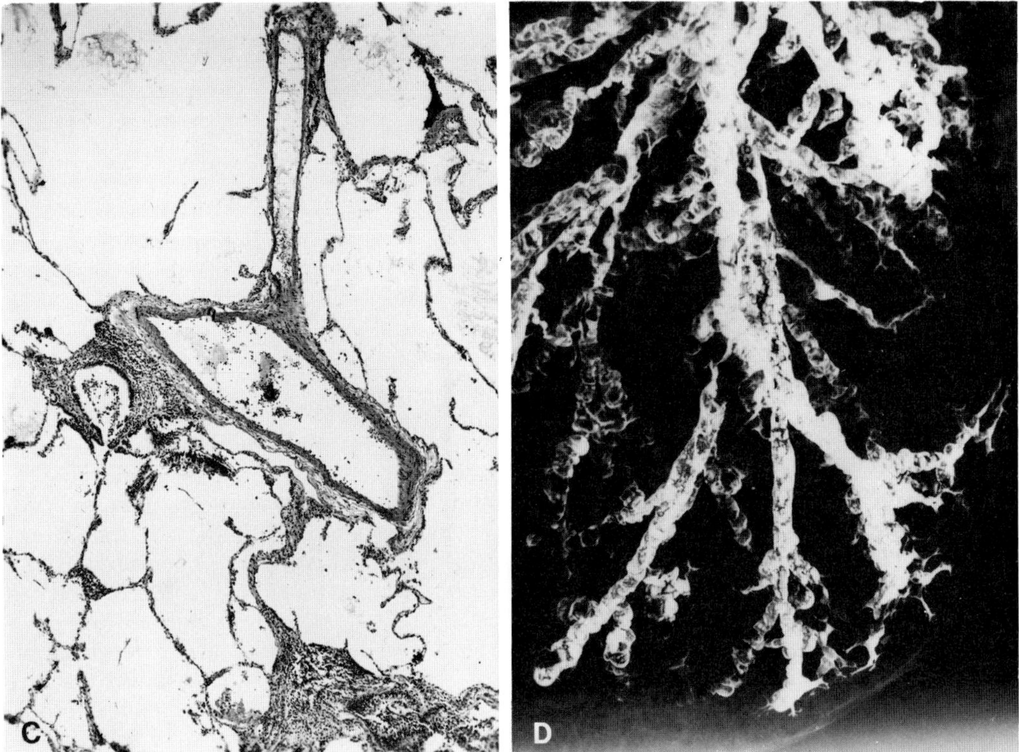

Fig. 2-13 Continued. Panlobular emphysema, with marked narrowing of the airways, seen in a histological specimen. *(D)* Panlobular emphysema, with narrowing of the small airways, seen in a bronchogram.

mechanism, stating that the decrease in elasticity, which is characteristic of emphysema, causes the small airways to be narrower at the particular lung volume than they normally would be.

The introduction of bronchial pressure measurements by Koblet and Wyss[56] enabled the lower airway resistance to be partitioned. Using such a technique, Macklem and co-workers[57] found that there were two sites of obstruction in patients with emphysema. The airways central to the segmental branches accounted for the increased resistance during forced expiration, and the airways beyond this point accounted for a fixed proportion of the resistance that was the same in both inspiration and expiration.

The contribution of large and small airways has also been studied in excised lungs; this study showed that the major site of obstruction was the peripheral airways (Figs. 2-12, 2-13) and that the resistance of these airways was the same on both inflation and deflation. It follows from the foregoing discussion of normal airways that the introduction of a fixed resistor in the small airways would result in markedly increased alveolar pressure to produce flow. This would be transmitted to the bronchial wall, causing dynamic compression of the large airways in forced expiration, which would severely limit maximum flow.

The nature of the peripheral-airways disease that is responsible for the fixed resistance in the small airways has been a subject of debate, and the various sites and mechanisms of obstruction that have been proposed are summarized in Figure 2-14. Leopold and Gough[42] were unable to demonstrate significant obstruction of airways leading to the centrilobular spaces. McLean[58] and Anderson and Foraker[59]

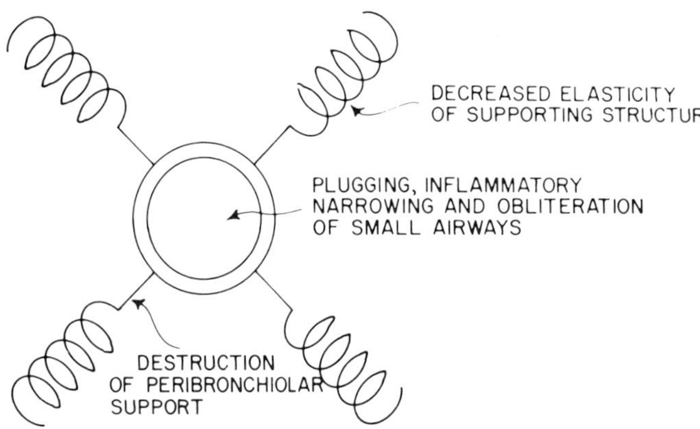

Fig. 2-14. The mechanisms that have been suggested for peripheral airways obstruction.

found evidence to support Laennec's original notion that organic obstruction of the small airways by mucous plugging and inflammatory narrowing and obliteration was important. Liebow[60] has been attracted by Dayman's hypothesis[21] that emphysema destroys peribronchial support, leading to a check-valve obstruction in the small airways. Butler and colleagues[55] postulated that diminished elastic recoil caused the peripheral airways to be narrower at a given lung volume than they would be in a normal lung at the same volume.

In our studies of postmortem lungs, the peripheral airways constituted the major site of airways resistance in both centrilobular and panacinar emphysema (Fig. 2-12, 2-13). These studies also showed that there was significant organic disease in the small airways to account for this increase in resistance, so that the original hypothesis of Laennec would seem to be the most correct. These findings suggest that the peripheral airways obstruction is fixed and that the marked increase in airways resistance seen on forced expiration during life is due to dynamic compression of the large airways rather than a check-valve mechanism in the small airways.

Cystic Fibrosis

Introduction. Cystic fibrosis is a disease of infancy and childhood, originally described by Andersen[61] in 1938 as being a rare, uniformly fatal, pancreatic disorder. The generalized nature of the disease was pointed out by Farber[62] in 1944, and he suggested the name *mucoviscidosis* because there seemed to be widespread involvement of the mucus-secreting glands. A recent review[63] of the advances in the understanding of the condition has shown that it is not rare; that survival into adulthood can be achieved; that it is transmitted as a Mendelian recessive; that it affects the respiratory system in all cases; and that the cause of death is most often related to pulmonary involvement. The term *mucoviscidosis* has now lost favor because abnormalities of the sweat glands have been demonstrated.

Pathological Anatomy of the Lung in Cystic Fibrosis. At autopsy, the trachea and bronchi are generally filled with mucopurulent material. The lungs are large and do not completely deflate, and bullae are sometimes seen on the lung surface. The cut surface of the lung shows widespread plugging of large and small airways with purulent mucus.[64] In a study of eighty-four autopsies on infants and children with fibrocystic disease, Esterly and Oppenheimer[65] reported that bronchiectasis was present in fifty-three cases and that hypertrophy and hyperplasia of the bronchial mucous gland layer, with evidence of chronic inflammation of bronchial walls with follicle formation, were common features in nearly all cases. They also found evidence of chronic inflammation of the bronchioles, which was severe and often obliterative in character. Evidence of emphysema in the children that Esterly and Oppenheimer studied, however, was sparse, and diffuse interstitial fibrosis was not an important feature.

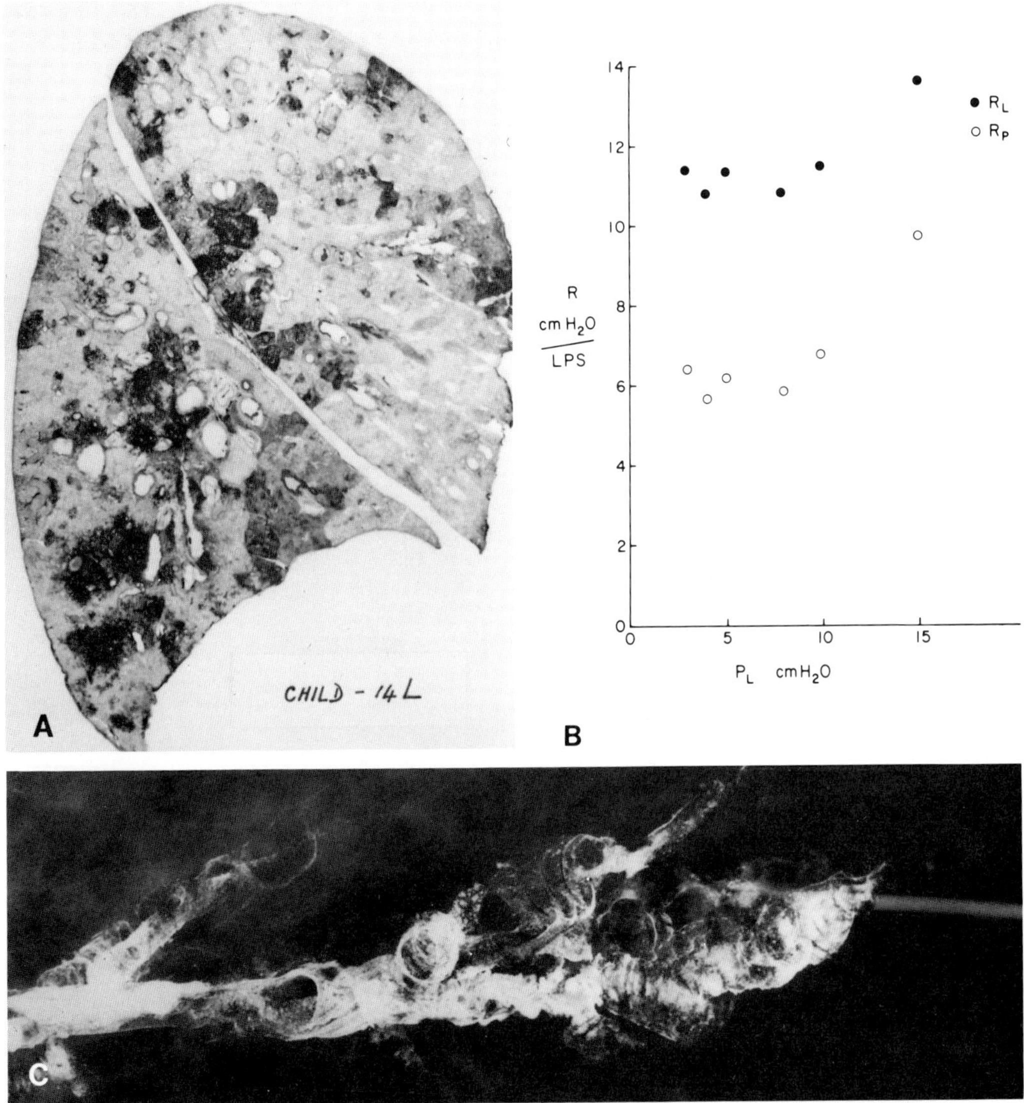

Fig. 2-15. From a case of fibrocystic disease of the pancreas. (*A*) Paper-mounted, whole lung section with marked bronchiectasis. (*B*) The marked increase in total airways resistance (R_L) is due to disease in the peripheral airways (R_P). (*C*) Bronchogram demonstrating marked bronchiectasis. (*B* modified from Hogg, J., *et al.*: Age as a factor in the distribution of lower airways conductance and in the pathologic anatomy of obstructive lung disease. N. Engl. J. Med., *282*:1283, 1970)

The major features of the pathology of the lung in fibrocystic disease of the pancreas are, therefore, bronchitis, obliterative bronchiolitis, and bronchiectasis, which is chronic and progressive in nature (Fig. 2-14). Atelectasis, pneumonia, and abscess formation, when present, are probably secondary to airway obstruction; whereas emphysema and diffuse pulmonary interstitial disease do not appear to be important features of the disease.

Mechanical Properties of the Lung in Cystic Fibrosis. The abnormalities in lung mechanics in fibrocystic disease have been studied by Mellins and co-workers.[66] Routine pulmonary function tests on patients with cystic fibrosis showed a reduction in vital capacity; a higher peak flow rate; increased air-flow resistance, on both inspiration and expiration, which is reflected in a reduced maximum breathing capacity; and a reduced dynamic compliance. They also presented cineradiographic evidence of dynamic collapse of the proximal portion of bronchiectatic airways and single-breath nitrogen washout curves, which would fit well with collapse of lower lobe airways because they have a markedly increased Phase IV. This is, however, not clearly interpretable in view of other evidence of airway disease.

Mellins and associates stressed the fact that patients with the abnormalities they have demonstrated have an ineffective cough, because the large airways collapse during cough, so that bronchial secretions are retained. They then interpreted their data to mean that cystic fibrosis is a patchy disease of large airways and that this is at variance with the pathological investigations[64,65] that showed the most severe disease in the small airways. Indeed, studies of the distribution of airways resistance carried out in our laboratories[18] on postmortem in lungs from patients dying with cystic fibrosis (Fig. 2-15) showed that the major site of airway obstruction in these lungs was in the small, not the large, airways. It therefore seems likely that the airway obstruction is primarily due to fixed organic disease in peripheral airways and that the larger airway collapse, which Mellins and colleagues demonstrated by cinebronchography, is due to dynamic compression of the central airways, brought on as a result of the peripheral-airways disease.

Bronchiectasis

Anatomical Types of Bronchiectasis. As the name implies, bronchiectasis occurs when there is a permanent dilation of one or more bronchi. The word *permanent* is important, because it excludes the acute reversible dilation of bronchi that often accompanies pneumonia.[67] Because an increase in the diameter of a bronchus can result from a variety of conditions, it is obvious that the term describes a disorder of anatomy rather than a single disease.

There have been many attempts to classify this condition, but none of these has been completely satisfactory. Lynne Reid[68] attempted to classify bronchiectasis on the basis of the appearance of the bronchi and on the number of branches of airways in the lung segment containing the bronchiectatic lesions. In the cylindrical form, she found that the number of branches identified in the specimen by dissection was within normal limits, although plugging of the airways by secretions often prevented the filling of the small airways on the bronchogram. In the varicose type of bronchiectasis, she found that the number of bronchi in the segment was reduced, both on the bronchogram and when the lung was dissected and the bronchi counted. She also found that discrete cords could be seen beyond the point at which the bronchial lumen was obliterated by fibrous tissue. In the saccular type, she found the least number of bronchial branches, with only a few generations of airway being demonstrable by careful dissection of the specimen.

Whitewell[69] classified bronchiectasis into follicular, saccular, and atelectatic forms on the basis of the pathology and clinical features of 200 surgically resected specimens. In follicular bronchiectasis (14% of his cases), the main lesion occurred in the smaller bronchi and bronchioles in the early stages, but as the condition became more severe, it extended towards the trachea, with gradual obliteration of the distal bronchial tree. The lesion initially consisted of thickening of the bronchiolar walls due to edema and lymph-follicle formation, with destruction of the elastic tissue near the follicles. More advanced lesions showed a diffuse mural bronchiolitis, with destruction of the elastic tissue. The clinical fact that this form of bronchiectasis usually begins in early childhood and either starts insidiously or follows illnesses thought to be associated with viral disease led Whitewell to speculate that this form of bronchiectasis was a sequel to acute viral infections.

Seventeen per cent of his 200 cases were

classified as saccular bronchiectasis, and he showed that the bronchial sacs were fibrous structures lined by cuboidal epithelium, without elastic tissue muscle or cartilage in their walls. No dilation occurred in the presaccular bronchi, but there was an inflammatory reaction in their walls, with polyposis of the bronchiolar epithelium. Although the dilations often ended blindly, atelectasis was not a feature of either follicular or saccular bronchiectasis; collateral ventilation apparently kept the parenchyma inflated. Ten per cent of Whitewell's cases were classified as atelectatic bronchiectasis, because the lung around the bronchiectatic sac was not well aerated. In these cases, there was a generalized distribution of collapse and bronchiectasis in the lobes, and no obstruction in the airways, but enlarged hilar nodes were always found around the lobar bronchus. Whitewell suggested that this condition was due to obstruction of the lobar bronchus, caused by external compression by the surrounding lymph glands, and that atelectasis occurred because collateral ventilation could not take place between lobes.

It is important to note that the majority of the cases that Whitewell described could not be classified under the headings that he chose. In fact, it seems that the capability to defy a particular classification is one of the most common features of any study of bronchiectasis. The disorder, however, seems to have many features that are common in a majority of individual cases. These include evidence of onset in early childhood, previous lower respiratory-tract infections that are often recurrent, chronic productive cough, and poor general health that extends over many years. The bronchial dilatations tend to involve the lung segmentally, with the segments of the left lower lobe being the most commonly affected. The lingula of the left upper lobe is involved more often than the right middle lobe. The reason for the tendency for involvement of the left side is presumably less adequate drainage, caused by the angle at which the left main bronchus branches off the trachea, but this has not been proven.

Mechanical Properties of the Lung in Bronchiectasis. In 1964, Bates and Christie[70] reviewed the available information on pulmonary function in bronchiectasis and concluded that there were insufficient data to establish a close correlation between structure and function. In their own cases, they usually found that the total lung capacity was close to the predicted value, but that there was a marked reduction in vital capacity, with increases in the residual volume and the functional residual capacity. Maximum expiratory flow rates were markedly reduced, and there was evidence of hypoxia, hypercapnia, and a reduced diffusing capacity in most cases. Cherniack and Carton[71] published an extensive study on pulmonary function in bronchiectasis in 1966 and demonstrated a reduced vital capacity, increased residual volume, and evidence of airway obstruction in more than half of their cases. This was directly proportional to the number of lobes involved.

Fraser and associates[72] studied twenty cases of bronchiectasis by combining bronchial-pressure measurements with cinebronchography. They clearly demonstrated that the marked reduction of flow seen on forced expiration in the varicose and cystic forms of the disease was associated with dynamic collapse of segmental airways. They also showed that the bronchial dilatations change little in size during forced expiration and cough, and they pointed out the deficiency in bronchial clearance that results because the dilated airways fail to narrow during cough. Figure 2-16 shows postmortem data from a case of varicose bronchiectasis seen in a 39-year-old female. The bronchogram demonstrates the severity of the bronchiectasis, whereas the physiological data show that the severity of the peripheral-airways disease resulted in a marked increase in peripheral resistance. These data showed that the obstruction in the peripheral airways was fixed on inspiration and expiration. Moreover, they appear to suggest that the marked increase in resistance seen in living persons during forced expiration is due to dynamic collapse of the central airways.

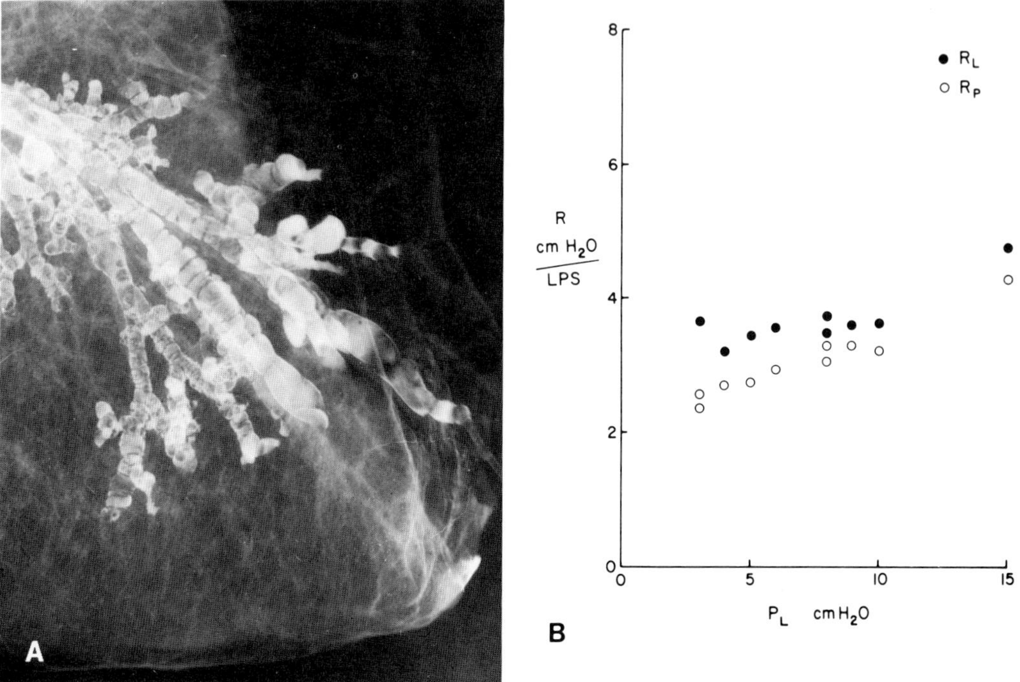

Fig. 2-16. (*A*) Bronchogram demonstrating severe varicose bronchiectasis. (*B*) The physiological data demonstrate a marked increase in peripheral airways resistance (R_P), causing a high total airway resistance (R_L).

SUMMARY

In considering obstructive lung diseases in total, it is apparent that there are many common features. For example, bronchiolitis in children and acute bronchitis in adults are quite similar morphologically, but their end results are very different. The fact that acute airways disease causes a life-threatening illness in the young child is, at least in part, related to lung development. The nature of this development puts the child at risk, because the development of the conducting airways seems to lag behind the development of the gas-exchanging portion of the lung in the first few years of life. Similarities are also seen among cystic fibrosis, bronchiectasis, bronchitis, and emphysema, where the major site of obstruction is in the peripheral airways, and this is due to inflammatory narrowing and plugging of these airways. As a consequence, these diseases all have a fixed peripheral-airways obstruction that is present on both inspiration and expiration. On forced expiration, this results in dynamic compression of the central airways, which causes collapse of the weakened airway wall in some cases. This causes the cough mechanism to be defective because the airways do not narrow properly, and increased mucus is retained.

The separation of bronchiectasis, bronchitis, and emphysema by age (Fig. 2-17) is of interest. Could it be that the age of the patient has something to do with the resulting anatomical disorder? For example, when chronic airways disease develops in a young person, as with fibrocystic disease and bronchiectasis, does the disproportion between conducting airways and parenchyma and the decreased collateral ventilation lead to alveolar collapse and infection,

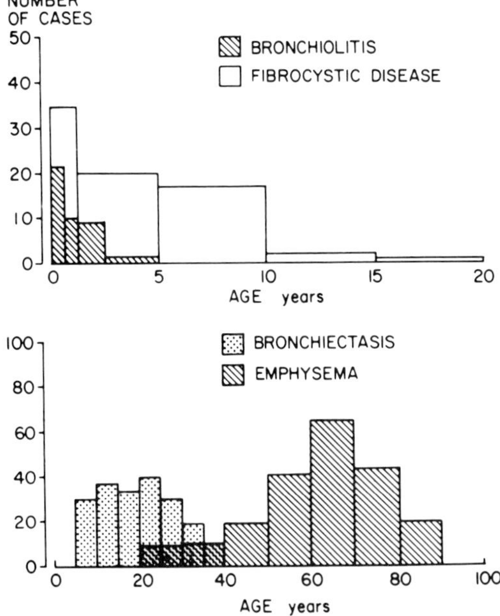

Fig. 2-17. Age distribution of obstructive lung diseases. Note that bronchiectasis (*bottom*) occurs primarily in the younger age period, whereas bronchitis and emphysema (*bottom*) occur primarily during the last third of life. Bronchiolitis (*top*) occurs primarily in the first few years of life, and fibrocystic disease (*top*) is seldom seen beyond 20 years of age.

so that the airways dilate and fill with secretions? Similarly, if the chronic disease starts after the lung is fully developed, does the obstruction and collateral ventilation of the obstructed units cause the pores of Kohn to fenestrate, so that emphysema develops? If this were so, one could think of the insult of airways disease in the same way that the orthopedic surgeon thinks of an insult such as a fall on the outstretched hand, where the nature of the fracture is determined by the age of the patient at the time the insult was received.

REFERENCES

1. Despas, P. J. M., Lerous, M., and Macklem, P. T.: Site of airway obstruction in asthma as determined by the maximal expiratory flow breathing air and a helium-oxygen mixture. J. Clin. Invest., *51*:3235, 1972.
2. Dosman, J., *et al.*: The use of a helium-oxygen mixture during maximum expiratory flow to demonstrate obstruction in small airways of smokers. J. Clin. Invest., *55*:1090, 1975.
3. Mead, J.: Lung—mechanical properties of the lungs. Physiol. Rev., *41*:281, 1961.
4. Otis, A. B., *et al.*: Mechanical factors in distribution of pulmonary ventilation. J. Appl. Physiol., *8*:427, 1956.
5. Clements, J., Sharp, J., Johnson, R., and Elam, J.: Estimation of pulmonary resistance by repetitive interruption of outflow. J. Clin. Invest., *38*:1262, 1959.
6. Mead, J., and Whittenberger, J.: Physical properties of human lungs measured during spontaneous respiration. J. Appl. Physiol., *5*:779, 1953.
7. Dubois, A., Brody, A., Lewis, D., and Burgess, B.: Oscillation mechanics of the lungs and chest in man. J. Appl. Physiol., *8*:587, 1956.
8. Dubois, A., Botelho, S., and Comroe, J., Jr.: A new method of measuring airway resistance in man using a body plethysmograph. J. Clin. Invest., *35*:327, 1956.
9. Dubois, A., *et al.*: A rapid plethysmographic method for measuring thoracic gas volume. J. Clin. Invest., *35*:322, 1956.
10. Fry, D.: Theoretical considerations of the bronchial pressure-flow-volume relationship with particular reference to the maximum expiratory flow volume curves. Phys. Med. Biol., *3*:174, 1958.
11. Fry, D., and Hyatt, R.: Mechanics—a unified analysis of the relationship between pressure-volume and gas flow in the lungs of normal and diseased human subjects. Am. J. Med., *29*:672, 1960.
12. Dubois, A.: The resistance of breathing. *In* Fenn, W. O., and Rahn, H. (eds.): American Physiological Society. Handbook of Physiology. section 3. vol. 1. Baltimore, Williams & Wilkins, 1964-1965.
13. Macklem, P., and Mead, J.: The resistance of central and peripheral airways measured by a retrograde catheter. J. Appl. Physiol., *22*:395, 1967.
14. Briscoe, W., and Dubois, A.: Relationship between airways resistance, airway conductance and lung volume in subjects of different age and body size. J. Clin. Invest., *37*:1279, 1958.
15. Cook, C., Helliesen, P., and Agathen, S.: Relation between mechanics of respiration,

lung size and body size from birth to young adulthood. J. Appl. Physiol., *13*:349, 1958.
16. Reid, L.: The Embryology of the Lung, in Development of the Lung. A CIBA Foundation Symposium. London, J. A. Churchill, 1967.
17. Hogg, J., Macklem, P., and Thurlbeck, W.: Site and nature of airways obstruction in chronic obstructive lung disease. N. Engl. J. Med. *278*:1355, 1968.
18. Hogg, J., *et al*.: Age as a factor in the distribution of lower airways conductance and in the pathologic anatomy of obstructive lung disease. N. Engl. J. Med., *282*:1283, 1970.
19. Weibel, E.: Morphometry of the Human Lung. New York, Academic Press, 1963.
20. Einthoven, U.: Ueber die Wirkung der Bronchialmuskeln nach einer neuen Methode untersucht und uber Asthma Nervosu. Arch. Ges. Physiol., *5*:367, 1892.
21. Dayman, H.: Mechanics of airflow in health and in emphysema. J. Clin. Invest., *30*:1175, 1951.
22. Dekker, E., Defares, J., and Hiemstra, H.: Direct measurements of intrabronchial pressure. Its application to the localization of the check valve mechanism. J. Appl. Physiol., *13*:35, 1958.
23. Mead, J., Turner, J., Macklem, P., and Little, J.: The significance of the relationship between lung recoil and maximum expiratory flow. J. Appl. Physiol., *22*:95, 1967.
24. Pride, W., Permutt, S., Riley, R., and Bromberger-Barnea, B.: Determinants of maximal expiratory flow from the lungs. J. Appl. Physiol., *23*:646, 1967.
25. Krogh, A., and Lindhard, J.: The volume of the dead space in breathing and the mixing of gases in the lungs of man. J. Physiol. (Lond.), *51*:59, 1917.
26. Rauwerda, P.: Unequal Ventilation of Different Parts of the Lung and the Determination of Cardiac Output. Theses Groningen, The Netherlands: University of Groningen, 1946.
27. Fowler, K.: Relative compliances of the well and poorly ventilated spaces in the normal human lung. J. Appl. Physiol., *19*:937, 1964.
28. Milic-Emili, J., *et al*.: Regional distribution of inspired gas in the lung. J. Appl. Physiol., *21*:749, 1966.
29. Dolfuss, R., Milic-Emili, J., and Bates, D.: Regional ventilation of the lung studied with boluses of xenon. Respir. Physiol., *22*:760, 1967.
30. Horsfield, K., and Cumming, G.: The morphology of the bronchial tree in man. J. Appl. Physiol., *24*:373, 1968.
31. Said, S.: Metabolic events in the lung. *In* Frohlich, E. D. (ed.): Pathophysiology: Altered Regulatory Mechanisms in Disease. ed. 2. Philadelphia, J. B. Lippincott, 1976.
32. Cohen, A., and Gold, W.: Defense mechanisms of the lungs. Annu. Rev. Physiol., *37*:325, 1975.
33. Satir, P.: How cilia move. Sci. Am., *231*:44, 1974.
34. High, R.: Bronchiolitis. Pediatr. Clin. North Am., *4*:183, 1957.
35. Coates, H., and Chanock, R.: The clinical significance of respiratory syncytial virus. Post-grad. Med., *35*:460, 1964.
36. CIBA Guest Symposium. Thorax, *14*:286, 1959.
37. Thurlbeck, W., and Angus, G.: A distribution curve for chronic bronchitis. Thorax, *19*:436, 1964.
38. Simonsson, B., and Tela, E.: Experimental studies on bronchial secretions [Int. Symposium]. Scand. J. Respir. Dis. [Suppl.], *90*, 1974.
39. Laennec, R.: A Treatise on the Diseases of the Chest and on Mediate Auscultation. ed. 3. New York, S. S. and W. Wood, pp. 167-168, 1838.
40. Strawbridge, H.: Chronic pulmonary emphysema (an experimental study). I. Historical review. Am. J. Pathol., *37*:161, 1960.
41. Gough, J.: Discussion on the diagnosis of pulmonary emphysema. Proc. R. Soc. Med., *45*:576, 1952.
42. Leopold, J., and Gough, J.: The centrilobular form of hypertrophic emphysema and its relation to chronic bronchitis. Thorax, *12*:219, 1957.
43. Heard, B., and Izukawa, T.: Pulmonary emphysema in fifty consecutive male necropsies in London. J. Pathol. Bacterol., *88*:423, 1964.
44. Thurlbeck, W.: Chronic Obstructive Lung Disease. Pathology Annual. New York, Appleton-Century-Crofts, pages 367-368, 1968.
45. ———: Measurement of pulmonary emphysema. Am. Rev. Respir. Dis., *95*:752, 1967.
46. Sweet, J., Wyatt, J., and Kinsella, P.: Correlation of lung macrosections with pulmonary function in emphysema. Am. J. Med., *29*:277, 1960.
47. Dunnill, M.: Quantitative methods in the study of pulmonary pathology. Thorax, *17*:320, 1962.

48. Pratt, P., Jtabha, O., and Klugh, G.: Quantitative relationship between structural extent of centrilobular emphysema and post mortem volume and flow characteristics of lungs. Med. Thorac., *22*:197, 1965.
49. Thurlbeck,W., *et al*.: A comparison of three methods of measuring emphysema. Hum. Pathol., *1*:215, 1970.
50. Restripo, G., and Heard, B.: The size of the bronchial glands in chronic bronchitis. J. Pathol. Bacteriol., *85*:305, 1963.
51. Thurlbeck, W.: Chronic bronchitis and emphysema. Med. Clin. North Am., *57*:651, 1973.
52. Christie, R.: The elastic properties of the emphysematous lung and their clinical significance. J. Clin. Invest., *13*:295, 1934.
53. Mead, J., Lindgren, I., and Gaensler, E.: The mechanical properties of the lungs in emphysema. J. Clin. Invest., *34*:1005, 1955.
54. Woolcock, A., Vincent, N., and Macklem, P.: Frequency dependence of compliance as a test for obstruction in small airways. J. Clin. Invest., *48*:1097, 1969.
55. Butler, J., Caro, C., Raphael, A., and Dubois, B.: Physiological factors affecting airway resistance in normal subjects and in patients with obstructive airway disease. J. Clin. Invest., *39*:584, 1960.
56. Koblet, H., and Wyss, F.: Das klinische und functionelle Bild des genuinem bronchial Kollapses mid lung Emphysem. Melv. Med. Acta. *23*:553, 1956.
57. Macklem, P., Fraser, R., and Brown, W.: Bronchial pressure measurements in emphysema and bronchitis. J. Clin. Invest., *44*:897, 1965.
58. McLean, K.: The pathogenesis of pulmonary emphysema. Am. J. Med., *25*:62, 1958.
59. Anderson, A., and Foraker, A.: Population of non-respiratory bronchioles in pulmonary emphysema. Arch. Pathol., *83*:286, 1967.
60. Liebow, A.: Pulmonary emphysema with special reference to vascular changes. Am. Rev. Respir. Dis., *80*:67, 1959.
61. Andersen, D.: Cystic fibrosis of the pancreas and its relation to celiac disease. Am. J. Dis. Child., *56*:344, 1938.
62. Farber, S.: Pancreatic function and disease in early life, pancreatic changes associated with pancreatic insufficiency in early life. Arch. Pathol., *37*:238, 1944.
63. Shwachman, H.: Cystic fibrosis. *In* Kendig, E. L., Jr. (ed.): Disorders of the Respiratory Tract in Children. Philadelphia, W. B. Saunders, 1967.
64. Esterly, J., and Oppenheimer, E.: Cystic fibrosis of the pancreas: structural changes in peripheral airways. Thorax, *23*:670, 1968.
65. ———: Observations in cystic fibrosis of the pancreas. III. Pulmonary lesions. Johns Hopkins Med. J., *122*:94, 1968.
66. Mellins, R., Levine, R., Ingram, R., and Fishman, A.: Obstructive disease of the airways in cystic fibrosis. Pediatrics, *41*:560, 1968.
67. Bachman, A., Hewitt, W., and Beekley, H. Bronchiectasis, a bronchographic study of sixty cases of pneumonia. Arch. Intern. Med., *91*:78, 1953.
68. Reid, L.: Reduction in the bronchial subdivisions in bronchiectasis. Thorax, *5*:233, 1950.
69. Whitewell, F.: A study of the pathology and pathogenesis of bronchiectasis. Thorax, *7*:213, 1952.
70. Bates, D., and Christie, R.: Respiratory Function in Disease. Philadelphia, W. B. Saunders, 1964.
71. Cherniack, N., and Carton, R.: Factors associated with respiratory insufficiency in bronchiectasis. Am. J. Med., *41*:562, 1966.
72. Fraser, R., Macklem, P., and Brown, W.: Airway dynamics in bronchiectasis, a combined cinefluorographic-manometric study. Am. J. Roentgenol. Radium Ther. Nucl. Med., *93*:821, 1965.

3 Ventilatory Function of the Lungs

Martin H. Welch, M.D.

EVALUATION OF THE PATIENT WITH VENTILATORY DYSFUNCTION

The clinical pulmonary-function laboratory offers help to the physician with patients in five basic categories (see list below). Tests of both ventilation and respiratory gas exchange are of importance in each of these circumstances. This section deals with the role of ventilatory tests in the evaluation of respiratory function.

Uses of the Clinical Pulmonary-Function Laboratory

1. Initial evaluation of the patient presenting with the complaint of breathlessness
2. Initial evaluation of the patient with known respiratory disease
3. Following the course of disease in a patient with an established diagnosis of respiratory disease
4. Preoperative evaluation of the patient with a high risk of respiratory complications
5. Screening for subclinical disease

Evaluation of Breathlessness. Ventilatory tests play an especially important role in the evaluation of the patient undergoing investigation of the complaint of shortness of breath, or dyspnea. This common symptom occurs in association with a wide range of conditions and defies a unifying concept of its pathogenesis.[1-3] It is a reasonable generalization to state that dyspnea, when it occurs as a manifestation of organic disease, correlates better with abnormal results of tests of ventilatory function than with respiratory gas exchange.

Factors Affecting Dyspnea. Dyspnea is a subjective sensation, by definition, and cannot be equated with any objective sign. It may be absent in the face of apparently labored, abnormally rapid, or deep breathing; and it may be present in a subject who appears normal. Breathlessness occurs as a normal phenomenon in exercise; and it is a common, benign manifestation of anxiety and excitement. To be considered a symptom worthy of investigation, it must occur with less exertion than is normally required to produce it. Some investigators require that a sensation of breathlessness be experienced as unpleasant to warrant application of the term *dyspnea*.

Dyspnea is best understood in terms of the relationship between the factors that stimulate tidal breathing and the resistances that must be overcome in the act of breathing. Some knowledge of the control of ventilation is therefore essential to a discussion of dyspnea. The reader is referred to Chapter 4 for details of neural and chemical control of ventilation.

In addition to those mechanisms that are of primary importance in the regulation of ventilation, a host of other neural influences are of secondary importance. Anxiety, excitement, pain, and the level of wakefulness are well known to influence ventilation. Stimulation of baroreceptors produces hyperventilation during hypotension from various causes. Stimulation of proprioceptors by movement of limbs is one of the mechanisms by which ventilation is increased during exercise.

All of these mechanisms of respiratory control, along with others not yet understood, play a role in producing or modifying the sensation of breathlessness in normal and abnormal persons.

Conditions that produce breathlessness as a symptom include those resulting primarily in an abnormally increased stimulus to breathe; a greater than normal effort required to breathe; and most mysteriously, an inability to respond to a ventilatory stimulus because of respiratory muscle weakness (see list below). Conditions in which dyspnea is primarily due to an increased effort required for ventilation are clinically the most frequent. These include a wide range of pulmonary diseases in which ventilatory abnormalities can be readily characterized by the pulmonary laboratory. The correlation between dyspnea and abnormal results of tests of ventilation is generally good in this category. Complex and poorly understood combinations of these three categories are probably common in clinical practice; but a simplified consideration of relatively pure examples is informative.

Some Factors Producing Dyspnea

Increased stimulus to breathe
- Exercise
- Anxiety
- Excitement
- Hypoxemia
- Acidosis
- CNS disease

Increased effort required to breathe
- Obstruction to air flow
- Decreased lung or chest-wall compliance

Decreased ability to exert effort required to breathe
- Disease of neural supply to muscles of respiration
- Primary muscle disease

Increased Ventilatory Stimulus. An abnormal respiratory drive in the presence of normal lungs and chest wall results in increased respiratory rate and depth; with a widely variable threshhold, individual persons may become aware of this change in ventilatory pattern and interpret this awareness as shortness of breath. Most surprising, perhaps, is the relative mildness of dyspnea of this sort in most circumstances. Indeed, some investigators would not apply the term *dyspnea* to this sensation, but would refer to it only as breathlessness, because it generally is not experienced as unpleasant. The hypoxemia incurred at high altitudes causes an increased drive to ventilation through stimulation of carotid and perhaps aortic body chemoreceptors; but if increased ventilation proceeds without mechanical hindrance, the subject breathes more rapidly and deeply with little awareness that he is doing so. Inadequate oxygenation of the brain causes confusion and euphoria, often before the drive to ventilate becomes intense enough to cause disproportion between sensed ventilatory need and ventilatory ability. Unconsciousness and death may therefore occur without apparent warning. This poor correlation between hypoxemia and dyspnea can result in death in aviators, underwater swimmers, and divers. Similarly, ignorance on the part of physicians and nurses can lead to the death of patients with hypoxemia, if lack of dyspnea is interpreted as proof of adequate oxygenation.

The hyperpnea of metabolic acidosis is another commonly encountered circumstance in which an increased ventilatory stimulus may occur in a subject with normal ventilatory reserve. In such a patient, increased hydrogen ion concentration produces increased ventilation through chemoreceptors in carotid and aortic bodies exposed to blood; and, in the floor of the fourth ventricle, exposed to acidotic cerebrospinal fluid. Objectively dramatic hyperpnea in a patient with metabolic acidosis often occurs with minimal or no awareness on the patient's part. When metabolic acidosis supervenes in a patient with impaired ventilatory reserve, it appears more likely to produce the subjective complaint of dyspnea.

Organic brain disease occasionally produces sustained hyperpnea, or the phasic ventilatory pattern of Cheyne-Stokes respiration. Again, this phenomenon is more likely to be noted by an observer than by the patient himself.

One of the most fascinating of respiratory aberrations associated with dyspnea is the "hyperventilation syndrome." This functional disturbance seems to be an exaggeration of the normal ventilatory response to anxiety and occurs acutely and sometimes chronically in susceptible subjects. The alkalosis of hyperventilation, which occurs so commonly in acute anxiety, may be accompanied by marked dyspnea and may produce dizziness, perioral and peripheral paresthesias, and sometimes bronchospasm and spasms of voluntary muscles, as discussed in Chapter 4.

Treatment consists of patient education, reassurance, and rebreathing from a reservoir such as a paper bag for several breaths during acute attacks. This maneuver returns arterial P_{CO_2} and pH toward normal and reduces symptoms. Most acute attacks of hyperventilation syndrome occur in normal but emotionally labile subjects under conditions of acute emotional stress, especially when hot weather and crowds of people induce an illusion of "suffocation." Such attacks respond promptly to treatment and most often do not recur. Occasionally, chronic anxiety states may be associated with chronic hyperventilation and respond poorly to treatment. Treatment of the underlying emotional disturbance is crucial to the management of these patients. The hyperventilation syndrome occasionally occurs in patients with underlying organic disease of the heart and lungs and complicates both diagnosis and management.

A disorder in which acute episodic dyspnea may mimic the hyperventilation syndrome is pulmonary embolism. Acutely, patients with this disorder often become severely dyspneic and hypoxemic, without an apparent mechanical hindrance to ventilation; in fact, respiratory alkalosis is usual. Correction of the hypoxemia is of only modest symptomatic benefit, suggesting that undefined humoral factors or a neurologic stimulus arising from lung tissue may be involved.

Increased Effort Required to Breathe. The dyspnea of most patients with organic respiratory disease has a mixed pathogenesis but is probably chiefly related to this mechanism. The effort required to breathe is known to be increased in these patients because of mechanical abnormalities of the lungs and chest wall. In diseases associated with obstruction to air flow through central or peripheral airways, the resistive work required to breathe is increased. In a wide range of disorders of the lung interstitium, pleura, and chest wall, stiffness (decreased compliance) of the diseased structures causes an increase in elastic resistance during breathing and, therefore, an increase in elastic work. Perhaps all mechanical disorders causing dyspnea have in common an increased work of breathing, and this increased work is somehow appreciated centrally and results in dyspnea.

An observation by Campbell,[1,2] in conjunction with a series of experiments involving detection of addition of mechanical loads to breathing in normal subjects, led to a modification of the "work of breathing" theory of the cause of dyspnea. He pointed out that dyspnea may not correlate so perfectly with the volume of air moved by the chest bellows or even with effort exerted in an attempt to accomplish ventilation, but that it may correlate better with the relationship between the volume of air moved and effort exerted. This relationship could well be expressed in terms of volume and pressure changes measured during ventilation. Because the relationship might most logically be expected to be sensed by intercostal muscle spindles, Campbell expressed it in terms of length and tension. Because his experiments demonstrated a remarkable ability of normal persons to detect changes from normal in the effort required to move a given volume of air, he formulated the theory that dyspnea is most closely related to changes from normal (inappropriateness) in the ratio of length to tension. His concept of length-to-tension inappropriateness has become the predominant unitary theory under consideration by investigators at present.

The clinical pulmonary laboratory of this decade offers no direct measurement of length-to-tension inappropriateness, and work of breathing is difficult to measure. The importance of this discussion to the clinician is to emphasize the relative importance of measurement of mechanical abnormalities, as opposed to arterial blood gases, in the assessment of patients with dyspnea. As a final example emphasizing this point, the patient with severe dyspnea at rest due to respiratory insufficiency should be considered. In many such cases, arterial Pco_2 is normal or even decreased, and hypoxemia is easily corrected or overcorrected by oxygen administration alone. In such cases, persistence of severe dyspnea is common and certainly is best explained in terms of mechanical abnormalities.

What measurements of abnormal ventilatory mechanics are readily available, and how well do they correlate with dyspnea.

Measurements of total or effective ventilation actually achieved during rest or exercise are rather easily accomplished but are of limited application. Normal values vary considerably, obscuring the slight changes that may occur because of inefficient ventilation in early lung disease. A significant, measurable decrease in total ventilation occurs chiefly in advanced disease, and serial measurements may be helpful in assessing the patient with severe respiratory failure, prior to the institution or discontinuance of mechanical ventilation.

A widely available, simple measure of ventilatory reserve, known as *maximum voluntary ventilation*, has broad application in the assessment of exertional dyspnea. This "sprint test" quantitates the amount of air that can be moved by the chest bellows during a brief (12 to 15 sec.) maximum effort. It normally exceeds the ventilation required under resting conditions by a factor of about twenty—a functional reserve so great that ventilation itself is not normally a limiting factor in exercise. Breathlessness is generally experienced by normal and abnormal subjects during exercise that requires a minute ventilation in excess of 50 per cent of the subject's maximum voluntary ventilation. This rule of thumb is useful in estimating the limitation of exercise tolerance due to decreased ventilatory reserve, if allowances are made for considerable normal variation and for the increased ventilation required in disease because of decreased efficiency of ventilation. Twenty to 30 liters of ventilation are generally needed each minute in normal subjects to provide 1 liter of oxygen for metabolic needs; the ratio may be as high as 40 to 1 in diseased subjects.[68]

Vital capacity is a limited measurement of ventilatory reserve that has a somewhat narrower application, because it correlates quite differently with maximum voluntary ventilation in restrictive, as opposed to obstructive, diseases. It is a simple measurement to perform and is of great value in following individual patients on successive occasions. In patients with neuromuscular disease, as well as other restrictive diseases of the lung and chest wall, it often correlates very well with dyspnea, and marked decreases may occur before blood gas abnormalities become evident.

The mechanical abnormalities that presumably are most directly responsible for dyspnea are increased airways resistance and decreased lung and chest-wall compliance. As pointed out in subsequent pages, these measurements can be carried out, but with some technical difficulty. Normal values for various populations are not well established. Consequently, measurements of airways resistance and compliance are not readily available or useful to clinicians in most communities.

Abnormalities in more readily available tests of lung mechanics generally accompany changes in airways resistance and compliance. Flow rate measurements during the maximum-effort expiratory maneuver have a close enough relation to airways resistance to be of great use. Most commonly available measurements of flow rates include the forced expiratory volumes, at 0.5 and 1.0 second, and the forced expiratory flow rate, from 25 to 75 per cent of the forced vital capacity. As described in more detail elsewhere, these measurements are theoretically imperfect reflectors of airways resistance, because the pressure differential generated to produce flow is not taken into account but is simply defined as *maximum* during the maximum-effort expiratory maneuver. This does not detract substantially from their practical usefulness.

Compliance changes in disease are rather well reflected by changes in the various compartments of lung volume. Reduction in vital capacity, particularly, is an easily measured change that usually accompanies reduced compliance. The lung diseases characterized by stiffness (decreased compliance) of lung parenchyma are characterized by a rather symmetrical decrease in lung volumes (restriction), except for residual volume and functional residual capacity, which may be normal or even increased. Likewise, the restrictive chest-wall diseases cause decreased lung volumes, except perhaps for residual volume and functional residual capacity. The obstructive diseases also show decreased vital capacity and increased RV and FRC but show normal total lung capacity, except for emphysema, in which TLC is increased, presumably owing to increased lung compliance.

It should be apparent, then, that measurement of lung volumes may serve as a helpful reflector of changes in lung or chest-wall compliance, but that interpretation must be made cautiously and with knowledge of the patient's clinical, radiological, and physiological profile. There can be no simple, quantitative relationship expressed between dyspnea and lung volumes, except perhaps for vital capacity in carefully defined circumstances.

Decreased Ability to Exert Effort to Breathe. Shortness of breath due to neuromuscular disease is intriguing in that it represents a third category of dyspnea that is not readily explained by an abnormal stimulus to breathe or by an increase in effort required to breathe; rather, it is explained by a decrease in the ability to respond to a stimulus. Distress in patients with respiratory muscle paralysis is usually prominent, with less weakness than that required to cause deterioration of arterial blood gases. Campbell has questioned whether the type or degree of distress in this setting is the same as that experienced by patients with mechanical hindrance to ventilation.[1,2] He has carried his curiosity to the point of inducing the two forms of distress in himself by curarization and by mechanical loading and found the former less unpleasant.

Whatever may be the nature or degree of distress in neuromuscular respiratory paralysis, it is clear that in patients with progressive disease such as Guillain-Barré syndrome, measurement of vital capacity is an excellent way to document deterioration or improvement. This measurement often correlates well with the patient's subjective complaints. Dyspnea and a decrease in vital capacity ordinarily occur before blood gas deterioration.

Evaluation of Patients With Respiratory Disease. A second important role of the pulmonary-function laboratory is the initial evaluation of patients with respiratory disease, regardless of the presence or absence of dyspnea. In such patients, quantitation of simple parameters of lung function is a desirable routine. Such an evaluation may be of some help in diagnosis, because most diseases produce characteristic, though not specific, physiological profiles of abnormalities. In addition, quantitation of the amount of dysfunction produced by a disease is often helpful in planning therapy, especially in providing a baseline for following the results of therapy.

Following the Course of Disease. Serial testing to follow progression of disease or results of therapy is a third valuable function of the pulmonary laboratory. Demonstration of stability or progression of physiological abnormality may be essential in such decisions as whether or not to treat pulmonary sarcoidosis with corticosteroids. Improvement in function may provide support for a decision to continue or discontinue such therapy. Similarly, the degree of success achieved with bronchodilators and other forms of therapy can be assessed with some objectivity by pulmonary-function testing. A change of 20 per cent from baseline spirometric values is often suggested as a minimum acute change in response to bronchodilator administration to be considered significant; but in an excellent laboratory, testing a cooperative and well-informed patient, reproducibility may be possible within 5 per cent for simple spirometric tests. Therefore, measurement of vital capacity and expiratory flow rates alone may be adequately discriminating to follow the course of diseases that affect them and the response to therapy in such diseases.

Preoperative Evaluation. Preoperative testing of patients at high risk of respiratory complications in association with the operative procedure is a fourth role of the pulmonary-function laboratory. Ventilatory failure may occur in patients with decreased ventilatory reserve following preoperative sedation or during recovery from anesthesia. Increased risk of this complication can be predicted by simple spirometry. Of course, patients with chronic carbon dioxide retention are at great risk of acute decompensation in this setting, so arterial blood gases should be measured in patients with decreased ventilatory reserve. Postoperative atelectasis with infection occurs with increased frequency in patients with obstructive lung disease, and its identification can enable the physician to provide appropriate measures to prevent it. Hypoxemia, when identified preoperatively, is in itself easily dealt with by oxygen administration. A history and physical examination, spirometry, and measurement of arterial blood gases, then, provide an adequate assessment for preoperative respiratory evaluation of most patients prior to surgery of virtually any kind, except thoracic and cardiovascular procedures. In fact, pulmonary resection is the only major procedure that commonly requires a more extensive workup, which may include evaluation of distribution of ventilation and blood flow, with reference to the portion of the lung to be resected. Preoperative pulmonary evaluation is discussed further in Chapter 9.

Screening of patients for subclinical disease is a fifth role of the pulmonary-function lab and may require more discriminating tests than simple ventilatory measurements. Populations at risk from special environmental hazards, such as miners, foundry workers, and others exposed to industrial hazards, may require periodic testing of a sort designed specifically to detect early effects of the injurious agent involved. Screening programs to detect early obstructive airways disease in the population at large have not as yet been proven useful. This subject is considered in greater detail on page 115.

Force and Resistance in Spontaneous Ventilation

The mechanical factors governing the flow of air into and out of the lungs during various spontaneous ventilatory maneuvers must be understood prior to undertaking a discussion of abnormalities of ventilation. Especially important is the recognition that factors that produce and limit air flow differ during resting tidal breathing, exercise, and maximum-effort ventilatory maneuvers that are widely used in pulmonary-function laboratories to assess ventilatory reserve (Table 3-1).

The Resting Expiratory State. The mechanics of the thorax and lungs during the resting expiratory state (Table 3-1A) are of basic interest.[4-6] At this level of inflation, referred to as *functional residual capacity*, a balance exists between two opposing forces: the tendency of the lungs to further collapse and the tendency of the chest cage to further expand. These forces are independent of effort on the part of the subject; they result from the elastic properties of the lungs and chest cage. This resting expiratory level of inflation will be assumed, then, at the bottom of a normal resting tidal breath, during deep anesthesia, or death. During these states, the respiratory muscles are relaxed, and elastic forces alone determine the level of lung inflation. The magnitude of the opposing elastic forces of the lungs and chest wall can be measured as intrapleural pressure, which is negative at functional residual capacity (FRC). The unopposed effect of these elastic forces is observed at surgery or autopsy, when the chest is opened: the lungs collapse further, and the chest inflates slightly, but perceptibly.

The volume of air in the chest at FRC, then, is determined by the elastic properties of the lungs and chest (which may be altered in disease) but is independent of

Table 3-1. Mechanical Characteristics of Spontaneous Ventilatory Maneuvers (Normal Subjects)*

	Volume per Breath	*Respiratory Rate*	*Minute Ventilation*	*Mechanical Forces at Work*	*Forces To Be Overcome*†	*Alveolar Pressure*‡	*Elastic Recoil Pressure*	*Pleural Pressure*	
A. Resting expiratory state	N/A	N/A	N/A	Elastic forces of chest tending to expand. Elastic forces of lungs tending to collapse.		0	+	−	100 TLC % 0 — FRC
B. Tidal breathing at rest	500 ml.	16/min.	8 L./min.	*Inspiration*: active, contraction of inspiratory muscles.	Air flow resistance. Elastic recoil.	−	+	−	
				Expiration: passive, elastic recoil of lungs and chest wall.	Air flow resistance.	+	+	−	100 TLC % 0 — FRC
C. Tidal breathing during heavy exercise	2000 ml.	50/min.	100 L./min.	*Inspiration*: active, contraction of inspiratory muscles.	Air flow resistance. Elastic recoil.	−	+	−	
				Expiration: may be passive or active. Elastic recoil of lungs and chest wall, and contraction of expiratory muscles.	Air flow resistance.	+	+	+ or −	100 TLC % 0 — FRC
D. Maximal voluntary ventilation	2000 ml.	80/min.	160 L./min.	*Inspiration*: active, contraction of inspiratory muscles.	Air flow resistance. Elastic recoil.	−	+	−	100 TLC % 0 — FRC
				Expiration: active, elastic recoil of lungs and chest wall, and contraction of expiratory muscles.	Air flow resistance.	+	+	+	
E. Maximal-effort expiratory maneuver	5000 ml.		N/A	Active contraction of expiratory muscle.	Air flow resistance.	+	+	+	100 TLC % 0 — FRC

*N/A = not applicable.
†Tissue viscous resistance and inertia must be overcome during any active ventilatory maneuver, but are negligible.
‡Pressures: O (atmospheric); − (negative); + (positive).

the subject's effort. Inflation or deflation above or below FRC requires contraction of the muscles of respiration and results in alterations in intrapleural and alveolar pressures, as discussed in the following paragraphs.

Tidal Breathing at Rest. Normal resting tidal breathing (Table 3-1B) consists of repetitive inflation to a level about 500 ml. above FRC (in the normal adult male), followed by deflation to FRC. Inflation is a result of active contraction of inspiratory muscles; deflation occurs passively, owing to elastic forces returning the chest to the resting level of inflation. During inflation, expansion of the chest cage produces increasingly more negative intrapleural pressure, which overcomes the elastic recoil pressure of the lung, and causes it to expand. During passive expiration, the lungs recoil, drawing the chest cage to FRC. During all phases of resting tidal breathing, intrapleural pressure remains negative (less than atmospheric), keeping the visceral and parietal pleura in intimate apposition.

Alveolar pressure, on the other hand, is less than atmospheric during inspiration, resulting in air flow into the lungs, and is greater than atmospheric during expiration, resulting in flow out of the lungs. Alveolar pressure during any phase of respiration is the algebraic sum of elastic recoil pressure of the lung and pleural pressure. Pleural pressure, in turn, is due to a combination of elastic forces and positive or negative forces created by contraction of the muscles of respiration.

These relationships are complicated by the fact that frictional as well as elastic forces must be overcome to produce lung inflation, and by the fact that frictional resistance must be overcome while elastic forces contribute to deflation. The frictional resistances to be overcome include viscous resistance of the tissues and resistance of the airways. Tissue viscous resistance and inertia are negligible in health and disease, whereas airways resistance is of major importance in normal and abnormal physiology. The latter topic has been extensively reviewed recently by Macklem.[7]

The chest bellows are capable of moving considerably larger volumes of air at much higher flow rates than those that occur during resting tidal breathing. In other words, the normal "ventilatory reserve" is great, and ventilation can increase to support a metabolic rate as much as twenty times the resting level.

Voluntary inflation of the lungs to levels above those reached during resting respiration can be readily attained by contraction of inspiratory muscles, achieving more negative pleural pressures. The maximum attainable level of inflation is referred to as *total lung capacity*. Deflation to FRC occurs passively, owing to elastic forces, when inspiratory muscles are relaxed. During such a passive expiration, pleural pressure remains negative. Expiration can be speeded up by voluntary contraction of expiratory muscles, in which case positive pleural pressures may be attained. Expiration below FRC requires contraction of expiratory muscles and results in positive pleural pressure, beginning at a level slightly below FRC. The minimum level of inflation that can be achieved by contraction of expiratory muscles is called *residual volume*.

Tidal Breathing During Exercise. During exercise, greatly increased flow rates, tidal volumes, and respiratory rates can be achieved (Table 3-1C). The mechanics of ventilation, as described previously, remain operative, with certain exceptions. Inspiration results in inflation greater than at rest, and expiration may result in deflation below FRC. Expiration may become active, rather than passive, with contraction of expiratory muscles increasing air flow. Normally, sustained exercise does not tax the ventilatory apparatus quite to its maximum, so that flow rates during inspiration and expiration remain below those that are the greatest achievable during a brief maximum voluntary effort.

Breathing During Maximal Voluntary Ventilation. Measurement of minute ventilation during a brief maximum effort is a useful test of ventilatory reserve (Table 3-1D). The mechanics of breathing in this "sprint" test are similar to those operative during exercise. The MVV is customarily carried out for only 12 to 15 seconds, however, so that higher values are obtained for minute ventilation than those that can be obtained for long periods or during maximal exercise.

Ventilatory Mechanics During the Maximal-Effort Expiratory Maneuver. Pulmonary-function testing that measures tidal ventilation at rest and during exercise may be diagnostically useful, because ventilation may become inefficient due to disease and because tidal ventilation required for a given level of exercise may increase. Ventilatory tests have been designed, however, that are more sensitive and discriminating. Measurement of certain ventilatory parameters during a single maximum expiratory effort can be used to tax the ventilatory apparatus to its mechanical maximum, thus contributing information ubout ventilation in health and disease that can be approached in no other way.

Analysis of the maximal-effort expiratory maneuver (Table 3-1E) has contributed to the basic understanding of normal and abnormal ventilatory function.[8,9] The maneuver consists of a full expiration from full inspiration, performed as rapidly and completely as possible. It has been recognized since the early use of clinical spirometry that this maneuver is quite reliable and reproducible and can be used to detect and quantitate obstructive lung disease. This knowledge has been refined, and special characteristics of the maneuver have been clarified in recent years.[10,11]

The most conventional analysis of the maximal-effort expiratory maneuver is carried out from a volume-time curve, as described in this book's section on clinical spirometry. More sophisticated equipment is needed for an analysis of flow-volume curves. Considerable experience with these techniques has shown that the midportion of a maximal-effort expiratory volume-time or flow-volume curve in any individual subject is remarkably reproducible and is sensitive to mild obstructive lung disease. The initial and terminal portions are effort-dependent, poorly reproducible, and less discriminating.

The relative effort-independence of flow during the midportion of a maximum-effort expiration can be demonstrated and quantitated by measuring both flow and effort during such a maneuver. Flow can be measured easily by use of a simple water-sealed spirometer. Effort can also be measured, indirectly, as esophageal pressure. The contraction of expiratory muscles during forced expiration contributes to air flow by producing a positive pleural pressure, which is transmitted to the alveolus, resulting in flow from the alveolus to the mouth. Pleural pressure cannot be measured without invasive techniques, but intra-esophageal pressure approximates pleural pressure. It can be measured by passing a small rubber balloon, connected by polyethylene tubing to a manometer, into the esophagus.

By this technique, it can be shown that increasing effort produces increasing expiratory flow up to only about one-fourth of maximum effort. Greater effort does not produce greater flow.[8,9] Maximum expiratory flow declines during the course of expiration; for a given lung volume, a maximum flow can be defined. Therefore, for any normal or abnormal person, the mid-portion of a volume-time or flow-volume curve performed with greater than one-fourth maximal effort is precisely reproducible. Current theory attempting to explain this phenomenon will be summarized on page 88.

Such a relationship between effort and flow does not exist during forced inspiration. Increasing effort, up to maximal for an individual person, produces increasing inspiratory flow.

Physical Findings in Ventilatory Dysfunction

- Shape of the thorax
- Character of movement of the thorax
- Movement of the diaphragm
- Percussion note
- Auscultatory findings
- Measurement of respiratory rate
- Estimation of tidal volume
- Estimation of expiratory flow rates

Bedside Evaluation of Ventilatory Function

Obstructive lung disease is often easily diagnosed at the bedside in the patient who is so severely afflicted that he is dyspneic at rest. Such a patient may assume a characteristic posture, usually the sitting position, bending slightly forward and bracing his hands or elbows against a table or upon his knees. His breathing may be obviously labored, with his chest moving poorly in spite of use of accessory muscles of respiration. A barrel-shaped chest, with intercostal and supraclavicular retraction on inspiration, is common. Expiration may be obviously prolonged, accompanied by wheezing, and carried out against pursed lips. The disordered ventilatory function in such a patient is easily appreciated.

Less severely diseased persons or those with a less classic clinical presentation may be difficult to assess. Early emphysema may produce dyspnea only on exertion, and cursory examination at rest may reveal no abnormalities. Dyspnea due to left ventricular decompensation may be accompanied by wheezing and may resemble obstructive or restrictive lung disease in clinical presentation. Mixed pulmonary and cardiac disease may be especially difficult to assess. The following paragraphs provide some suggestions to assist in the detection and identification of ventilatory dysfunction, especially that due to obstructive lung disease.

Observation of respiratory rate and depth are basic to physical diagnosis, but they are often misused and misinterpreted. Rapid rate and increased tidal volume in the hyperventilation syndrome or in severe metabolic acidosis are easily recognized but are often interpreted as respiratory distress due to heart or lung disease. Rapid rate and diminished tidal volume in lung disease with decreased alveolar ventilation can easily be mistaken for overbreathing, because the adventitious sounds in such a case may create the illusion that normal or increased volume is being exchanged with each breath. Often such a patient is described as "hyperventilating," when, in fact, his alveolar ventilation is diminished, or at least inadequate for his metabolic rate, as reflected by an elevated arterial carbon dioxide tension. Observation of breathing rate and depth should always be carried out, but with the knowledge that tidal volume is difficult to quantitate in this fashion.

The shape of the chest and the extent and character of its movement during respiration is another basic but deceptive part of the clinical examination. There is general agreement that the "barrel chest" configuration of the thorax, with increased anteroposterior diameter of the chest, is a classic finding in advanced chronic obstructive lung disease, but that this finding is not a sensitive indicator of mild disease and may be seen in persons without obstructive disease, especially elderly persons.

Related findings referable to the thorax have been examined in a study to detect correlation with presence and severity of airway obstruction.[12,13] One study was carried out on a group of patients with "stable" obstructive disease. Airway obstruction was quantitated as "specific conductance," a measurement that is the reciprocal of airway resistance, corrected for lung volume. Rhonchi and rales at the bases, and diminished breath sounds, although frequently present, were not correlated significantly with specific conductance. Other signs that did not correlate were paradoxical inward movement of the costal margin with inspiration; loss of lateral and upward bucket-handle movement of the upper ribs, with exaggeration of forward and upper (pump handle) movement; and shortening of the length of the trachea, from cricoid cartilage to sternal notch. These findings do occur in obstructive lung disease but are not sensitive indicators or reliable indicators of severity of disease.

In the same study, correlation was found between specific conductance and the time required to perform a complete forced expiration from maximum inspiration. This finding was not unexpected, because velocity of air flow is inversely proportional to airways resistance. Correlation of specific conductance was also found with a group of signs related only indirectly to resistance of airways *per se*. Increased resonance to percussion showed significant correlation, though it is due to the secondary effect of increased lung volume. Another secondary effect, disordered muscle activity, produces tracheal descent (due to downward pull of the depressed diaphragm) and contraction of the scalene and sternomastoid muscles during inspiration. These findings correlated with specific conductance, as did excavation of the supraclavicular fossae on inspiration, a result of wide intrathoracic pressure swings required to produce air flow through a highly resistant system of airways.

A more recent study examined the reliability of subjective complaints and physical findings in assessing the severity of acute attacks of bronchial asthma.[14] The investigators studied subjective dyspnea and wheezing at rest, retraction of the sternocleidomastoid muscles, and wheezing audible through the stethoscope during tidal breathing. These complaints and findings were correlated with plethysmographic measurements of airways resistance and lung volumes and with spirometric measurements of forced expiratory flow rates. The results are interesting and useful.

Only retraction of the sternocleidomastoids correlated closely with severity of functional derangement. When this sign was present, specific conductance, maximum mid-expiratory flow rate, and forced expiratory volume at 1 second were always severely reduced, the latter usually to less than 1 liter. Subjective wheezing and dyspnea, and wheezing audible through the stethoscope on tidal breathing were always present with functional derangement but did not correlate well with its severity.

During improvement, a definite order of disappearance of signs and symptoms was the rule. Retractions disappeared first, then symptoms, then wheezing on stethoscopic examination. At the time of disappearance of signs and symptoms, lung function remained abnormal, with most parameters only 60 to 70 per cent of normal.

The findings of these two studies serve well to remind us that the classic symptoms and physical findings of obstructive lung disease, although useful, are not perfectly discriminating. A more sensitive technique is often needed for detection of mild obstructive disease. Even in moderate disease, more quantitative techniques may be needed to distinguish obstructive disease from other causes of dyspnea, such as cardiac decompensation.

One popular bedside test that roughly quantitates the severity of obstructive airways disease is the match test. Several variations of this test of ability to extinguish a match with a forced expiration have been described.[15-17] Snider and colleagues described a technique in which the subject was directed to blow out a match held 6 in. from his open mouth.[15] Ability to perform this test correlated well with a maximum voluntary ventilation of 60 liters per minute and a forced expiratory volume at 1 second of 1.6 liters.

Of the 52 subjects who could not blow out the match, 80 per cent had a maximum voluntary ventilation below 60 liters per minute, and 85 per cent had a forced expiratory volume at 1 second below 1.60 liters. Of the 74 who could extinguish the match, 80 per cent had a maximum voluntary ventilation above 60 liters per minute, and 85 per cent had a forced expiratory volume at 1 second above 1.60 liters.

In a similar study, Olsen found that 94.8 per cent of 327 subjects who could blow out a match 3 in. from the open mouth had MVV values of 40 liters per minute or greater.[16] Eighty-nine per cent of the 26 subjects who could not extinguish the match had MVV values below 40 liters per minute.

Approaching the match test somewhat differently, Carilli and Henderson studied 146 subjects, including normal persons and those with assorted forms of ventilatory defect.[17] They determined the maximum distance at which a match could be extinguished with a forced expiration through a standard mouthpiece and 3 inches of Collins spirometer tubing. They found that the predicted MVV in percentage was approximately equal to the match distance in centimeters.

Another useful bedside technique for clinical estimation of severity of airway obstruction is the measurement of forced expiratory time.[18,19] To perform this test, the subject is instructed to inspire maximally, then exhale as rapidly, forcefully, and completely as possible to residual volume, as when performing a forced vital-capacity maneuver. The cessation of expiratory flow can best be detected with a stethoscope placed at the lung base or over the trachea; and the duration of time required for the maneuver can be measured with a second hand of a conventional watch or more precisely with a stopwatch. Rosenblatt and Stein[18] and Lal and associates[19] have correlated the forced expiratory time with clinical spirometric indices in two separate studies. It appears that virtually all normal subjects can complete the forced expiratory maneuver in less than 4 seconds, whereas most subjects with moderate to severe obstructive disease require more than 6 seconds. More precise quantitation of airway obstruction appears impractical by this technique, and it should be emphasized that the subject must be vigorously coached in order to perform the test well.

Regional alterations of ventilation may also be recognized clinically. The findings are summarized in Chapter 4.

LABORATORY EVALUATION OF VENTILATORY FUNCTION

Volume-Time Analysis of Air Flow

In the preceding section, we considered parameters of chest-wall and lung mechanics according to a classification designed to help the reader better understand ventilatory function. Not all of the parameters considered are equally susceptible to measurement in the usual clinical pulmonary-function laboratory. Subsequent discussion will consider measurements of ventilatory function in a more practical way, with reference to their availability to the clinician.

A group of measurements of ventilatory function that are easily performed with inexpensive equipment will be discussed first. This group of measurements, performed and displayed in a stereotyped fashion, is highly recommended as a basic ventilatory profile with which the clinician should become thoroughly familiar, and which should be obtained on all patients entering the laboratory. This battery of tests can be performed with a simple recording spirometer that is inexpensive enough to be standard equipment in the diagnostic laboratory of even the smallest hospital caring for patients with respiratory disease. Recommended criteria for a satisfactory spirometer have recently been published by the American College of Chest Physicians.[20] Normal values have been established for these parameters in a spectrum of subjects of both sexes, varying ages, and varying sizes.[21-31] Patterns of abnormality in a wide range of diseases have been characterized during the past 20 years.

The tests are heavily dependent on patient understanding and cooperation and must be carried out by an informed technician who is able to communicate instructions well. Extensive training however, is not required. Properly performed and interpreted, the ventilatory profile thus obtained provides a large return in information essential for diagnosis and patient care, with a very small investment.

Clinical spirometry for volume-time curve analysis consists of the recording of volume change plotted against time during a series of ventilatory maneuvers by the patient. This permits the determination that the patient has either normal ventilatory reserve or an abnormal pattern characteristic of obstructive, restrictive, or mixed ventilatory abnormalities. Although most diseases are rather predictable in the type of ventilatory defect that they produce, it should be emphasized that such patterns are nonspecific. Spirometry alone is never sufficient to enable a physician to make a diagnosis of a specific disease; however, the volume-time curve is sufficiently reproducible to be useful in following the course of many disease processes. An estimation of the degree of exercise limitation due to a ventilatory defect is possible from volume-time studies; and the patient who is likely to incur ventilatory failure can be identified.

As with any clinical measurement, sensible interpretation of ventilatory testing requires a clear understanding of its limitations. Spirometry does not provide a measurement of the amount of air contained in the chest at the completion of a full expiration (residual volume) and therefore does not permit calculation of the other lung compartments containing residual volume (functional residual capacity, total lung capacity). Likewise, it does not provide direct assessment of the resistance to breathing (lung and chest-wall elastance and airways resistance). It provides no information about control of ventilation, distribution of ventilation, or respiratory gas exchange. Because it is effort-dependent, it cannot be performed usefully on patients who are unable or unwilling to cooperate. Furthermore, the range of normal values for volume-time indices is high. Nevertheless, in combination with measurement of arterial blood gases, spirometry provides sufficient information for intelligent care of patients with respiratory disease in almost every case. More sophisticated tests, requiring far more complicated instrumentation, often provide a fuller understanding of pathophysiology. They certainly have provided a rich fund of knowledge for our current understanding of disease in general. Therefore, the information to be gained from simple volume-time curve analysis is emphasized in this chapter. Tests that require additional instrumentation are described subsequently in detail, and the supplementary information that they provide is discussed.

In obtaining volume-time curves, the patient breathes in and out through a mouthpiece, with a nose clip in place, displacing the air within a reservoir of some sort. The excursions of the reservoir are recorded as volume change (on a vertical axis) against time (on a horizontal axis). Many satisfactory devices are commercially available for carrying out simple spirometry. Water-sealed spirometers are inexpensive and reliable. Air is displaced from a container suspended in a water seal, and an attached pen inscribes vertical movement on a drum that revolves at a predetermined speed. The patient is instructed to perform three breathing maneuvers: (a) the vital capacity maneuver, (b) the forced expiratory maneuver, and (c) maximum voluntary ventilation.

Vital Capacity and Other Static Lung Volumes. Early in the development of clinical spirometry, only static lung volumes were measured. The usefulness of dynamic ventilatory measurements in obstructive disease was recognized later. Of the static lung volumes defined by the Pappenheimer Committee in 1950,[32] vital capacity was most routinely measured as a clinical reflection of ventilatory reserve.

In the vital capacity maneuver, the patient is instructed to inhale as deeply as possible and then exhale fully, taking as much time as he requires. The measurement sought from this maneuver is a single volume measurement. An alternative way of arriving at this measurement is to add two of its components. The patient first exhales maximally from resting expiration, to record expiratory reserve volume. After a few breaths, he then inspires fully from resting expiration, to record inspiratory capacity. These two measurements are added, giving a "combined vital capacity." Normally, and in most patients, the vital capacity and the combined vital capacity are equal. Occasionally, a severely obstructed patient is unable to complete a conventional vital capacity maneuver without interrupting it because of air hunger or fatigue. In this case, the combined vital capacity appears larger than the vital capacity.

The pathophysiological significance of the vital capacity can best be appreciated by referring to the diagram of the subdivisions of lung volume defined by the Pappenheimer report (Fig. 3-1). This 1950 report summarized the terminology agreed upon by the country's leading respiratory physiologists.

Consideration of this diagram readily reveals that each of the volumes here defined can be recorded and measured by a simple spirometer as described earlier, except those containing residual volume. This volume, remaining in the thorax at the end of a maximum expiration, can be measured only by indirect means (e.g., helium dilution, nitrogen washout, or body plethysmography). Also readily apparent

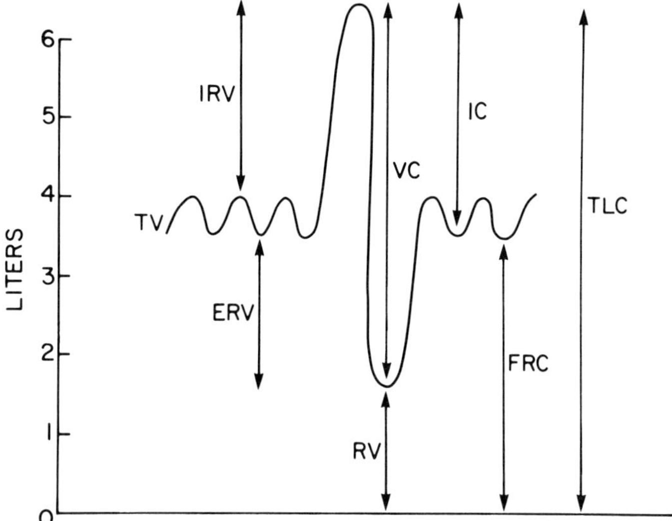

Fig. 3-1. Subdivisions of lung volume. Key: TV–tidal volume, IRV–inspiratory reserve volume, ERV–expiratory reserve volume, RV–residual volume, VC–vital capacity, IC–inspiratory capacity, FRC–functional residual capacity, TLC–total lung capacity.

is the fact that vital capacity can be reduced in two different ways: reduction of total lung capacity and increase in residual volume. These two mechanisms can be differentiated clearly only by measurement of residual volume and calculation of total lung capacity. Subsequent experience has shown that significant elevation of residual volume is the mechanism by which vital capacity is limited in the "obstructive diseases": asthma, chronic bronchitis, and emphysema. Diseases that cause infiltration or edema of the interstitium, or volume displacement of lung tissue cause a decrease in vital capacity chiefly by a decrease in total lung capacity. The demonstration of marked reduction in expiratory flow rates may support a clinical diagnosis of one of the obstructive diseases and may permit the clinical interpretation that vital capacity is limited by high residual volume. Conversely, relatively normal flow rates may rule out obstructive disease and may permit a presumption that a severe decrease in vital capacity is due to decreased total lung capacity.

The measurement of reduced vital capacity alone, then, provides a very inadequate, nonspecific assessment of decreased ventilatory reserve. The performance of complete clinical spirometry provides additional clarification of the mechanism and severity of a ventilatory defect with satisfactory clinical accuracy. The additional measurement of residual volume, at greater inconvenience and expense, provides convincing proof of the presence or absence of lung overinflation or underinflation.

The Maximal-Effort Expiratory Maneuver. During the years following 1950, interest in physiology began to move toward clinical application. It soon became apparent that measurement of vital capacity had severe limitations in the assessment of ventilatory abnormalities. In particular, patients with significant disability from obstructive lung disease were often noted to have a relatively normal vital capacity. Demonstration of decreased flow rates during breathing, especially during forced expiration, correlated well with clinical disability, however. The maximal-effort expiratory maneuver was therefore developed. Extensive literature soon appeared that centered on the analysis of measurements obtained during performance of this maneuver by normal subjects and by patients with various respiratory diseases. Efforts to extract information from this simple maneuver by a host of different analytical approaches continue to the present.

In performing the maximal-effort expiratory maneuver, the subject is instructed to exhale as rapidly and forcefully as possible, from a full inspiration. When this maneuver is performed as a part of conventional clinical spirometry, volume is recorded on the vertical axis of recording paper, and time is recorded on the horizontal axis; the curve so obtained is referred to as a *forced vital capacity curve*.

In analyzing the volume-time curve obtained during a maximal-effort expiratory maneuver, three types of measurements can be readily performed. The volume exhaled during a defined time interval (forced expiratory volume, timed) following initiation of the maneuver can be measured; the ratio of such a volume to the total forced vital capacity can be computed; and average flow rates during defined portions of the curve can be obtained. During the early years of clinical spirometry, many variations of these three types of measurements were performed and their relative merits touted. Terminology was confusing and poorly standardized.

In 1963, the Section on Pulmonary Function Testing, Committee on Pulmonary Physiology, American College of Chest Physicians, outlined a format for clinical spirometry that incorporated an analysis of the maximal-effort expiratory volume-time curve and maximal voluntary ventilation, in addition to vital capacity.[33] Table 3-2 summarizes the committee report concerning definitions and terminology, which has since been reviewed and confirmed.[34]

"To warrant diagnostic acceptance, the expiratory spirogram should exhibit a reproducible configuration which reflects the underlying physical state of the respiratory tract."[35] Various portions of the curve have differing diagnostic characteristics. The mid-portion of the maximal-effort expiratory curve is the most effort-independent portion, and it may be most sensitive to early disease of peripheral airways. Ths early portion of the curve is more effort-dependent; is less sensitive to mild airways disease; and is perhaps more sensitive to obstruction in large central airways, as due to tumor in the trachea or tracheomalacia. The terminal portion is sometimes poorly recorded when a dyspneic patient terminates the maneuver prematurely because of air hunger.

More recently, analysis of flow-volume curves has been popularized as a method of studying the maximal-effort expiratory maneuver and is discussed in more detail below. This method requires somewhat more complex instrumentation but is thought by some investigators to contribute superior diagnostic information in certain cases.

Forced Expiratory Volume, Timed. The forced expiratory volume at 1 second (FEV 1.0 sec.) is the dynamic volume (or flow) measurement that has been most often used, along with the vital capacity, in an abbreviated form of spirometry. It incorporates the early, effort-dependent portion of the curve but also enough of the mid-portion to make it reproducible and sensitive enough to be clinically useful. It has an advantage of simplicity, because it can be easily read from a permanently recorded spirogram, or it can be read automatically by a variety of inexpensive spirometers with timing devices. The literature indicates a large experience with this measurement. Normal values for a variety of populations are available, as well as correlation with the degree of clinical disability and long- and short-term prognoses for impairment due to a variety of disorders. Forced expiratory-volume measurements at 0.5 sec. and 0.75 sec. incorporate more of the effort-dependent portion of the curve and that portion which has been alleged to better reflect large central-airway obstruction. The latter property is not reliable enough to be of clinical value. Therefore, the FEV 1.0 sec. is more useful than the FEV 0.5 sec. or FEV 0.75 sec., and the addition of one of the latter measurements serves chiefly as a validity check to the complete spirogram. The FEV 2.0 sec. and FEV 3.0 sec. add very little additional information.

Forced Expiratory Volume, Timed, as a Percentage of Forced Vital Capacity. The forced expiratory volumes expressed as a percentage of the total forced vital capacity have a limited value. Prior to the availability of satisfactory prediction tables for the

Table 3-2. Terms Used for Spirometric Measurements*

Description	*Term Used*	*Symbol*	*Other Previously Used Terms*
The largest volume measured on complete expiration after full inspiration	Vital capacity	VC	
The vital capacity performed with expiration being as forceful as possible (i.e., forced)	Forced vital capacity	FVC	Timed vital capacity Fast vital capacity
The volume of gas exhaled over a given time interval during the performance of a forced vital capacity	Forced expiratory volume (qualified by subscript indicating the time interval in seconds)	FEV_t (e.g., $FEV_{1.0}$)	Timed vital capacity
FEV_t expressed as percentage of the forced vital capacity (i.e., $\frac{FEV_t}{FVC} \times 100$)	Percentage expired (in t sec.) (e.g., $FEV_{1.0}$)	$FEV_t\%$	Timed vital capacity
The average rate of flow for a specified volume segment of the forced expiratory spirogram. (Most commonly used segment in adults is between 200 and 1200 ml.)	Forced expiratory flow qualified by subscript indicating volume segment	$FEF_{V1\text{-}V2}$ (e.g., $FEF_{200\text{-}1200}$)	Maximal expiratory flow rate
The average rate of flow during the middle two quarters of the volume segment of the forced expiratory spirogram (i.e., from 25–75% of the volume)	Forced mid-expiratory flow	$FEF_{25\text{-}75\%}$	Maximal mid-expiratory flow
The volume of air that a subject can breathe with voluntary maximal ventilatory effort for a given time	Maximal voluntary ventilation	MVV	Maximum breathing capacity

*Adapted from Kory, R.C.: Clinical spirometry: recommendations of the Section on Pulmonary Function Testing, Committee on Pulmonary Physiology, American College of Chest Physicians. Dis. Chest, 43:214, 1963.

volumes themselves, these ratios were useful as crude indicators of airways obstruction. Normally, the FEV 0.5/FVC should exceed 50%, and the FEV 1.0/FVC should exceed 75%. (A recent study by Morris and associates[31] defined the latter ratio more precisely in normal subjects and indicated decline with age.) Lower values reliably indicate airways obstruction. Normal or greater ratios, however, do not reliably exclude airways obstruction, especially when the FVC is reduced. When reduction of the FVC is due to interstitial disease or chest-wall restriction, with the airways being normal, FEV/FVC ratios are increased. Failure of the ratio to increase in this clinical setting may actually result from concomitant airways disease. Interpretation of the spirogram in mixed disease may then be facilitated by looking at the forced expiratory volumes in absolute terms as a percentage of predicted, rather than as a percentage of FVC. Flow rates are volume-dependent and do decrease in restrictive disease without airways obstruction, but precise quantitation of this phenomenon in various pure restrictive diseases is not available. Measurement of airways resistance may be helpful in sorting out this kind of problem.

In summary, then, a decreased FEV/FVC ratio reliably indicates airway obstruction; a normal ratio does not reliably exclude it if the FVC is reduced.

Average Forced Expiratory Flow Rates. Two measurements of average flow rate over portions of the expiratory curve have been widely used. The forced expiratory flow between the first 200 and 1200 ml. of the forced vital capacity ($FEF_{200\text{-}1200}$) was originally called the *maximal expiratory flow rate* (MEFR) and was introduced to evaluate that portion of the curve that is most affected by obstruction of the larger airways and that is most responsive to bronchodilation. These properties have not stood the test of time well, and the test is declining in popularity. The forced expiratory flow between 25 and 75 per cent of the forced vital capacity was introduced by Leuallen and Fowler as the maximal mid-expiratory flow rate (MMF). It was intended to select the most effort-independent portion of the curve and that portion most sensitive to obstructive disease of the smaller airways. These properties have gained support from both clinical experience and recent theory, and the $FEF_{25\text{-}75\%}$ is currently widely used, especially as an indicator of early disease of peripheral airways in asymptomatic subjects with otherwise normal spirometry. It should be noted that both the $FEF_{200\text{-}1200}$ and $FEF_{25\text{-}75\%}$ demonstrate wide variation in normal populations studied. Therefore, 95 per cent confidence limits for normal values are wide.

Peak Expiratory Flow Rate and Other Instantaneous Flow Measurements. Instantaneous flow-rate measurements cannot be read from a conventional volume-time spirometric tracing. The moment of most rapid expiratory flow occurs early in the maximum-effort expiration and is brief. Peak flow as an isolated measurement is easily assessed with a Wright peak flow meter.[36] Because the peak flow occurs during an effort-dependent portion of the expiratory maneuver, it is not optimally reproducible. Great effort by a patient with obstructive disease can produce a relatively normal peak flow by expulsion of air from compressible airways, creating an impression of better ventilatory ability than is actually the case. Peak expiratory flow rate has, therefore, declined in popularity as a single measure of ventilatory ability.

The peak flow rate and the flow rates when 25, 50, or 75% of forced vital capacity have been exhaled can be easily read from a flow-volume curve, and will be discussed in more detail later in this chapter.

Relative Effort-Independence of the Maximal-Effort Expiratory Maneuver. It has been mentioned that certain portions of the FVC curve are remarkably effort-independent and reproducible in the same person. This is a rather surprising observation and deserves further comment. Recent experimental data support the observation, and recent theory provides an intriguing explanation.[8-11]

Expiratory flow rate from the lungs during a FVC maneuver can be viewed as resulting from driving force created by lung elastic recoil and intrapleural pressure. That is, air is expressed from the lungs by the tendency of the lungs to collapse, owing to their elastic properties, and by pressure exerted on them by the thoracic cage (during active expiration)—measured as intrapleural pressure. These forces are opposed by the resistance of the airways and, of less importance, the resistance and inertia of lung tissue, opposing deformation. The degree of patient effort in a FVC maneuver is reflected by pleural pressure, and close approximation of pleural pressure can be obtained by measurement of intra-esophageal pressure. This can be done by having the patient swallow a tiny balloon, connected by polyethylene tubing to a manometer. It can be shown that increasing effort creates increasing expiratory flow rates only up to about one-fourth the effort that can be exerted by a normal person. This is true over the lower two-thirds of vital capacity. Maximum flow for a given lung volume may be reached by effort resulting in as little as 10 or 20 cm. of water pleural pressure. Increases in pressure to as high as 60 or 80 cm. of water do not result in further increases in flow rate.[10,11] Thus, the clinical observation of relative effort-independence of a portion of the FVC curve is firmly supported and quantitated.

It has been suggested that critical narrowing or collapse of airways occurs at the flow maxima, to account for this phenomenon.[10,11] Intrapleural pressure created during active expiration not only creates flow by elevating alveolar pressure, but it also is transmitted to the walls of intrathoracic airways, tending to collapse them. Collapse is prevented by airway pressure, which gradually drops from alveolus to mouth, as well as by stiffness of the walls of the airways themselves. At some point along the airways, the pressure inside is equal to the pressure outside, and narrowing or collapse may occur. The location of these "equal pressure points"[10] is a function of the mechanical properties of the subject's lungs: elastic recoil, as well as airways resistance. The location of the equal pressure points changes during the course of expiration; but so long as they occur within the thorax, flow maxima may occur. Increasing intrapleural pressure results in increased driving force to create flow, but also in equal force to narrow airways and oppose flow.

It can be readily imagined that disease might alter any of the determinants of expiratory flow rate, as hypothesized by this model, and therefore might alter the maximum flow achievable at any lung volume. Bronchospasm, edema, and obstructing secretions might increase the magnitude and alter the location of resistance limiting to air flow. Emphysema might contribute to the collapsibility of airways by the loss of supportive alveolar walls. Infiltrative interstitial diseases might increase recoil pressure and decrease airway collapsibility, with a resultant increase in maximum flow rates. For a detailed theoretical discussion, see Chapter 2.

Maximal Voluntary Ventilation (MVV). This test was introduced in 1933 by Hermannsen[37] and was known for many years as the *maximal breathing capacity*. It is defined as the maximal volume of air in liters that can be moved by voluntary effort during 1 minute. Patients are instructed to breathe as rapidly and deeply as possible for 12 to 30 seconds; the ventilatory volumes are recorded; and the result is expressed in liters per minute. When the longer periods of time are used, fatigue may result in diminution in ventilation toward the end of the test in patients with cardiopulmonary or other disease. If the test is carried out for longer periods, even normal persons are unable to maintain the initial levels of ventilation, because of fatigue. Diagnostic usefulness of the test may be increased by analyzing the breathing frequency chosen by the patient.

The MVV is a performance test that is heavily dependent on patient cooperation and effort. It is sensitive to loss of muscular coordination, musculoskeletal disease of the chest wall, neurologic disease, and deconditioning from any chronic illness. Values are reduced in patients with airways obstructive disease, but less so with mild or moderate restrictive disease, because a rapid, shallow breathing pattern can be chosen that compensates effectively for the mechanical defect.

In spite of these serious drawbacks, the MVV can be useful in special circumstances. It correlates well with subjective dyspnea; it is useful in evaluating exercise tolerance; and it has prognostic value in the preoperative workup, because the extrapulmonary factors to which it is sensitive are important in the patient's recovery from a surgical procedure.

Table 3-3. Commonly Used References for Predicted Normal Values for Ventilatory Tests

Year of Publication	*Ref. No.*	*Authors*	*TLC*	*FRC*	*RV*	*VC*	*FEV 1.0*	*FEF 25–75*	*MVV*	*Age* (years)*	*Sex*	*Smokers Specifically Excluded*	*Method for RV and FRC*	*Comments*	*Number of Subjects*
1948	21	Baldwin, et al.	✓	✓	✓	✓			✓	16–69	Both	No	Nitrogen washout	Regression equations incorporating height and age for VC and MVV	92
1955	22	Leuallen and Fowler						✓		Men 20–79 Women 17–62	Both	No		Normal values for men and women grouped according to age by decade	140
1959	23	Goldman and Becklake	✓	✓	✓	✓			✓	Men—mean, 44.3 (SD, 16.6) Women—mean, 38.5 (SD, 16.3)		No	Helium dilution	Regression equations incorporating height and age	94
1961	24	Kory, et al.				✓	✓	✓	✓	18–66	Males	No		Regression equations incorporating height and age, except for $FEF_{25\text{-}75\%}$	468
1962	25	Bates, et al.	✓	✓	✓	✓		✓			Males			Regression equations incorporating height and age	
1965	26	Ferris, et al.				✓	✓			25–74	Both	Smokers and nonsmokers tested and compared		Regression equations incorporating height and age	1,167
1966	27	Cotes, et al.				✓	✓			20–64	Males	No		Regression lines incorporating height and age	275

1969	28	Weng and Levison	✓	✓	✓	✓	✓	✓	✓	4–18	Both	No	Helium dilution	Regressions are for height, with boys and girls combined	139
1971	29	Morris, et al.				✓	✓	✓		20–80	Both	Yes		Regression equations incorporating height and age	988
1972	30	Cherniack and Raber				✓	✓	✓	✓	15–79	Both	Yes		Regression equations incorporating height and age	1,331
1966	67	Boren, et al.	✓	✓	✓	✓	✓		✓	20–66	Males	Partially excludes smokers	Nitrogen washout and helium dilution	Regression equations incorporating height and age	422

*SD = standard deviation.

Interpretation of Volume-Time Studies

The range of normal values for spirometric indices is rather wide[21-31] (Table 3-3). For static lung volumes and forced expiratory volumes (timed), there are good correlations with sex, age, and height. Larger values are normally seen in males and in taller subjects, and values normally decline with age after adulthood. When these variables are taken into account, a mean value for a normal population can be found that has 95 per cent confidence limits (approximately two standard deviations), extending 20 to 30 per cent above and below the mean. That is, for a group of normal persons of a stated sex, age, and height, 95 per cent have lung volumes and expiratory flow rates that are within a range of no more than 20 per cent above and below the mean value for that measurement.

The range of normal for certain of the mid-flow measurements has been even more difficult to define. Correlations with sex, age, and height are poor, and even a recent study that was confined to healthy nonsmoking adults demonstrated wide variation in normal subjects.[29]

This wide range of normal values places certain limitations on spirometric interpretation.[38,39] If the spirometric values of a person studied at a given point in time are in the very low normal range, they may represent normality for that subject, or they may represent significant functional derangement in a person whose vital capacity or flow rates were higher than average prior to the onset of disease. A discrepancy between static and dynamic volume measurements, expressed as a percentage of that predicted, can be a clue to this sort of circumstance. For instance, a normal person seldom would have a vital capacity of 115 per cent of predicted and a forced expiratory volume of 85 per cent of predicted. A person with such values probably has obstructive airways disease. Statistical data to support such an interpretation are not available, however, and in general it is wise to avoid over-interpretation of spirometric measurements. As with all laboratory tests, sensible clinical correlation is essential if spirometry is to be helpful rather than misleading.[38,39]

Although the range of normal values is wide, reproducibility of spirometric measurements in the same subject is possible within very close limits. Beyond the point of a modest learning effect, spirometry in a cooperative subject should be reproducible to within at least 5 to 10 per cent of the initial values obtained. Gaensler[38] has indicated that with optimal cooperation, variation as small as 2 to 3 per cent can be achieved. If a subject is unable or unwilling to cooperate fully, a valid spirogram cannot be obtained. Certain patterns of abnormality are characteristic of poor effort, and malingering or inability to cooperate can be suspected from such patterns, as will be described later.

There are two basic patterns of spirometric abnormality in disease: restrictive and obstructive. Typical examples of these two patterns are easily recognized and interpreted. From a classic spirogram demonstrating predominant obstruction or restriction, it may be possible to infer validity and adequate patient cooperation, and even to predict exercise tolerance and likelihood of supervening ventilatory failure with some degree of confidence. Mixed patterns are common and may be difficult to interpret, because a combination of slow flow rates and reduced vital capacity may occur in many clinical settings. Muscular weakness and suboptimal patient effort and cooperation may contribute to such a mixed pattern and may be difficult to recognize.

Restrictive Ventilatory Defect. "Restriction" to ventilation, as defined spirometrically, is simply reduction in vital capacity; that is, limitation of the extent of excursion of the chest bellows. A classic "restrictive pattern" on spirometry consists of reduced vital capacity (to less than 80% of the predicted values); little or no reduction in expiratory flow rates; and relative preservation of the maximum voluntary ventilation (see list below and Fig. 3-2). A patient whose spirogram shows a restrictive pattern can be considered to be suffering from one of the *restrictive diseases*—conventionally referring to a group of disorders in which the vital capacity is reduced, primarily due to reduction in total lung capacity rather than to increase in residual volume.

The Restrictive Pattern

Characteristics of restrictive ventilatory defect
- Decreased vital capacity
- Relatively normal expiratory flow rates
- Relatively normal maximal voluntary ventilation

Supplementary data confirming restriction
- Decreased total lung capacity

The "restrictive diseases," which result in a typical restrictive spirometric pattern and reduction in vital capacity due to low total lung capacity, are quite variable in etiology and pathology (see list below). They include a variety of interstitial lung diseases: the diffuse interstitial pneumonias, pulmonary edema, interstitial granulomas, and fibrosis, which can result from any of the foregoing. Any localized parenchymal disorders that occupy volume and displace lung tissue, such as tumors, may be included. Pleural diseases (including effusion, pneumothorax, and fibrosis) limit chest bellows expansion and are included in the group of restrictive disorders. Numerous diseases of the central and peripheral nervous system, muscle, joints, and bone interfere with movement of the chest wall and diaphragm and are classified as restrictive disorders. Although the ventilatory defect as demonstrated by spirometry may be identical in these diseases, the effects on blood-gas exchange may be quite variable. It should be kept in mind that some degree of slowing of expiratory flow rates is seen in severe examples of pure restrictive disorders of all sorts. This decrease in flow rates is minimal and is easily recognized as being secondary to low lung volumes, unless the restrictive disorder is extremely severe or airway obstruction coexists. Several causes for the slowing of expiratory flow, other than obstructive airways disease, may be operative in the restrictive diseases. Altered action of respiratory muscles and smaller diameter of airways at low lung volumes; altered tissue viscous resistance and elastance; and decreased fitness of respiratory muscles may all play a part.

The relative preservation of the maximal voluntary ventilation in restrictive disease may be diagnostically helpful. Reduction of vital capacity can be moderately severe before it impinges upon the volume of the tidal breath that the patient usually adopts when instructed to breathe as rapidly and deeply as possible. In addition, a subject with decreased vital capacity has the option of selecting a very rapid and shallow breathing pattern in order to perform a MVV maneuver, if his maximum flow rates are not reduced. The MVV helps to distinguish most patients with true restriction from subjects who have muscular weakness or who are not cooperating fully, because the latter usually have reduced vital capacity and MVV, with relatively normal flow rates.

A subject with restrictive disease, then, characteristically has a reduced vital capacity but relatively normal expiratory flow rates and MVV.

Common Causes of Restrictive Ventilatory Defect

- Interstitial lung diseases
  - Interstitial pneumonitis
  - Fibrosis
  - Pneumoconiosis
  - Granulomatosis
  - Edema
- Space-occupying lesions
  - Tumors
  - Cysts
- Pleural diseases
  - Pneumothorax
  - Hemothorax
  - Pleural effusion, empyema
  - Fibrothorax
- Chest-wall diseases
  - Injury
  - Kyphoscoliosis
  - Spondylitis
  - Neuromuscular disease
- Extrathoracic conditions
  - Obesity
  - Peritonitis
  - Ascites
  - Pregnancy

Obstructive Ventilatory Defect. Although the diagnosis and quantitation of airway obstruction is one of the most important uses of clinical spirometry, it is important to realize that airway resistance cannot be directly measured by spirometry. The spirometric parameters used to infer elevated airway resistance are simply expiratory flow rates that are achieved with an effort that is presumed to be the patient's maximum. Since the "maximum" effort is not quantitated, the observer can only presume, without solid evidence, that a decrease in flow is due to increased resistance to flow rather than to a decrease in the driving force that creates flow.

Nevertheless, reproducible patterns of spirometric values in normal subjects (Fig. 3-3) and in diseased persons are sufficiently characteristic that a valid maximum effort can usually be assumed. The diagnosis of increased airway resistance can be made with reasonable assurance, and correlation is reasonably good with body plethysmographic measurement of airways resistance in bronchitis and asthma, as well as in obstruction of the trachea or upper airways due to tumor, stenosis, collapse, or foreign body.

In subjects with emphysema, a decrease in maximum expiratory flow rates is thought to be chiefly due to decreased elastic recoil of the lungs and, therefore, to decreased driving force rather than increased resistance to flow. Nevertheless, it is customary to speak of emphysema (along with bronchitis, bronchiectasis, asthma, and bronchiolitis) as one of the *obstructive* lung diseases. According to one school of thought, there is a collapse of the airways in emphysema due to loss of elastic recoil of the alveolar tissue that normally supports the walls of the airways by radial traction. To the extent that this actually occurs, emphysema may truly be an obstructive disease in the more usual sense.

In emphysema and in other diffuse "obstructive" diseases, it is common for a decrease in expiratory flow rates to be accompanied by a decrease in vital capacity.

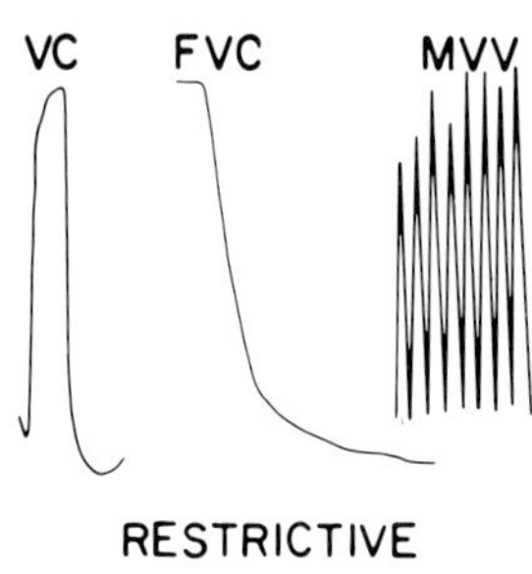

Interpretation: Mild Restrictive Ventilatory Defect

	Predicted Normal	Performed	Percent of Predicted
VC	3.72 L.	2.84	76
FVC	3.72 L.	2.84	76
$FEV_{0.5}$	2.21 L.	2.28	103
$FEV_{0.5\ (\%FVC)}$	50%	80%	
$FEV_{1.0}$	2.92 L.	2.50	86
$FEV_{1.0\ (\%FVC)}$	75%	88%	
$FEF_{25\text{-}75\%}$	3.6 L./sec.	4.33	
MVV	129 L./min.		

Fig. 3-2. Restrictive ventilatory pattern. Age, 51; sex, M; height, 63½″.

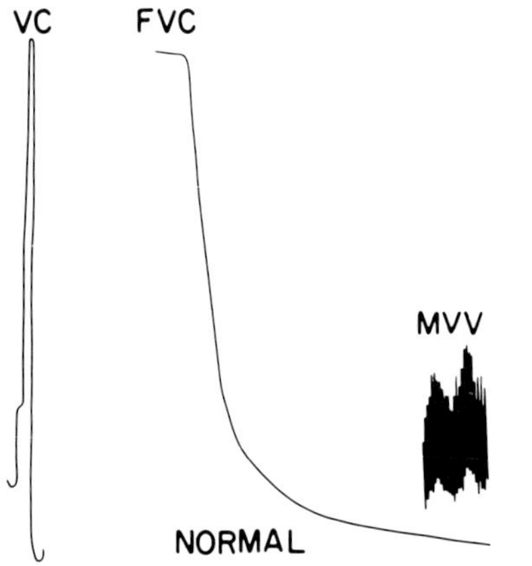

Interpretation: Normal Ventilatory Study

	Predicted Normal	Performed	Percent of Predicted
VC	4.52 L.	4.89	108
FVC	4.52 L.	4.89	108
$FEV_{0.5}$	2.60 L.	2.67	103
$FEV_{0.5\ (\%FVC)}$	50%	55%	
$FEV_{1.0}$	3.55 L.	3.82	108
$FEV_{1.0\ (\%FVC)}$	75%	78%	
$FEV_{25\text{-}75\%}$	4.3 L./sec.	4.11	
MVV	152 L./min.		

Fig. 3-3. Normal spirogram. Age, 47; sex, M; height, 69″

Interpretation: Very Severe Obstructive Ventilatory Defect

	Predicted Normal	Performed	Percent of Predicted
VC	4.60 L.	2.33	51
FVC	4.60 L.	2.33	51
$FEV_{0.5}$	2.70 L.	0.54	20
$FEV_{0.5\ (\%FVC)}$	50%	23	
$FEV_{1.0}$	3.68 L.	0.85	23
$FEV_{1.0\ (\%FVC)}$	75%	36	
$FEF_{25\text{-}75\%}$	4.3 L./sec.	0.39	
MVV	158 L./min.		

Fig. 3-4. Obstructive ventilatory pattern. Age, 41; sex, M; height, 68½″

This decrease is a result of increased residual volume, that is, an inability to normally empty the lungs. Measurement of residual volume is necessary to unequivocally document that this "air trapping" phenomenon is the mechanism of decreased vital capacity, rather than a decrease in total lung capacity, which occurs in the "restrictive" diseases. Typically, however, the decrease in vital capacity in obstructive diseases is relatively less severe than the decrease in flow rates. This relation can be readily observed by comparing the values recorded in the column labeled *percent predicted* on the display form recommended. The observation of this "obstructive pattern" of ventilatory defect permits the inference that the relatively mild decrease in vital capacity is due to increased residual volume (see list below and Fig. 3-4). This inference is usually correct.

The Obstructive Pattern

Characteristics of obstructive ventilatory defect
- Normal or decreased vital capacity
- Decreased maximum expiratory flow rates
- Decreased MVV

Supplementary data confirming obstruction
- Increased residual volume
- Increased airway resistance

The obstructive pattern is relatively nonspecific, however, und usually permits no inference to be made as to the disease process producing it (see list below). A relatively greater decrease in flow rates over the early portion of the curve may suggest major airway obstruction, whereas diffuse peripheral obstruction may be reflected by a more severe decrease in mid-flow rates. These findings are not entirely clinically reliable, however. When central airway obstruction is suspected, repeated studies may establish reproducibility, suggesting adequate patient cooperation. Because central airway obstruction is manifested by a considerable decrease in inspiratory as well as expiratory flow rates, performance of a forced inspiratory maneuver may be of help in distinguishing central from peripheral airway obstruction. The ratio of the forced expiratory volume at 1 second to the forced inspiratory volume at 1 second is approximately 0.85 in normal subjects. The ratio is decreased in peripheral airways obstruction and is increased in central obstruction. A ratio greater than 1 in a subject with a decreased $FEV_{1.0}$ suggests that the obstruction may be central.[40] This topic is discussed below, along with other aspects of flow-volume relationships.

Common Causes of Obstructive Ventilatory Defect

Upper airway disease
- Pharyngeal and laryngeal tumors, edema, infections
- Foreign bodies
- Tumors, collapse, and stenosis of trachea

Peripheral airway disease
- Bronchitis
- Bronchiectasis
- Bronchiolitis
- Bronchial asthma

Pulmonary parenchymal disease (loss of airway support and of elastic recoil)
- Emphysema

Another convenient index of central airway obstruction can be obtained by measurement of the peak expiratory flow rate (PEFR) with a Wright peak flow meter and comparison with the forced expiratory volume at 1 second. The ratio of the FEV_1 (in milliliters) to PEFR (in liters per minute) usually exceeds 10 in upper airway obstruction and is less than 10 in normal subjects or those with diffuse peripheral obstruction.[41]

Assessment of reversibility of impaired expiratory flow rates may be useful. Diagnostically, reversibility implies exclusion of emphysema, at least as a cause of the reversible component of the impairment. Reversibility may occur acutely in response to bronchodilator administration; chronically in response to an assortment of treatment modalities; or spontaneously during remissions of bronchial asthma. Reversibility implies a better prognosis than fixed impairment of expiratory flow and may have considerable significance in planning a therapeutic program.

Laboratory techniques for assessment of acute reversibility of airways obstruction in response to bronchodilator administration must vary according to the needs of the individual patient and laboratory logistics. Ideally, chronic bronchodilator administration should, of course, be discontinued several hours before testing; but this may not be feasible in some patients. An aerosol bronchodilator should be administered in the appropriate dose, which varies from one patient to another, and testing should be carried out after an interval appropriate to the time of onset and duration of action of the drug selected. No amount of care in standardizing dose and route of administration can really insure that each patient will receive a maximally effective nontoxic dose, or a comparably effective dose, so individualization is necessary. Interpretation of test results should be made rather cautiously, appropriate to the difficulties inherent in standardizing such a test.

The Committee on Emphysema of the American College of Chest Physicians has suggested that the forced vital capacity, the forced expiratory volume at 1 second, and the maximal mid-expiratory flow rates are the simplest and most available tests reflecting severity of airways obstruction.[42] The committee members have recommended that a significant change in two of these three tests be required as evidence of improvement. A 15 to 25 per cent change is considered slight reversibility; 25 to 50 per cent improvement is moderate reversibility; and a greater than 50 per cent change reflects marked reversibility (see list below).

These rather rigorous criteria are useful as guidelines for interpretation and are certainly appropriate for comparison of populations for investigative purposes. For clinical purposes in individual patients, bronchodilator therapy should not be withheld simply on the basis of failure of one spirometric test to meet arbitrary criteria. Bronchodilator therapy is commonly useful in patients with less demonstrable acute response than these criteria demand. The forced vital capacity is sometimes the only spirometric parameter that shows improvement (reflecting a decrease in residual volume) in patients who have subjective and arterial blood-gas improvement from a bronchodilator.

The "Poor-Effort" Pattern of Spirometric Abnormality. Spirometry is heavily dependent on the cooperation of the subject being tested. For this reason, excellent laboratories have traditionally demanded that the physician who is responsible for interpretation of the test results observe the patients as they perform effort-dependent tests. In addition, some such laboratories have considered that interpretation of pulmonary-function tests should be carried out by specialists in pulmonary disease only as a part of a complete clinical evaluation, including history and physical examination.

Criteria for Reversibility of Airways Obstruction

Significant improvement in two of these three parameters indicates reversibility
- Forced vital capacity
- Forced expiratory volume at 1 second
- Forced expiratory flow rate from 25–75% of forced vital capacity

Degree of reversibility
- Slight: 15–25% change
- Moderate: 25–50% change
- Marked: greater than 50% change

Such requirements place undesirable restrictions on the use of the pulmonary-function laboratory, and the benefits of wider application of simple ventilatory tests outweigh the disadvantages of less careful quality control. When a competent and conscientious technician carries out the test procedures and when a recording of the tracings obtained accompanies the battery of measurements recommended, interpretation of the data may render a satisfactory judgment as to validity in most cases. The "poor-effort" spirogram can usually be identified (see list below).

"Poor-Effort" Pattern

Characteristics of "poor-effort" ventilatory defect
- Decreased vital capacity
- Relatively normal expiratory flow rates
- Decreased maximum voluntary ventilation

Supplementary data confirming invalid test results
- Uneven, slurred, or notched curve on direct examination
- Poor reproducibility on repeated testing

Interpretation should be carried out with some caution, avoiding terms that imply that a morphological or etiological diagnosis can be made from these test results alone. A specific diagnosis must be made in the final analysis by the physician caring for the patient, using all the available knowledge at his disposal, interpreting test results in the light of other clinical findings.

Certain portions of the data collected during performance of spirometry are more likely to be abnormal with poor effort than others. The vital capacity and maximal voluntary ventilation are rather heavily effort-dependent. Early portions of the forced vital capacity curve are somewhat less effort-dependent, and the mid-portion of the forced vital capacity curve is much less effort-dependent and highly reproducible. As would be expected from this, a poor effort in a normal subject commonly results in a reduced vital capacity; a somewhat reduced forced expiratory volume at 0.5 second; and a less reduced volume at 1.0 second, since the latter measurement incorporates relatively more of the effort-independent portion of the curve. A poor-effort spirogram almost invariably shows a reduced maximal voluntary ventilation.

A submaximal effort is poorly reproducible and is characterized by an uneven, slurred forced expiratory curve, which may be terminated before reaching a plateau. Whether the poor effort is due to inadequate understanding, muscular weakness, neurasthenia, or malingering often cannot be determined readily for examination of test data.

A valid restrictive spirogram generally differs from the "poor-effort" test in being reproducible; showing relatively normal forced expiratory volumes at both 0.5 and 1.0 second, with expiratory curves appearing smooth on direct examination; and demonstrating a normal or nearly normal maximum voluntary ventilation.

The validity of any normal spirogram can be inferred from close reproducibility on repeated performance and from the appearance of smooth expiratory curves, without continued notching or slurring, until a plateau is achieved. Comparable decrease in forced expiratory volumes at 0.5 and 1.0 second usually accompanies the appearance of a smooth curve when obstruction is present, except that central airway obstruction or central airway collapse may produce a greater decrease in the volume at 0.5 second than at 1.0 second. In a normal or abnormal subject, a maximum effort produces a value for maximal voluntary ventilation that is about 40 times the forced expiratory volume at 1.0 second. Achievement of this value for the MVV is excellent evidence of validity of the spirogram in terms of patient cooperation.

The Mixed Pattern of Ventilatory Impairment. In most cases of ventilatory impairment, a decrease in vital capacity and a decrease in expiratory flow rates coexist, but one or the other often clearly predominates. If decreased vital capacity predominates, restriction is inferred, and obstruction need not be considered in order to explain a milder decrease in flow rates. A predominant decrease in expiratory flow rates suggests obstruction, with an accompanying decrease in vital capacity due to increased residual volume. Restriction need not be considered in order to explain the decreased vital capacity in such a case.

Clear guidelines are not available to suggest what degree of predominance must be present in order to infer pure obstruction or restriction and exclude a mixed pattern of impairment. For purposes of uniformity and simplicity, it is suggested that the forced expiratory volumes at 1.0 second, expressed as a percentage of predicted values, be used as an index of obstruction, and that vital capacity be used as an index of restriction. When the percentage of predicted values differs by more than 15 per cent, the more severely abnormal one indicates predominance of obstruction or restriction. A smaller difference often indicates a mixed ventilatory defect (see list below). The observation of a mixed or indeterminate defect is an indication for further pulmonary-function testing if the defect is to be more precisely defined.

An impression of the overall severity of the defect in terms of its impairment of the patient's ventilatory function can be

Mixed or Indeterminate Pattern

Characteristics of Mixed Ventilatory Defect
- Decreased vital capacity
- Decreased expiratory flow rates
- Decreased maximal voluntary ventilation
- Lack of predominance of obstruction or restriction

Supplementary tests
- Lung volume determination
- Repeat tests after bronchodilator administration
- Diffusing capacity
- Compliance
- Airways resistance

gained from the forced expiratory volumes, whether or not the character of the defect is clearly defined. The forced expiratory volumes at 0.5 second and at 1.0 second, expressed as a percentage of predicted normal values, may be used to categorize the severity of a ventilatory defect.[43] Arbitrarily, values from 65 to 79 per cent of predicted reflect a mild defect; 50 to 64 per cent characterize a moderate abnormality; and 35 to 49 per cent reflect severe impairment. Values below 35 per cent are categorized as very severe ventilatory impairment (see list below).

Criteria for Severity of Ventilatory Defect*

Tests utilized to reflect overall severity of ventilatory defect
- Forced expiratory volume at 0.5 second
- Forced expiratory volume at 1.0 second

Degree of severity
- Mild: 65–79% of predicted value
- Moderate: 50–64% of predicted value
- Severe: 35–49% of predicted value
- Very severe: below 35% of predicted value

*Adapted from data in Snider, G. L., Kory, R. C., and Lyons, H. A.: Grading of pulmonary function impairment by means of pulmonary function tests. Recommendations of the Committee on Pulmonary Physiology, American College of Chest Physicians. Dis. Chest, *52*:270, 1967.

If better characterization of a mixed defect than can be obtained from spirometry is desired, measurement of lung volumes, airways resistance, and compliance may be indicated (see The Restrictive Pattern, p. 96, and The Obstructive Pattern, p. 99).

Tests of Lung Mechanics That Supplement Volume-Time Analysis

As described previously, volume-time curve analysis provides an inexpensive, simple approach to pulmonary-function testing that can be provided by small hospital laboratories or even in the physician's office. Along with arterial blood-gas and pH measurements, volume-time curves provide sufficient physiological information for sensible care of patients with clinically significant respiratory disease in virtually every instance. Normal values for measurements obtained from volume-time curves are available, obtained from relatively large populations of varying ages and both sexes.

Additional measurements of lung mechanics require substantially more expensive and complex instrumentation. The information obtained often provides additional insight into the pathophysiology of disease in the patient tested and occasionally may result in significant alterations in therapy. Normal values for many of these measurements are inadequately established, however, and in some cases, the techniques are sufficiently cumbersome to cast doubt on the accuracy of results obtained in laboratories that perform the tests infrequently.

Table 3-3 summarizes references containing normal values for both volume-time parameters of ventilatory function and the more complex measurements of lung mechanics described subsequently.

Flow-Volume Relationships. *Flow-Volume Curves and Loops in Normal Subjects.* Conventional spirometric analysis has been developed around the plot of volume against time, because this sort of spirogram can be obtained with simple, inexpensive equipment. The development of sophisticated electronic gadgetry has led to an interest in analysis of various other parameters, plotted in numerous ways. One of the most popular has been the flow-volume curve,[8,9,44-49] which is obtained by having the subject inspire and

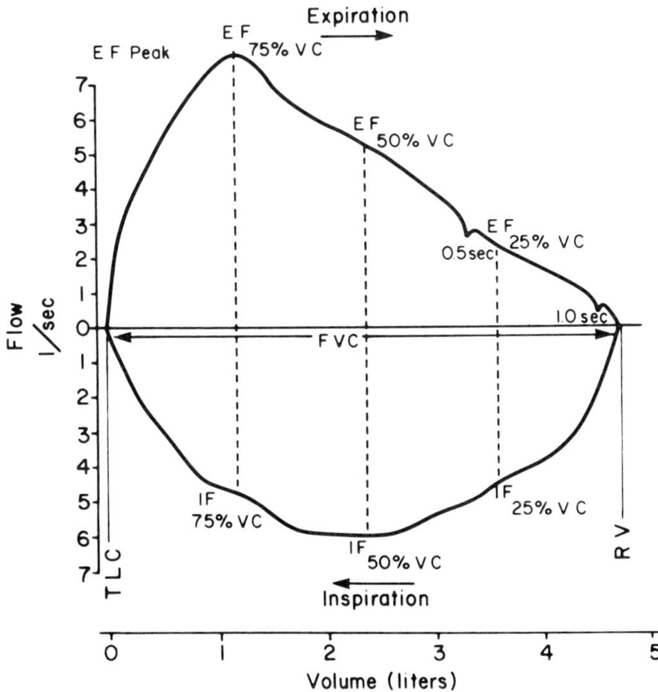

Fig. 3-5. Normal maximal-effort flow-volume loop. Note that the recorded maneuver begins after a maximal inhalation. The subject is asked to exhale as rapidly and forcefully as possible, and the expiratory curve is inscribed by the recording pen. Expiratory flow (EF) can be measured at its peak, or at various volumes of expired air (e.g., 75%, 50%, 25% of the vital capacity). Furthermore, the volume exhaled in 0.5 second or 1.0 second can be plotted as indicated by the time markers on the expiration curve. The total air exhaled is, of course, the vital capacity (VC). Immediately following the maximal expiration, the subject is asked to inhale as quickly and deeply as possible, and then inspiratory flow (IF) is measured.

expire fully, with maximum effort, into an instrument that measures flow and volume change simultaneously. These parameters are plotted on the two axes of an X-Y recorder or oscilloscope. Such a curve actually presents no information not contained in a conventional display of volume plotted against time, because flow, after all, is simply a function of these two parameters. Consideration of similar data displayed in a different fashion, however, often leads to advances in understanding. Accordingly, flow-volume curve analysis has contributed to our basic understanding of the mechanical events that occur during ventilatory efforts. In particular, it has emphasized the dependence of maximum achieveable flow on lung volume. For every point on the lower two-thirds of the volume axis of an expiratory curve, a maximum flow exists that cannot be exceeded, regardless of the effort exerted (see also Chap. 2). It logically follows from this observation that maximum flow must be dependent on mechanical characteristics of the lungs. Elucidation of some of these mechanical characteristics has resulted from flow-volume curve analysis. In addition, flow-volume curves constitute an informative way of displaying ventilatory data for clinical diagnostic purposes,[50] and some investigators predict that this type of analysis of the maximal-effort expiratory maneuver will prove to be more useful than conventional spirometry as more experience with it is accumulated.

The initial portion of a flow-volume curve during a forced expiratory maneuver describes flow during exhalation of approximately the first one-third of the vital capacity (Fig. 3-5). The curve shows a rapid ascent to "peak flow" and then begins a slow descent. This initial portion of the curve is effort-dependent; that is, increasing transpulmonary pressure results in increasing flow. It can be readily demonstrated that as a subject exerts increasing effort during exhalation, this is reflected by increasing intrathoracic pressure, and therefore increasing flow is generated, as displayed on the initial phase of the flow-volume curve. This portion of the curve is of limited diagnostic use, then. Its appearance depends chiefly on the subject's muscular effort rather than on the mechanical characteristics of the lung as altered by disease.

Shortly after the development of peak flow, a remarkably reproducible portion of the flow-volume curve can be identified as a slow descent continues to residual volume. As discussed in the section on volume-time analysis, this portion of the curve has been shown to be relatively effort-independent. For each point on the volume axis, a maximum flow exists, which cannot be exceeded, regardless of the pressure generated. Maximum flow is reached at about one-quarter of the maximum muscular effort that can be generated. In fact, flow at a given volume may decrease as pressure increases above a certain value. In such a situation, which may exist in health or disease, the maximum-effort expiratory flow-volume curve may not demonstrate maximum flow.

The effort-independent portion of the expiratory curve is very reproducible in a given subject from time to time but is altered in a characteristic way as disease changes the mechanical properties of the lung.

The recording of flow plotted against volume during forced inspiration as well as expiration is referred to as a *maximal-effort flow-volume loop* (Fig. 3-5). The inspiratory limb of this loop is entirely effort-dependent; that is, no maximum flow has been defined for any portion of it. The shape of the inspiratory limb is rather symmetrical, with flow increasing to a peak about midway through inspiration, then decreasing as inspiration proceeds to total lung capacity.

The inspiratory limb of the maximal-effort flow-volume loop is more sensitive to major central airway obstruction than is the expiratory limb. The inspiratory limb is relatively little influenced by diffuse peripheral airway or parenchymal disease. Flow-volume loops including the inspiratory limb therefore have major practical usefulness when central airway obstruction is suspected, and ordinary spirometry demonstrates a nonspecific obstructive pattern.

Flow-Volume Analysis in Screening for Asymptomatic Obstructive Disease. Abnormalities of flow-volume loops in clinically manifested disease have been well defined, and this type of analysis is comparably useful to conventional spirometry in the usual types of obstructive and restrictive pulmonary disease. It has been hoped that special advantages might become apparent with further experience, especially in the area of screening for early asymptomatic obstructive disease, because maximum expiratory flow rates at low lung volumes are thought to be sensitive to resistance in small peripheral airways. In order for subtle abnormalities to be identifiable in flow-volume loops, normal values for these parameters must be established, with rather narrow confidence limits. The studies accomplished up to the present have been unable to provide sufficiently narrow confidence limits for this purpose, and studies of larger populations are needed.[49,51,52]

The Flow-Volume Loop in Airways Obstruction. Normally, the descending limb of the curve is relatively linear, with only a slight upward concavity. In patients with obstructive lung disease[45,46,48,53-55] and indeed in some normal persons, especially when initiating the forced expiration from a low lung volume, this linearity is disrupted by an initial sharp, downward deflection of the curve. This deflection corresponds to a "tracheobronchial collapse" pattern sometimes seen on a conventional spirogram. More consistently, obstructive disease produces simply an exaggerated upward concavity of the descending limb of the curve (Fig. 3-6). The descending limb usually follows a diminished peak flow in subjects with obstructive disease. Peak flow is often less impaired than flows at lower lung volumes, because peak flow appears to occur before the flow-limiting mechanism becomes operative. In addition, it is probable that abrupt emptying of the airways, during a vigorous expiratory maneuver that causes them to collapse, can result in a very brief period of high flow.

Emphysema seems to have the greatest tendency to produce early downward bow-

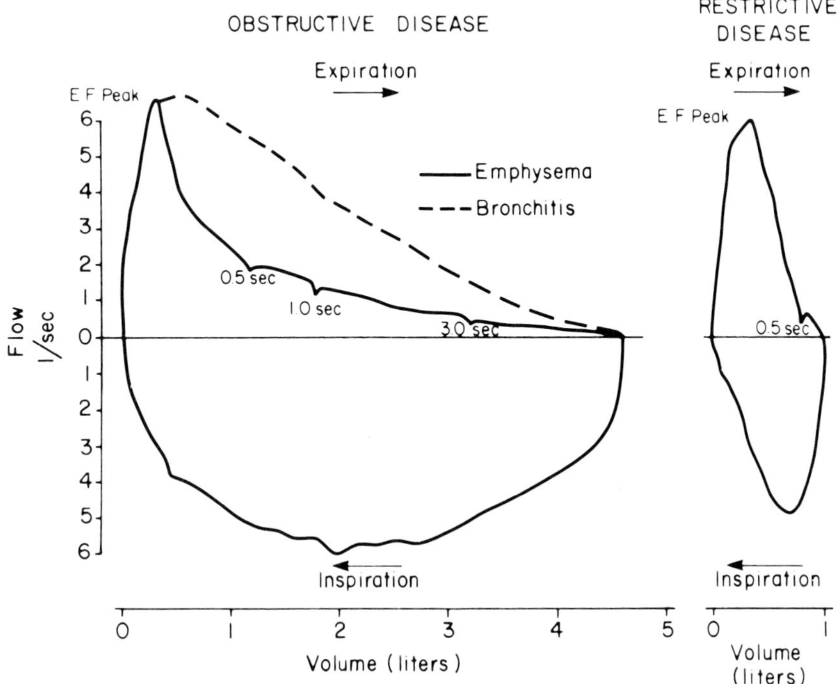

Fig. 3-6. Maximum-effort flow-volume curves in obstructive and restrictive disease. Typical flow-volume loops for a patient with obstructive disease (*left*) and a patient with restrictive disease (*right*). Note that patients with obstructive disease have reduced expiratory flow rates, particularly at low lung volumes. In emphysema, with obstruction primarily due to loss of elastic recoil, there is an early peak flow as the airways collapse, followed by severely reduced flow rates during sustained expiratory effort. This "collapsing" expiratory flow curve is typical of advanced emphysema.

ing of the descending limb of the curve. This tendency is not entirely consistent, however, and downward bowing relates to severity of obstruction as well as type of disease.

Shortening of the volume axis of the curve in both obstructive and restrictive disease indicates decreased vital capacity. This shortening is relatively less in obstructive than restrictive diseases, so that the characteristic obstructive flow-volume loop appears oriented along the horizontal axis.

Flow-volume loops may be especially helpful in identifying tracheal or upper-airway disease as a cause of obstruction. Central airway obstruction tends to produce a blunted, upwardly bowed appearance of the descending limb of the maximum-effort expiratory flow-volume curve. This appearance of a high flow "plateau" takes the place of the usual rapid rise to and descent from peak flow.[56-58] When a characteristic expiratory curve or clinical information such as an audible inspiratory stridor suggests central airway obstruction, particular attention should be given to the inspiratory limb of a flow-volume loop.

Miller and Hyatt[57,58] described characteristic flow-volume loop abnormalities occurring in central airway obstructions of three types: fixed obstruction, variable extrathoracic obstruction, and variable intrathoracic obstruction. The type of pattern produced depends on the location and character of the lesion, as well as the rigidity of the adjacent tracheal wall.

In fixed obstruction, the diameter of neither the obstructed lumen nor the proximal or distal trachea is altered by changes in transmural pressure. Such an obstruction, whether intrathoracic or extrathoracic, produces a similar decrease in inspiratory and expiratory flow rates. This proportionate obstruction to both phases of respiration is in contrast to the predominant expiratory slowing seen with diffuse peripheral airways obstruction. Ths ratio of mid-vital capacity flow rate during expiration to that during inspiration permits quantification of this phenomenon. When central airway obstruction is variable, the flow-volume loop produced depends on location of the lesion.

The extrathoracic trachea has a negative intraluminal pressure (relative to atmospheric) during inspiration and a positive pressure during expiration. This may result in a tendency to collapse during inspiration and to dilate on expiration. Extrathoracic obstruction is therefore commonly worse during inspiration than expiration. The intrathoracic trachea, however, is subjected to the intrathoracic pressure swings. These tend to dilate the trachea during inspiration and to collapse it during expiration. Obstructing lesions of the intrathoracic trachea, therefore, impair inspiration to a lesser degree than expiration.

The pattern of variable extrathoracic obstruction, then, consists of a predominant decrease in inspiratory flow rates. Variable intrathoracic obstruction predominantly affects expiratory flow, in a pattern similar to that of diffuse peripheral obstruction, but often characterized by a plateau following a peak flow, rather than by downward bowing of the expiratory limb.

Flow-Volume Loops in Restrictive Ventilatory Disorders. Because restrictive disorders are characterized by a predominant decrease in vital capacity and less impaired flow rates, the typical flow-volume curve in restriction is tall and narrow[54,55] (Fig. 3-6). Peak expiratory flow is relatively preserved, and the descending portion of the expiratory limb is straightened, falling sharply downward from peak flow to residual volume. The loop often maintains a nearly normal shape, appearing miniaturized in all dimensions.

Measurement of Lung Volumes. Conventional terminology for the subdivisions of lung volume has been discussed elsewhere (see p. 84, and Fig. 3-1).[34] All of these subdivisions can be measured directly with simple spirometry, except those containing residual volume. Residual volume is the quantity of air contained in the lungs at the end of a full expiration and can be measured only by special techniques. These generally utilize the body plethysmograph or inert gas dilution or washout,[4,5,59-62] or planimetric measurement of chest roentgenograms[63-66] (see list below). Functional residual capacity and total lung capacity both contain residual volume and therefore cannot be measured without these techniques.

Methods for Measurement of Subdivisions of Lung Volume

Methods that underestimate lung volume in obstructive disease and bullous disease
- Nitrogen washout[59]
- Helium dilution[61]

Methods that accurately measure lung volume in obstructive disease and bullous disease
- Plethysmography[60]
- Planimetry of chest roentgenograms[63-65]

These techniques can be adapted to measure any quantity of gas contained in the lungs at the time the test is initiated. That is, one could measure RV by initiating the test at maximum expiration; FRC by initiating the test at resting expiration; or TLC by initiating the test at full inspiration. One such measurement would be sufficient, because vital capacity, inspiratory capacity, and expiratory reserve volume, measurable from simple spirometry, can be added or subtracted to compute the remaining volumes.

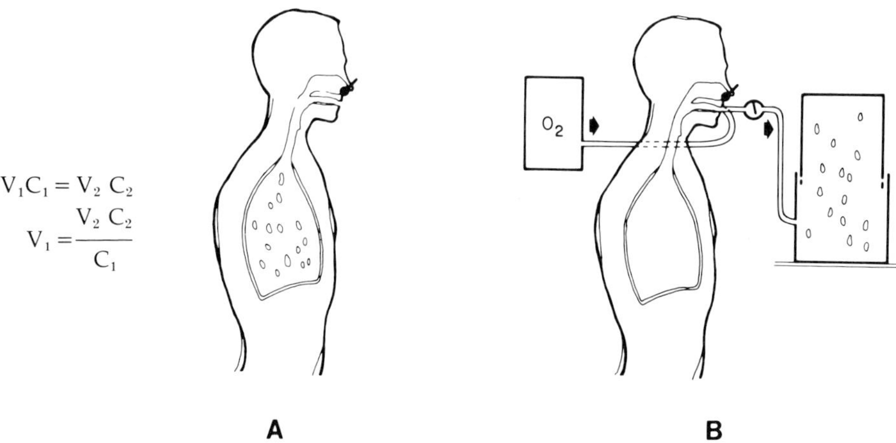

Fig. 3-7. Lung volume determination by nitrogen washout. (*A*) Resting expiration prior to test. (*B*) Resting expiration at end of test. V_1= volume of lungs (to be determined); C_1= concentration of nitrogen in lungs at beginning of test (assumed to be 79%, as in room air); V_2= volume of gas in spirometer at end of test (measured); C_2= concentration of nitrogen in spirometer at end of test (measured).

By convention, FRC is selected for measurement by inert gas or body box; RV is calculated by subtracting ERV; and TLC is calculated by adding IC. The reason for this selection is simple: FRC is the most effort-independent and reproducible of the volumes. To achieve RV by exhaling fully requires effort, understanding, and cooperation. To achieve TLC by inhaling fully also requires effort, understanding, and cooperation. FRC is attained normally at the end of each tidal breath and requires no patient cooperation. An alert technician can initiate the test at the end of a normal breath simply by observing the patient.

Inert gas techniques usually used to measure FRC are nitrogen washout[4,59] (Fig. 3-7) and helium dilution[4,61] (Fig. 3-8). These two gases are harmless and are neither produced nor utilized by the body. Their concentrations can be measured simply and rapidly by equipment that is commercially available at moderate cost.

Nitrogen normally represents 79 per cent of the total gaseous atmospheric constituents. It exists within the lungs at approximately the same level (approximate because oxygen utilization and carbon dioxide production slightly alter the concentration, but not the amount, of nitrogen). To measure FRC by nitrogen washout, pure oxygen is inhaled in order to wash the nitrogen from the lungs. The exhaled gas is collected and its volume measured, and the nitrogen concentration is analyzed. Knowing the amount of nitrogen that was washed out and the concentration in which it was present in the lungs, one can calculate the lung volume in which it was contained. To determine FRC accurately by this technique, the washout process must be initiated properly at resting expiration by a quick turn of a valve in the circuit. The washout must be continued until nitrogen is emptied from all parts of the lung. This process is normally completed in less than 7 minutes but may require 20 or 30 minutes in patients with obstructive disease who have abnormal distribution of ventilation. The washout must take place within a completely closed system, with a well-fitting mouthpiece and a nose clip in place; and it must be uninterrupted, because the addition of nitrogen to the system from room air invalidates the calculation.

Helium dilution is performed by introducing the patient into a circuit containing

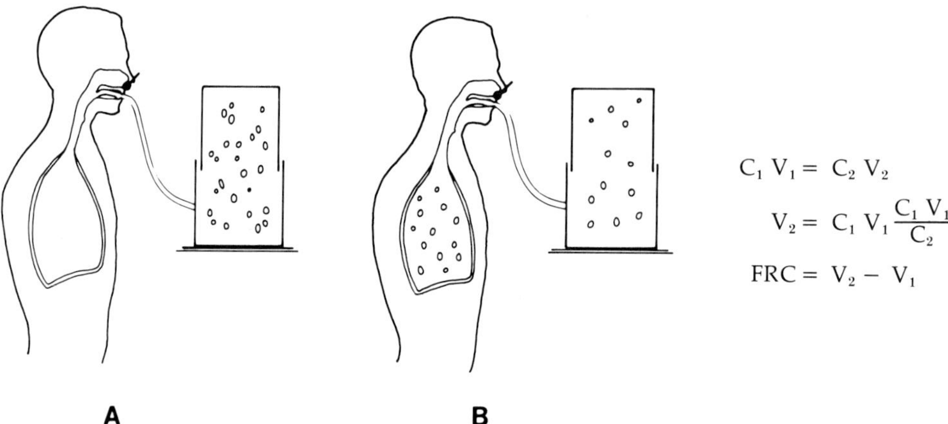

Fig. 3-8. Lung volume measurement by helium dilution. (*A*) Resting expiration at beginning of test. (*B*) Resting expiration at end of test. Helium is now evenly distributed throughout lungs and spirometer. $C_1 =$ concentration of helium in spirometer at beginning of test (measured); $V_1 =$ volume of gas in spirometer (measured); $C_2 =$ concentration of helium in spirometer and in patient's lungs at end of test (measured); $V_2 =$ volume of gas in spirometer and in patient's lungs combined (to be calculated).

a known volume and concentration of helium. Carbon dioxide is removed from the system by an adsorbent, and oxygen is added at the rate at which it is consumed. After an appropriate time for equilibration of helium throughout the system (7 to 30 minutes), the study is terminated. Equilibration is assumed to have occurred when the helium concentration within the circuit, which is continually monitored, stabilizes. The helium concentration at the end of the test is lower than the initial concentration, in proportion to the volume of the FRC by which it has been diluted.

These two techniques, nitrogen washout and helium dilution, have similar limitations. Patients with blebs or bullae that are very poorly ventilated may not have equilibration of these areas of the lung with the helium or nitrogen circuit during the time the test is carried out, and therefore falsely low values for FRC may be obtained.

Plethysmography. The body plethysmograph overcomes this handicap by utilizing Boyle's law, and measurements of pressure and volume change during ventilatory efforts against a closed shutter to measure FRC[4,60] (Fig. 3-9). This technique employs more expensive instrumentation than the inert gas techniques. Total gas volume within the chest at the initiation of the test sequence is measured, however, and air spaces in poor communication with airways are included. Prior to surgery to remove bullae, FRC determined by inert gas techniques can be subtracted from FRC determined by plethysmography, in order to provide an estimate of the volume occupied by bullae that are functionally not in communication with the airways. A discrepancy between values obtained by the two techniques does not prove the presence of discrete bullae, however, because diffuse emphysema or small-airways disease may produce such a discrepancy.

For determination of FRC by plethysmography, the subject is placed in a large, sealed chamber, with a mouthpiece in place that can be occluded by a remotely operated shutter. A sensitive pressure transducer measures pressure at the mouth, proximal to the shutter. This pressure, under conditions of no air flow, is assumed to reflect pressure within the thorax. Another pressure transducer measures pressure in the chamber, outside the subject's thorax. As inspiratory and ex-

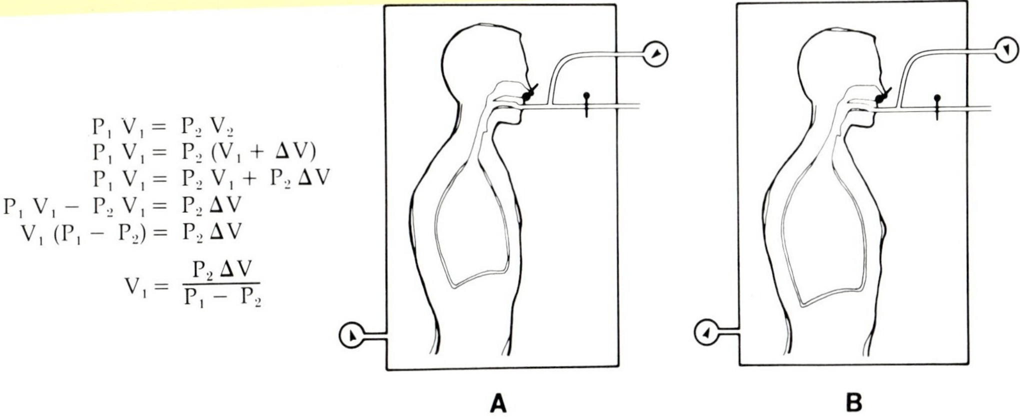

Fig. 3-9. Measurement of lung volume by plethysmograph. (*A*) Resting expiration. (*B*) Inspiratory effort. P_1 = alveolar pressure during resting expiration (measured at the mouth); V_1 = volume of lungs during resting expiration (to be determined); P_2 = alveolar pressure during inspiratory effort (measured at the mouth); V_2 = volume of lungs during inspiratory effort (unknown); $\Delta V = V_1 - V_2$ (measured as box pressure change).

piratory efforts are made by the subject against the closed shutter, volume changes within the thorax cause volume changes in the chamber and are reflected by pressure changes in the chamber. Pressure change in "the box" is thus employed to measure volume change within the thorax. We thus have a system in which a subject can attempt to breathe against a closed shutter, expanding and contracting the air within his chest. Two parameters can be measured during this maneuver: pressure in the chest and volume change within the chest. Note that pressure, referenced to atmosphere, can be measured during both attempted inspiration and attempted expiration. Volume in the chest cannot be measured, but volume change from inspiratory to expiratory effort can be measured. These data are sufficient to calculate lung volume at the initiation of the test according to Boyle's formula, relating pressure change to volume change. This system, a constant-volume, variable-pressure plethysmograph, is replaced by a constant-pressure, variable-volume unit in some laboratories.[9]

Roentgenography. Planimetric measurement of total lung capacity, using posteroanterior and lateral chest roentgenograms, has been demonstrated to be an acceptable substitute for inert gas and plethysmographic methods.[63-66] Logistical considerations may favor the selection of a roentgenographic method in some hospitals (Fig. 3-10).

Measurement of the subdivisions of lung volume is of greatest interest when a ventilatory defect is mixed or indeterminate, as demonstrated by simple volume-time spirometry. Extreme elevations of residual volume and an increase in total lung capacity strongly support a diagnosis of an obstructive disorder, especially emphysema. A decrease in residual volume and total lung capacity defines a restrictive defect and may force strong consideration of a group of disease processes of entirely different etiology. The additional information gained from measurement of compliance and airways resistance may complete the physiological profile in a subject with mixed disease, clarifying the relative contributions of each disorder to the ventilatory dysfunction.

Satisfactory estimation of predicted values for normal populations has been carried out in order to facilitate the interpretation of measurements performed in individual patients.[23,28,67]

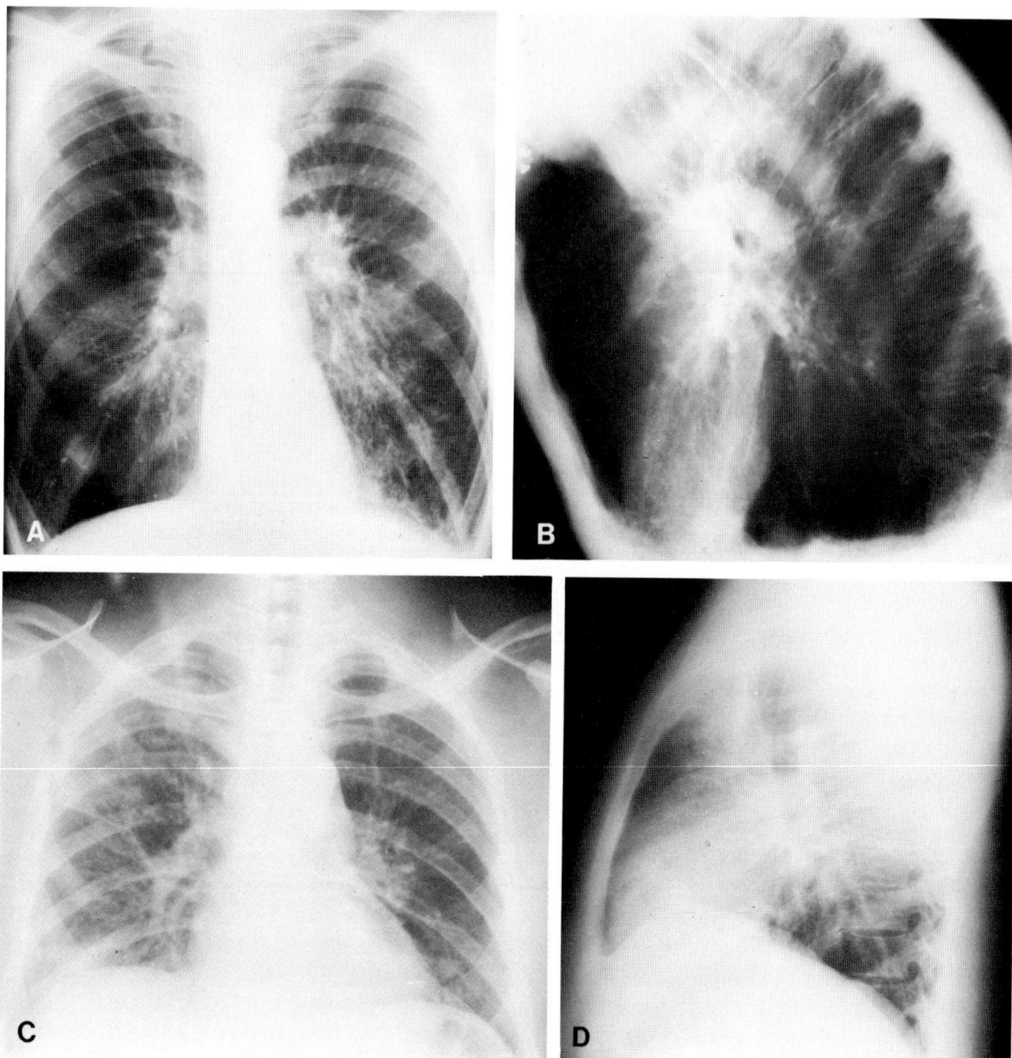

Fig. 3-10. Chest radiographs of patients with abnormally large and small lung volumes. (*A, B*) Patient with emphysema. Total lung capacity = 14.6 L. (194% predicted). (*C, D*) Patient with sarcoidosis. Total lung capacity = 4.5 L. (71% predicted).

Abnormalities of Ventilation at Rest and During Exercise. Tidal breathing at rest requires far less than a normal person's maximum ability to ventilate. Therefore, ventilatory impairment due to disease must be extremely severe before it significantly reduces minute ventilation at rest. Disease can alter mechanics sufficiently, however, to change the pattern of tidal breathing. Obesity tends to produce a reduced tidal volume and increased rate, as do interstitial edema, fibrosis, and other parenchymal and chest disorders that decrease compliance of the lungs or thorax. Disorders that increase airways resistance often produce a relatively slow, deep breathing pattern, though not consistently. Disorders of regulation of respiration produce characteristic patterns of breathing which may be diagnostic and

Table 3-4. Methods of Assessing Ventilatory Impairment as a Factor Limiting Exercise Tolerance

Method	*Requires Measurement of*
1. Efficiency of ventilation	
Ventilatory equivalent of oxygen consumption	Minute ventilation and oxygen consumption
Ventilation required for exercise	Minute ventilation and exercise load (treadmill, bicycle ergometer)
Oxygen extraction	Oxygen concentration of inspired and expired air
2. Maximum exercise load clinically tolerated	Exercise load, observation of clinical distress, pulse, blood pressure. If available, electrocardiogram, arterial blood gases, and oxygen consumption may be useful
3. Maximum voluntary ventilation	Minute ventilation during brief stint of maximum effort
4. Maximum oxygen consumption (impractical for most clinical purposes)	Oxygen consumption at increasing exercise loads until plateau is reached
5. Predicted maximum oxygen consumption	Ventilatory equivalent of oxygen consumption at submaximal exercise and maximum voluntary ventilation

which are discussed in detail in Chapter 4. The rapid, deep pattern of central hyperventilation or of metabolic acidosis, referred to as *Kussmaul's respiration*, may be readily recognized. Alveolar hypoventilation due to extensive central nervous system disease or to drug depression may be characteristic, usually producing a shallow pattern, with a normal initial rate, and a slowing of rate as depression deepens. Patients with idiopathic central hypoventilation may show a remarkable variation in depth and rate from moment to moment but usually have a notably slow rate. The phasic, concurrent increase and decrease in rate and depth in Cheyne-Stokes respiration are well known and easy to recognize at the bedside. This pattern may be associated with circulatory failure and an assortment of cerebral disorders. The irregular irregularity of rate and depth of "ataxic" or Biot's respiration is less common and is related to brain lesions at the level of the medullary respiratory centers.

Ventilatory efficiency also can be altered by disease, so that increased minute ventilation at rest is required for normal gas exchange (Table 3-4). Normal variation in ventilatory patterns and efficiency is so great, however, that the diagnostic usefulness of such alterations is limited.[4-6] Alterations in ventilation during exercise may be somewhat more informative.[6,39,68]

An average-sized normal adult male at rest breathes about 16 to 18 times each minute, exchanging about 500 ml. of air during each breath. Of each breath, about 150 ml. is "wasted," ventilating only airways (anatomical dead space) and poorly perfused areas of lung (alveolar dead space). The total of this wasted ventilation is referred to as *physiological dead space* ventilation. The remainder of each breath takes part in gas exchange by coming into intimate contact with pulmonary capillaries, contributing oxygen to and removing carbon dioxide from the blood. This portion is referred to as *alveolar ventilation*.

Because there is considerable normal variation in blood flow and ventilation distribution, the amount of physiological dead space varies from person to person,

Table 3-5. Relationship of Dead Space to Alveolar Ventilation*

Total Minute Ventilation	*Respiratory Rate*	*Tidal Volume*	*Physiological Dead Space*	*Alveolar Ventilation*
(A) 8 l./min.	16	500 ml.	150 ml.	5.6 l./min.
(B) 8 l./min.	8	1,000 ml.	250 ml.	6.0 l./min.
(C) 8 l./min.	16	500 ml.	250 ml.	4.0 l./min.

*Note that the same minute ventilation may result in widely varying alveolar ventilation. A normal relationship of about one-third dead space ventilation is illustrated in A. This is contrasted with a larger tidal volume in B. Dead space increases normally with increased tidal volume, but not directly proportionately. In C, an abnormally high dead space results in reduced alveolar ventilation.

and the amount of each breath that contributes to gas exchange (alveolar ventilation) varies. Variation in depth of respiration also varies normally from person to person. For purposes of gas exchange, slow ventilation is more efficient than rapid, shallow ventilation, because a greater portion of each breath contributes to alveolar ventilation (Table 3-5).

Because of these factors (variation in physiological dead space and variation in ventilatory pattern), efficiency of ventilation varies from one normal person to another. Minute ventilation required to provide adequate gas exchange for a given metabolic demand is therefore inconstant.

Efficiency of ventilation can be expressed conveniently in terms of minute ventilation required per liter of oxygen consumed (ventilatory equivalent of oxygen consumption). The normal ventilatory equivalent ranges from 20 to 30 liters of ventilation for each liter of oxygen consumed.[68] A reciprocal of this measurement, percentage of oxygen extraction, is an equally convenient expression of ventilatory efficiency. Ventilatory equivalent or oxygen extraction can be assessed simply by measuring minute ventilation and oxygen consumption; or the latter can be estimated rather closely, knowing body size and level of activity and referring to tables readily available.[69] As mentioned previously, however, the wide range of normal values limits the diagnostic usefulness of such information. Change in ventilatory efficiency, especially during exercise, can be demonstrated in an individual person over a period of time, however. Improvement due to breathing retraining and physical conditioning can be demonstrated and quantitated in this way.[70]

The deterioration in ventilatory efficiency that occurs in disease is chiefly due to the mechanism of ventilation perfusion imbalance. Increased physiological dead space occurs whenever redistribution of ventilation and perfusion results in decreased blood flow to well-ventilated areas or in increased ventilation to poorly perfused areas. Ventilation in excess of perfusion is wasted ventilation, because it does not result in increased gas exchange. Therefore, total minute ventilation for a given metabolic demand is increased, to provide adequate alveolar ventilation in the face of increased wasted ventilation. When altered mechanical characteristics of the lung and chest wall result in a rapid, shallow breathing pattern, efficiency of ventilation is further reduced, owing to the increased proportion of dead space per breath. Ventilation perfusion imbalance results to some extent from most disorders that alter the mechanical properties of the lungs: airways disease, interstitial disease of various sorts, pneumonia, and neoplasms. Chest-wall diseases may alter ventilatory patterns to such an extent that ventilation perfusion imbalance occurs. Chronic obstructive lung disease is one of the most common and most important of the diseases that cause increased physiological dead space. Improvement in this physiological dysfunction occurs whenever the basic disease process is reversed; but even in the face of irreversible disease, some physiological improvement may occur. Breathing training, with development of a slow, deep ventilatory pattern, may be especially useful.

Ventilatory efficiency is, in fact, the major ventilatory parameter that can consistently be demonstrated to improve over time through rehabilitation programs that incorporate breathing retraining and physical conditioning.[70] For simplicity of measurement in such a program, minute ventilation is usually measured during a given level of exercise without measurement of oxygen consumption. Standardized exercise on a treadmill or bicycle ergometer is carried out on successive occasions. Minute ventilation is measured; a decrease in the ventilation required for a specified work load reflects improved efficiency.

The pulmonary laboratory is often called upon to quantitate exercise capacity in a patient with ventilatory impairment. Direct and indirect means are available to carry out this request. A simple, direct approach consists of observing the subject perform standardized exercise on a treadmill or bicycle ergometer. Pulse rate, respiratory rate, and the patient's appearance and subjective complaints of distress usually provide a reasonable guide as to the maximum amount of exercise he is able to perform and sustain. It has been suggested[69] that exercise testing not be pressed to levels of intensity that result in heart rates above 170 per minute for subjects aged 20 to 29 years, decreasing to 130 per minute for subjects age 60 to 69. Signs or symptoms of circulatory insufficiency, including inappropriate bradycardia for a given level of exercise, should signal cessation of the test. The level of exercise achieved can be related to various activities of daily living by reference to published tables.[71] The specific physiological function that limits exercise in a given patient may not be readily apparent; hypoxia, ventilatory insufficiency, cardiovascular insufficiency, or musculoskeletal dysfunction may be operative.[72,73] Malingering is usually easy to recognize, though it may be difficult to prove.

A simple, indirect approach to assessing ventilatory impairment during exercise is the measurement of maximal voluntary ventilation.[39] This measurement reflects a subject's ability to perform a brief stint, not a sustained level of ventilation. It is a reasonable rule of thumb that most persons can sustain a level of exercise requiring a minute ventilation of 35 to 50 per cent of their MVV. Considering that 30 liters of ventilation is the upper limit of normal required to sustain a liter of oxygen consumption and that diseased persons may have somewhat less efficient ventilation, it is possible to roughly estimate the degree of exercise limitation, in terms of oxygen consumption, by a known limitation in ventilatory capacity. The oxygen requirements for common activities of daily living can then be obtained from tables such as those available through the American Heart Association.[71] In this way, exercise limitation can be translated into readily understandable terms. It is evident that a person with a normal MVV may have severe exercise impairment due to other causes, such as heart failure (see list below).

Some Factors That May Limit Exercise Tolerance in Disease

- Decreased ventilatory reserve
- Hypoxemia
- Cardiovascular disease: angina, limited cardiac output
- Musculoskeletal disorders
- Dyspnea in absence of objective ventilatory impairment
- Malingering

Measurement of maximum oxygen consumption in the sense intended by physiologists implies repeated measurement of oxygen consumption at successively increasing exercise loads until a plateau is reached, above which increased exercise no longer results in increased oxygen consumption. This sort of measurement is neither safe nor practical for clinical purposes in patients with cardiorespiratory disease. Measurement of oxygen consumption at a maximum exercise load that is clinically well tolerated, however, is a practical and useful measurement.

Armstrong and colleagues,[74] using data compiled by Wright, have described a precise, objective, and safe approach to quantitating exercise impairment due to ventilatory limitation. Their technique consists of the measurement of the ventilatory equivalent of oxygen consumption at a submaximal exercise level, and the measurement of maximum voluntary ventilation. A predicted maximum oxygen consumption is then calculated from the following formula:

$$Vo_2 \text{ max} = 0.018 \text{ MVV (liters/min.)} - 0.044 \text{ } O_2 \dot{V}_E + 2.14$$

Sophisticated techniques are now available to assess cardiac output, oxygen delivery, anaerobic metabolism, in addition to ventilatory function. Many research-oriented laboratories routinely perform these evaluations.[72,73]

Airways Resistance. Air flow into and out of the airways of the lungs, like flow of fluid through any system of tubes, is dependent on driving pressure across the system and on the resistance of the system. In the case of the respiratory tract, driving pressure is the difference between pressure in the alveoli and the atmospheric pressure at the mouth; and resistance of the system of tubes is airways resistance as defined by the formula:

$$\text{airway resistance (cm. } H_2O\text{/L./sec.)} = \frac{\text{alveolar pressure (cm. } H_2O) - \text{mouth pressure (cm. } H_2O)}{\text{flow (L./sec.)}}$$

Tissue viscous resistance is quantitatively small but contributes to the total frictional resistance of the lungs. Resistance of such a system in turn depends on length and cross-sectional area, as well as on flow characteristics of the fluid.[4,9,75] Theoretical concepts that have application to air flow in the pulmonary airways are considered in depth in Chapter 2.

The usual clinical approach to diagnosis and quantitation of obstructive disease of the airways is the measurement of expiratory flow during maximum effort. It is tacitly assumed that effort, hence the alveolus-to-mouth pressure gradient, is constant and that decreased flow is evidence of increased resistance of airways. With some qualifications, this simplified approach can be clinically useful, but of course it is not physiologically correct. Determination of actual airways resistance is more informative but requires measurement of alveolar pressure, and this measurement presents technical problems.

Methods of Measuring Air-Flow Resistance

Techniques used to measure total pulmonary resistance
- Transpulmonary pressure (esophageal balloon)[76]
- Forced oscillations[77]

Techniques used to measure only airways resistance
Estimation of alveolar pressure by:
- Momentary flow interruption[78]
- Panting technique with plethysmography and sustained shutter closure[79]

In fact, analysis of pressure-flow characteristics of breathing presents complications beyond the technical problem of measuring alveolar pressure.[75] The diameter and length of the airways are not constant; they are continually changing during respiration. In addition, the intricate branching of the system of airways results in a changing combination of laminar and turbulent flow, which influences pressure-flow relationships. In spite of these problems, the measurement of airways resistance has been tackled with some degree of success by techniques briefly described below. In each case, the description concentrates on the problem of measurement of alveolar pressure, because flow can be easily obtained by flow meters or as volume change per unit of time, measured with a conventional spirometer.

Techniques of Assessing Airways Resistance. Alveolar pressure in any phase of respiration is the algebraic sum of pleural (esophageal) pressure and lung elastic recoil pressure. This relationship is true throughout the respiratory cycle but is most easily understood by considering active expiration. During a forced expiration, the positive alveolar pressure that drives air from alveolus to mouth is the sum of elastic recoil pressure (tending to deflate the lungs) and positive pleural pressure (compressing the lungs). Elastic recoil pressure can be measured as the reciprocal of negative pleural (esophageal) pressure when there is no air flow. During active expiration, positive pleural pressure is created by respiratory muscle contraction and is measured as positive esophageal pressure. Therefore, alveolar pressure at any level of lung volume during a forced expiratory maneuver is the sum of two different pressures: elastic recoil pressure (measured under static conditions at that lung volume) and pressure created by active muscle contraction under dynamic conditions. To arrive at alveolar pressure, then, two separate measurements must be carried out. A static pressure-volume curve must be constructed from numerous measurements of esophageal pressure at different levels of inflation. A dynamic pressure-volume curve must be traced during forced expiration. The alveolar pressure at any level of inflation can be obtained by adding the two pressure measurements taken at that level during the two maneuvers. Alveolar pressure during tidal breathing can be calculated by measuring compliance as "dynamic" compliance, taking esophageal pressure measurements at points of no flow, at end inspiration and expiration.[76] This technique actually measures total flow resistance, including tissue viscous as well as airways resistance. A newer method of measuring flow-resistive forces, utilizing forced oscillations generated from a loudspeaker,[77] is described in Chapter 2.

Another technique (simpler, but perhaps not entirely valid) is the flow-interruption technique, in which a forced expiration is carried out through a mouthpiece, and momentary shutter closure interrupts flow.[78] Pressure at the mouth is measured during flow interruption and is assumed to equal alveolar pressure. In patients with airways obstruction, it is believed that equilibration of pressure from alveolus to mouth may be sufficiently delayed to invalidate this technique. This technique measures only the resistance of the airways.

A fourth technique, using the body plethysmograph, is currently popular, and commercially available automated instrumentation has been designed around it.[79] It consists of a two-part test, carried out during a rapid, shallow, panting maneuver in order to minimize phase lag and the changes in airways resistance that occur with change in the level of inflation. Panting is carried out with similar effort with an open shutter, and then against a closed shutter. The entire test is carried out within a sealed cabinet. Pressure change within the chamber is monitored during the maneuver, as chest expansion and contraction displace volume and alter chamber pressure. With the shutter open, flow is plotted against chamber pressure on an X-Y recorder or oscilloscope. With the shutter closed, mouth pressure is plotted against chamber pressure. Under conditions of no flow, imposed by the shutter, mouth pressure is assumed to be equal to alveolar pressure. In this way, two relationships are measured: flow to chamber pressure, and alveolar pressure to chamber pressure. From these two relationships, a third relationship can be calculated: flow to alveolar pressure. This third relationship is, in fact, airways resistance. This method of measuring airways resistance appears to be theoretically valid; is reproducible; and changes predictably with diseases and drugs that would be expected to alter airways resistance. It provides a single estimate, at only one lung volume, of airways resistance during the artificial circumstance of the panting maneuver.

It has been demonstrated that in the normal lung, most of the resistance to flow is in airways central to those that are 2

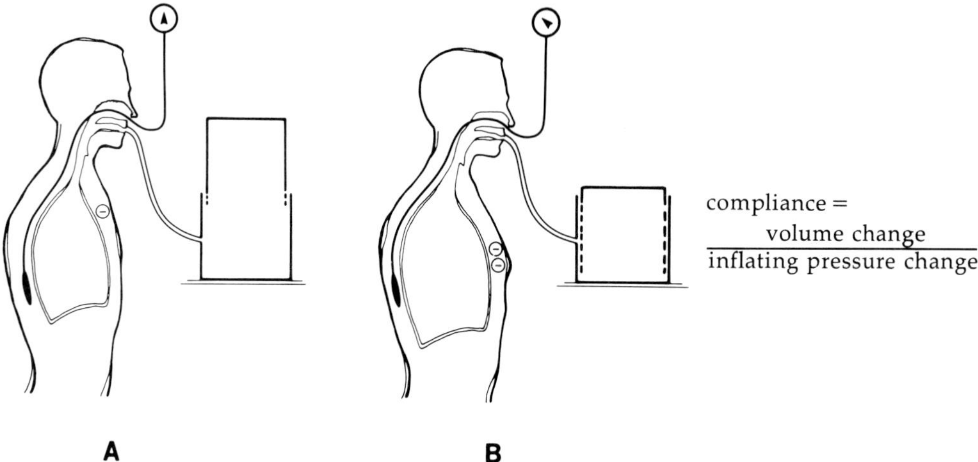

Fig. 3-11. Lung compliance. (*A*) Resting expiration. (*B*) Breath-holding during inspiration, with glottis open. Change in lung volume is measured with a conventional spirometer. Change in inflating pressure (intrapleural pressure) is measured with an intraesophageal balloon.

millimeters in diameter and less.[80] So little resistance occurs in the smaller peripheral airways that considerable narrowing due to disease must occur before total airways resistance is significantly altered. Because these airways appear to be the site of most of the pathological changes in chronic obstructive lung disease, airways resistance is an insensitive test for identifying early disease of this sort (see page 115). Severe asthma and bronchitis, however, are associated with elevation of airways resistance, which improves with bronchodilator drugs. It appears that emphysema without bronchospasm or bronchitis can cause significant slowing of maximum expiratory flow rates without causing elevation of airways resistance. Two factors may explain this phenomenon. The major cause of slowed flow in this situation may be the loss of the contribution of elastic recoil to lung deflation, and the airways may be unaffected. On the other hand, loss of elastic support may permit the airways to collapse, and pressures in the alveoli distal to the collapsed segments may not be transmitted to the mouth, thereby invalidating the alveolar pressure measurement.

Compliance of the lungs and chest wall is, for most clinicians, a rather nebulous physiological concept, with little application to practice. In fact, compliance is a rather simple mechanical property that undergoes major alterations in disease and can be easily measured.[4,9,75,81-85]

Compliance is simply distensibility. Physiologically, it is defined as volume change (in milliliters) produced by pressure change (in centimeters of water). By definition, compliance is a static quality or measurement and is not influenced by frictional forces or inertia. Compliance of the lungs, or lungs and thorax, might be defined as the pressure required to maintain a given level of inflation, because frictional forces and inertia must be overcome in order to obtain it but not to maintain it. Elastance, or elastic recoil, is the reciprocal of compliance and is the tendency of the lungs, or lungs and thorax, to return to a given level of inflation. Physically, compliance is a measure of the ease with which a body or substance may be deformed, and elastance is a measure of its tendency to resist deformation.

Because elastic forces are stored, an inflated chest contains energy to return it to

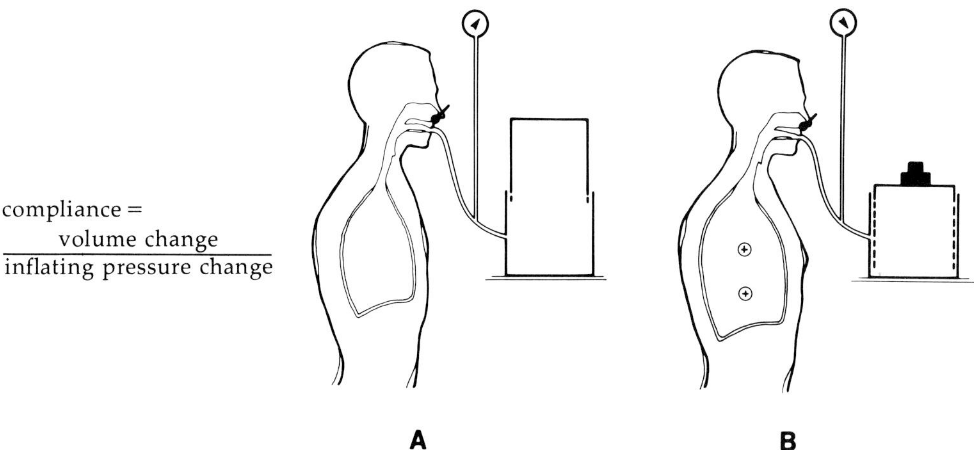

Fig. 3-12. Total respiratory compliance. (*A*) Resting expiration, with weightless spirometer. (*B*) Resting expiration with weighted spirometer. Change in lung volume is measured with a conventional spirometer as change in the level of FRC. Change in inflating pressure is measured as positive alveolar (mouth) pressure created by weights on the spirometer bell.

FRC; hence, active work is not usually required for tidal exhalation. Exhalation is ordinarily passive, requiring little or no contraction of muscles of respiration, except to overcome resistive forces, which are normally small during tidal breathing.

Compliance of the lungs can be measured clinically with the use of an esophageal balloon (Fig. 3-11); compliance of the lungs and chest wall in concert can be measured by assessing the difference between alveolar pressure and atmospheric pressure required to maintain a known level of inflation (Fig. 3-12). These techniques will be described subsequently. Chest compliance cannot be measured directly but can be calculated from the difference between reciprocals of lung and total thoracic compliance, according to the formula:

$$\frac{1}{\text{total compliance}} = \frac{1}{\text{lung compliance}} + \frac{1}{\text{chest-wall compliance}}$$

Measurement of Static Compliance of the Lung. As the lungs are suspended within the chest at any given level of inflation, it is the difference between alveolar pressure and pleural pressure that maintains that level of inflation. Whether the negative pleural pressure or the relatively positive atmospheric pressure in the alveoli is viewed as being responsible is immaterial; the difference between them is the same. Intrathoracic pressure is measured by an intra-esophageal balloon, which reflects intrapleural pressure with reasonable accuracy[81,82]; this measurement is plotted against chest volume. The volume change created by a given change in negative intrathoracic pressure, measured under conditions of no flow, is compliance. Although data for the prediction of normal values for lung elasticity are somewhat limited,[84] normal lung compliance over the tidal volume range is about 200 ml. per centimeter of water. At higher levels of inflation, near the elastic limits of the lungs, compliance is reduced. Interpretation of a compliance measurement therefore requires knowledge of the level of inflation at which it is taken. An abnormally high value results when emphysema destroys alveolar walls; an abnormally low value reflects "stiffness" of the lung, caused by infiltrative diseases of the lung parenchyma, such as interstitial fibrosis.

Elastance is the reciprocal of compliance and, of course, has similar significance; specific compliance and specific elastance are those measurements, corrected for the level of inflation at which they are obtained. A compliance curve can be constructed over the vital capacity range to provide a complete representation of elastic properties of the lung, or a single simplified but less informative measurement called *elastic recoil* can be obtained. Elastic recoil is a term commonly applied to the maximum negative esophageal pressure that can be generated at the end of a full inspiration.

Measurement of total respiratory compliance requires knowledge of the difference between alveolar pressure and atmospheric pressure at various levels of inflation. This can be obtained in a trained subject by maintaining inflation at various levels of a passive deflation against a closed shutter or by maintaining inflation with negative pressure outside the chest, as with a Drinker respirator. These techniques require a trained and relaxed (or anesthetized) subject, to avoid interference with the test by respiratory-muscle activity. An alternative technique involves the use of a water-sealed spirometer with a weighted bell.[83] The subject is directed to breathe normally, and changes in FRC are noted to occur as the weights on the bell are changed. Because FRC occurs at a moment of chest-muscle relaxation and no flow, pressure at the mouth at FRC is equal to alveolar pressure. The change in FRC in response to changes in alveolar pressure induced by the weighted bell is in effect a measure of total thoracic compliance. Normal total compliance over the tidal volume range is about 100 ml. per centimeter of water pressure.

Abnormalities of Compliance. Clinically significant abnormalities of compliance are common in disease of the lungs and chest wall.[9,85] Pulmonary emphysema is the major recognized cause of abnormally increased lung compliance. At first glance, increased compliance would not appear to be a physiological disadvantage, because it implies less effort required to inflate the lungs; however, increased compliance involves loss of the ability to store elastic energy, thus impairing the ability of the lung to recoil passively to FRC. In addition, the loss of elastic support of the airways permits them to collapse during expiration, which further interferes with lung emptying.

Interstitial diseases (whether resulting in edema, inflammatory infiltrate, granulomas, or fibrosis) cause a decrease in lung compliance. In these disorders, increased effort is required to inflate the lungs, but emptying occurs readily. A shallow, rapid, ventilatory pattern results, and severe exertional dyspnea may be a concomitant of decreased compliance, as chest-wall stretch receptors recognize the increased tension required for ventilation.

Unfortunately, these approaches to the assessment of compliance involve an averaging effect. Almost certainly, variations in compliance of some lung units take place in disease, long before the average changes, thereby limiting the diagnostic usefulness. Similarly, when certain lung units (e.g., large emphysematous bullae) occur, they may reduce the average lung compliance when many lung units are normal. Assessment of regional lung compliance is not yet possible.

A measurement known as *dynamic compliance* can be made during tidal breathing. This measurement and its significance are discussed further under the heading, Laboratory Screening for Subclinical Respiratory Disease (p. 115).

Distribution of Ventilation. Even in the normal young adult, ventilation is not entirely equal throughout all areas of the lungs.[86] In the upright posture, the lower, dependent lung zones are best ventilated during tidal breathing at rest. The reason for this is that the lung parenchyma in the upper zones supports the weight of the lung beneath it, producing a more negative pleural pressure in the upper thorax and stretching the lung nearer to its elastic limit. A given change in intrapleural pressure during respiration therefore produces little change in the volume of the already distended upper lung zones but produces greater change in the volume of the lower zones. Interesting phenomena occur with deeper breathing above and below the tidal volume range, however.

During an inspiration to TLC, ventilation is distributed preferentially to upper zones, beginning at some point above tidal volume after the lower zones have been filled. During exhalation below FRC, ventilation to and from dependent lower zones ceases, owing to functional, if not anatomical, closure of the airways. The volume at which this occurs is referred to as *closing volume*. The principles underlying this measurement are discussed in detail on page 48.

In the recumbent posture, airway closure occurs chiefly in the posterior lung zones, which are now dependent.[87] Closing volume increases with age[88,89] after maturity, and with the onset of chronic obstructive lung disease. The increase is more functionally significant in the recumbent posture than in the upright posture, because FRC is less in the supine position than in the sitting position. When airway closure occurs above FRC (that is, within the tidal volume range), dependent lung zones cease to be ventilated but continue to be perfused, and ventilation-perfusion imbalance ensues, with physiological shunting and arterial hypoxemia. Closing volume above FRC occurs with normal aging, first in the recumbent and later in the upright posture, accounting for at least part of the drop in arterial oxygen tension that occurs with age. Obstructive lung disease accelerates these changes with age, which presumably are related to loss of elastic recoil, at least in part.

In addition to these changes in regional distribution of ventilation, patchy unevenness of ventilation occurs in emphysema, bronchitis, and asthma, owing to uneven changes in compliance and airways resistance. These changes have long been recognized and studied by single-breath[90,91] and multiple-breath nitrogen washout techniques.[92] Single-breath nitrogen washout is carried out by continuous measurement of nitrogen concentration at the mouth during a full exhalation from total lung capacity, following a single inhalation of pure oxygen. Normal distribution of ventilation results in an "alveolar plateau" of uniform nitrogen concentration in the gas leaving all portions of the lung parenchyma. Uneven distribution disrupts the alveolar plateau. The closing volume measured by the nitrogen washout technique is a modern refinement of the traditional single-breath technique and appears to be sensitive to early, asymptomatic obstructive disease (see Fig. 2-7B, p. 49). During multiple-breath nitrogen washout, the nitrogen concentration is monitored at the mouth during tidal breathing of pure oxygen, which slowly replaces nitrogen. Normal distribution of ventilation is indicated by a smooth, rapid (exponential) decrease in expired nitrogen concentration; uneven ventilation is indicated by a delayed and irregular decrease. The decrease in nitrogen concentration with each succeeding breath proceeds slowly and unevenly in obstructive disease, contrasted with the smooth, rapid washout in a normal person. Multiple-breath washout is rather insensitive to mild disease.

Radioactive-isotope-ventilation studies provide an especially graphic way of evaluating regional ventilation. Radioactive xenon may be inhaled and its distribution mapped out by quantitating radioactive counts over the surface of the thorax. Numerical counting or scintiphotography may be used. Patchy distribution of ventilation occurs in most forms of obstructive lung disease, and a defect in ventilation predominantly affecting the lower zones is characteristic of panacinar emphysema.[93] As carried out in most clinical isotope laboratories, these techniques provide reliable topographical mapping of distribution of ventilation, but quantitation in absolute terms of ventilation to each zone may be performed for investigative purposes. Regional distribution of ventilation, especially with reference to matching of ventilation and perfusion, is discussed in Chapter 4.

Laboratory Screening for Subclinical Respiratory Disease

Laboratory detection of early, subclinical pulmonary dysfunction has been of interest in past years chiefly to physicians practicing industrial medicine. The usefulness of detecting functional changes due to industrial disease early in its course, prior to the development of crippling pneumoconiosis, is evident. Programs for the detection of these diseases have used rather specialized techniques, such as determination of diffusing capacity at rest and with exercise. Until recently, the detection of early asymptomatic emphysema and chronic bronchitis has been given little attention. Simple laboratory techniques have not been available, and the usefulness of early detection of this group of diseases has not been evident.

Recently, techniques for the detection of obstructive lung disease have been sufficiently refined and simplified for wide clinical use by informed physicians. Aberrations in lung function can now be detected in smokers who do not have disabling pulmonary disease, at a stage when normal values are obtained in conventional tests of ventilation, such as vital capacity and forced expiratory volumes.[94] Furthermore, evidence now available indicates that these subtle abnormalities can be reversed by treatment.[94,95]

This knowledge is exciting to the physician interested in preventive medicine. It raises the possibility of detecting obstructive lung disease early in susceptible persons and of instituting preventive measures in a selective and intensive way, with special emphasis on interdiction of smoking. Such an approach implies, however, a link, as yet unproven, between these subtle laboratory findings and crippling obstructive lung disease. Are the asymptomatic patients who have laboratory evidence of airways obstruction those who will develop severe chronic bronchitis and emphysema? If so, can the course of the disease be altered if detected early? Only carefully designed, prospective, longitudinal studies can answer these questions; and such studies are urgently needed.[96,97]

The place that screening tests for airways obstruction may ultimately find in clinical practice, then, remains unclear. A description of currently available techniques is warranted, however, because the need for widespread clinical evaluation of their usefulness is clear. It is notable that the discussions below deal with sensitivity and avoid the question of specificity, because this problem has not yet been solved conclusively. Pathological correlations are not available for the physiological abnormalities in very early peripheral airways obstruction, and long-term follow-up is not available, of course. Correlation among decreased maximum mid-expiratory flow rate (MMF), abnormal closing volumes, and frequency dependence of compliance has been demonstrated, however[94,96]; and these parameters have been shown to coexist in many cases with elevated residual volume,[95,96] physiological dead space to tidal volume ratio, and alveolar-arterial oxygen tension difference.[95] When frequency dependence of compliance is due to changes in the elastic properties of the lung, altered static compliance might be expected. Therefore, normal static compliance in a subject with frequency dependence of dynamic compliance is generally interpreted as evidence of obstructive disease of small peripheral airways. A recent morphological study of the lungs of young (average age, 25 years) smokers and nonsmokers, who died from traumatic causes, provides support for this interpretation.[98] The smokers had a characteristic finding: respiratory bronchiolitis associated with clusters of pigmented alveolar macrophages. The investigators suggested that this lesion may be a precursor of centriacinar emphysema and may cause the changes in dynamic compliance and closing volume that have been found in some young smokers.

The evidence is attractive, then, though not conclusive, that physiological tests may be capable of detecting emphysema or small airways obstructive disease very early in its course. The prognostic implications for the patient with such physiological abnormalities are uncertain. Evidence has recently been cited to show that if the forced expiratory volume at 1 second is normal in a 40-year-old patient, he will never be seriously disabled by chronic obstructive lung disease, so slow is the progression of this disorder.[97] A similar analysis[99] has suggested that the FEF_{25-75}

will probably be abnormal by age 30 in a subject who will be severely disabled at age 50. If this is true, then more sensitive screening tests would need to be performed in subjects under the age of 30 in order to justify their use.

Frequency Dependence of Dynamic Compliance. The cumbersome technique of measuring frequency dependence of dynamic compliance has gained acceptance as being the most sensitive physiological indicator of obstructive disease involving airways smaller than 2 millimeters in diameter.[94,100,101] Because the measurement is difficult to carry out, it is impractical for widespread use. It is, however, regarded as the standard to which simpler techniques for detection of early obstructive disease are compared. The concept of dynamic compliance requires some explanation, because compliance is ordinarily defined as a static measurement, taken under conditions of absence of flow rather than during tidal breathing.

When esophageal pressure and lung volume are plotted against each other during normal respiration, with no attempt to interrupt flow, the relation becomes nonlinear, and a pressure-volume (P-V) loop is traced. Because flow stops momentarily at the end of inspiration and at the end of expiration, the line drawn through these points normally has a slope identical to a compliance slope that is constructed from a series of no-flow points. This slope remains identical over a wide range of breathing frequencies in normal lungs of a normal person. Therefore, the measurement expressed as *compliance* is identical whether it is obtained from a series of points taken during breath holding (static compliance) at several levels of inflation or whether taken from the tangent drawn through a P-V loop inscribed during breathing (dynamic compliance) over a wide range of frequencies.

This tendency of dynamic compliance to be independent of breathing frequency is due to uniformity of the mechanical properties of the normal lung and, hence, synchronism of all portions of the lung on inflation and deflation. When disease alters the lung nonuniformly, rapid breathing rates may result in failure of some portions to fill and empty. Dynamic compliance is then measurably reduced, progressively so with each increase in respiratory rate. This may occur when disease alters the elastic or resistive properties nonuniformly. Dynamic compliance is then "frequency dependent."

It seems likely that when nonuniform changes in elastic properties of the lung become severe enough to result in frequency dependence of dynamic compliance, static compliance will also be altered. On the other hand, there is evidence to show that it is possible for nonuniform alterations of small airways resistance to occur and to result in frequency dependence of dynamic compliance, without causing any measurable changes in other physiological parameters. Small airways normally contribute so little to total airways resistance that such early changes might be expected not to affect measurements of total airways resistance or maximum expiratory flow rates.[7]

On the basis of hhsss considerations, persons with normal static pressure-volume curves, airways resistance, and conventional spirometry, who exhibit frequency dependence of dynamic compliance are thought to have early obstructive disease of small peripheral airways.

Mid-Expiratory Flow Rate. It has been recognized since early in the development of the technique of simple spirometry that the midportion of the forced expiratory volume-time curve has the special characteristic of relative independence of patient effort, as compared with the initial portion of the curve. More recently, another special characteristic of the midportion of the curve has appeared: it is relatively sensitive to alteration caused by obstructive disease in small peripheral airways.[95]

The maximum mid-expiratory flow rate (MMF) or "forced expiratory flow rate from 25 to 75 per cent of forced vital capacity" has been most extensively studied.[22,29] (See the section on volume-time curve analysis, p. 85.) This measurement is simple to carry out, with inexpensive equipment and minimal patient discomfort. The patient is instructed to perform a forced expiratory maneuver into a spirometer (i.e., he exhales completely from full inspiration, as rapidly as possible). Volume is usually plotted on the vertical axis and time on the horizontal axis of the recording device. The portion of the curve from 25 to 75 per cent of the volume expired (forced vital capacity) is chosen for analysis. Ths average rate of flow over this portion of the curve is calculated by drawing a straight line between the two points, defining its extent and determining its slope.

A recent study[95] has focused on a group of smokers with normal spirometry, except for a reduction in MMF, and with normal airways resistance and static compliance. These persons had frequency dependence of dynamic compliance, supporting the interpretation that they did have obstructive disease of small peripheral airways. Bronchodilator therapy and cessation of smoking resulted in improvement of these functional abnormalities in many, and return to normal in some of these subjects.

It seems clear from these investigations and others that this simple test can detect peripheral airways disease earlier than most other spirometric indices, sometimes at a stage of complete reversibility. Other evidence suggests, however, that this test detects only half of the subjects identified as abnormal by demonstration of frequency dependence of compliance.[94] The wide range of values for this determination in normal subjects may account for this relative insensitivity.[29] If Bates' analysis of the time course of the disease[99] is correct, however, insensitivity may not be a serious handicap to the use of the MMF for practical clinical screening. Perhaps the abnormalities detected only by more sensitive tests are of no importance as a cause of disabling disease, at least if they do not occur until after the age of 30 or 40.

Flow-Volume Curves. When expiratory flow is plotted against volume (Fig. 3-5) during a maximum-effort expiratory maneuver, the flow rate rapidly reaches its peak, dependent to a large extent on effort; then as lung volume decreases, the flow rate approaches zero at RV.

Expiratory flow rates late in the maneuver, at low lung volumes, have characteristics that would suggest that their measurement would provide a useful means of identifying mild peripheral small airways obstruction.[51] Flow rates during the later portion are relatively effort-independent and are more sensitive to narrowing in small airways, where the changes of chronic obstructive pulmonary disease are most marked.

Either flow-volume or volume-time curves can be used to evaluate abnormalities of this sort. Flow-volume curves, however, logically provide a more convenient and potentially more precise method, because a reproducible maximum flow rate can be defined for each point on the volume axis of such a curve for a given person. This maximum flow rate is dependent on elastic and resistive properties of the lung at each lung volume.

The full potential usefulness of flow-volume curves in the quantitation of peripheral airways obstruction cannot be realized until normal values are well established. Further studies of flow-volume curve parameters in larger normal populations are needed.[49,52] As such data become available, it should be expected that flow-volume curve analysis will be more widely used.

Closing Volume. The currently most promising techniques for identifying early obstructive airways disease, which combine simplicity and sensitivity, are those that determine closing volume.[102-107] This determination has been defined as "the lung volume at which the dependent lung zones cease to ventilate presumably as a result of airway closure." Alterations in closing volume occur with obstructive disease of small airways and can be detected with a sensitivity approaching that of frequency dependence of dynamic compliance. The mechanisms that cause alterations in closing volume are a matter of some debate, as is the significance of such alterations. This topic has been recently well reviewed.[103]

Techniques for determining closing volume utilize any of a group of inert gases that can be inspired without harm and whose concentration can be easily measured. Changes in the expired concentration of any of these gases can be plotted during a vital capacity maneuver and can be interpreted in light of the knowledge of regional differences in ventilation summarized below.

Ventilation to or from dependent lung zones is greater during normal tidal breathing than that of upper zones. A given change in intrapleural pressure during breathing therefore produces little change in the volume of the already distended upper lung zones, but a greater volume change in the lower zones.[86]

At low lung volumes, however, functional closure of small airways in dependent lung zones occurs, and ventilation of these zones ceases. The level at which this closure occurs is called *closing volume* and is detected as the lung volume at which an abrupt shift in ventilation from dependent to upper lung zones occurs.

Closing volume can be detected by any of several variations of this technique: a patient is connected via a mouthpiece to a spirometer, and a detector sensitive to argon concentration is placed at the mouthpiece. The patient is instructed to exhale maximally and then slowly inhale maximally.

As inhalation begins, a bolus of argon is introduced into the mouthpiece. Because the dependent airways are closed at the beginning of the inspiration, the argon is distributed mostly to the upper zones. As the dependent airways open, the subsequently inspired room air enters the dependent lung zones. As full inspiration is reached, the recording of volume and argon concentration on two axes of an X-Y recorder is begun, and the patient is instructed to begin a slow, full expiration. Argon concentration at the mouthpiece rises in four stages during expiration (see Fig. 2-7, p. 49).

1. Dead space gas contains little argon.
2. Mixed dead space and alveolar gas contains a higher concentration.
3. Alveolar gas from lower lung zones contains a slightly higher concentration, which gradually increases (slope of Phase III).
4. Near the end of expiration, airway closure occurs in the dependent lung zones, and the final portion of the breath contains a high concentration of argon from the upper lung zones.

This final sharp rise in argon concentration is interpreted as coinciding with dependent airway closure, and the volume at which it occurs is recorded as closing volume.

Variations in the closing volume technique utilize argon detected by a mass spectrometer; xenon (Xe^{133}) detected by its radioactivity; helium detected by conventional rapid analyzers available in most pulmonary laboratories; and nitrogen concentration as altered by breathing pure oxygen and detected with a conventional rapid nitrogen analyzer.

Closing volume increases with advancing age and increases in obstructive diseases of small peripheral airways. As normal values for closing volume in different age groups continue to be developed, and as further data are collected about alterations in disease, this measurement may find great usefulness as a screening technique for early obstructive lung disease.[103-107]

A further variant, analysis of the slope of the "alveolar plateau" or Phase III of the single-breath test, may also be used to study airways function. Abnormal results of this analysis are believed to be an early manifestation of airways disease.

REFERENCES

1. Howell, J. B. L., and Campbell, E. J. M. (eds.): Breathlessness: Proceedings of an International Symposium. Oxford, Blackwell Scientific Publications, 1966.
2. Howell, J. B. L., and Campbell, E. J. M.: Breathlessness in pulmonary disease. Scand. J. Respir. Dis., *48*:321, 1967.
3. Lukas, D. S.: Dyspnea. *In* MacBryde, C. M., and Blacklow, R. S.: Signs and Symptoms: Applied Pathologic Physiology and Clinical Interpretation. ed. 5. pp. 341-357. Philadelphia, J. B. Lippincott, 1970.
4. Comroe, J. H., Jr., *et al*.: The Lung. Chicago, Year Book Medical Publishers, 1962.
5. Comroe, J. H., Jr.: Physiology of Respiration. ed. 2. Chicago, Year Book Medical Publishers, 1974.
6. Dejours, P.: Respiration. New York, Oxford University Press, 1966.

7. Macklem, P. T.: Airway obstruction and collateral ventilation. Physiol. Rev., *51*:368, 1971.
8. Hyatt, R. E.: Dynamic lung volumes. *In* Fenn, W. O., and Rahn, H. (eds.): Handbook of Physiology. Section 3: Respiration. Baltimore, Williams & Wilkins, 1964, 1965.
9. Bates, D. V., Macklem, P. T., and Christie, R. V.: Respiratory Function in Disease. Philadelphia, W. B. Saunders, 1971.
10. Mead, J., Turner, J. M., Macklem, P. T., and Little, J. B.: Significance of the relationship between lung recoil and maximum expiratory flow. J. Appl. Physiol., *22*:95, 1967.
11. Pride, N. B., Permutt, S., Riley, R. L., and Bromberger-Barnea, B.: Determinants of maximal expiratory flow from the lungs. J. Appl. Physiol., *23*:646, 1967.
12. Campbell, E. J. M.: Physical signs of diffuse airways obstruction and lung distension. Thorax, *24*:1, 1969.
13. Godfey, S., Edwards, R. H. T., Campbell, E. J. M., and Newton-Howes, J.: Clinical and physiological associations of some physical signs observed in patients with chronic airways obstruction. Thorax, *25*:285, 1970.
14. McFadden, E. R., Kiser, R., and DeGroot, W. J.: Acute bronchial asthma: clinical and physiologic relations. N. Engl. J. Med., *288*:221, 1973.
15. Snider, T. H., Stevens, J. P., Wilner, F. M., and Lewis, B. M.: Simple bedside test of respiratory function. J.A.M.A., *170*:1631, 1959.
16. Olsen, C. R.: The match test: a measure of ventilatory function. Am. Rev. Respir. Dis., *86*:37, 1962.
17. Carilli, A. D., and Henderson, J. R.: Estimation of ventilatory function by blowing out a match. Am. Rev. Respir. Dis., *89*:680, 1964.
18. Rosenblatt, G., and Stein, M.: Clinical value of the forced expiratory time measured during auscultation. N. Engl. J. Med., *267*:432, 1962.
19. Lal, S., Ferguson, A. D., and Campbell, E. J. M.: Forced expiratory time: a simple test for airways obstruction. Br. Med. J., *1*:814, 1964.
20. Morgan, W. K. C., and Branscomb, B. V.: The assessment of ventilatory capacity. Statement of the Committees on Environmental Health and Respiratory Physiology, American College of Chest Physicians. Chest, *67*:95, 1975.
21. Baldwin, E. deF., Cournand, A., and Richards, D. W., Jr.: Pulmonary insufficiency. I. Physiological classification, clinical methods of analysis, standard values in normal subjects. Medicine (Baltimore), *27*:243, 1948.
22. Leuallen, E. C., and Fowler, W. S.: Maximal midexpiratory flow. Am. Rev. Tuberc., *72*:783, 1955.
23. Goldman, H. I., and Becklake, M. R.: Respiratory function tests: normal values at median altitudes and the prediction of normal results. Am. Rev. Tuberc., *79*:457, 1959.
24. Kory, R. C., Callahan, R., Boren, H. G., and Sizner, J. C.: The Veterans Administration Army Cooperative Study of Pulmonary Function. I. Clinical spirometry in normal men. Am. J. Med., *30*:243, 1961.
25. Bates, D. V., Woolf, C. R., and Paul, G. I.: Chronic bronchitis. A report on the first two stages of the co-ordinated study of chronic bronchitis in the Department of Veterans Affairs, Canada. Med. Serv. J. Canada, *18*:211, 1962.
26. Ferris, B. G., Jr., Anderson, D. O., and Zickmantel, R.: Prediction values for screening test of pulmonary function. Am. Rev. Respir. Dis., *91*:252, 1965.
27. Cotes, J. E., Rossiter, C. E., Higgins, I. T. T., and Gilson, J. C.: Average normal values for the forced expiratory volume in white caucasian males. Br. Med. J., *1*:1016, 1966.
28. Weng, T. R., and Levison, H.: Standards of pulmonary function in children. Am. Rev. Respir. Dis., *99*:879, 1969.
29. Morris, J. F., Koski, A., and Johnson, L. C.: Spirometric standards for healthy nonsmoking adults. Am. Rev. Respir. Dis., *103*:57, 1971.
30. Cherniack, R. M., and Raber, M. B.: Normal standards for ventilatory function using an automated wedge spirometer. Am. Rev. Respir. Dis., *106*:38, 1972.
31. Morris, J. F., Temple, W. P., and Koski, A.: Normal values for the ratio of one-second forced expiratory volume to forced vital capacity. Am. Rev. Respir. Dis., *108*:1000, 1973.
32. Pappenheimer, J. R. (committee chairman): Standardizations of definitions and symbols in respiratory physiology. Fed. Proc., *9*:602, 1950.
33. Kory, R. C. (committee chairman): Clinical spirometry: recommendations of the Section on Pulmonary Function Testing, Committee on Pulmonary Physiology,

American College of Chest Physicians. Dis. Chest, *43*:214, 1963.
34. Burrows, B. (committee chairman): Pulmonary terms and symbols. Chest, *67*:583, 1975.
35. Dayman, H.: The expiratory spirogram. Am. Rev. Respir. Dis., *83*:842, 1961.
36. Wright, B. M., and McKerrow, C. B.: Maximum forced expiratory flow rate as a measure of ventilatory capacity. Br. Med. J., *2*:1041, 1959.
37. Hermannsen, J.: Untersuchungen über die maximale Ventilationsgrosse (Atemgrenzwert). Z. Gesamte Exp. Med., *90*:130, 1933.
38. Gaensler, E. A.: Clinical pulmonary physiology. N. Engl. J. Med., *252*:177-184, 221-228, 264-271, 1955.
39. Gaensler, E. A., and Wright, G. W.: Evaluation of respiratory impairment. Arch. Environ. Health, *12*:146, 1966.
40. Clark, T. J. H.: Inspiratory obstruction. Br. Med. J., *3*:682, 1970.
41. Empey, D. W.: Assessment of upper airways obstruction. Br. Med. J., *3*:503, 1972.
42. Snider, G. L., Woolf, C. R., Kory, R. C., and Ross, J.: Criteria for the assessment of reversibility in airways obstruction. Report of the Committee on Emphysema, American College of Chest Physicians. Chest, *65*:552, 1974.
43. Snider, G. L., Kory, R. C., and Lyons, H. A.: Grading of pulmonary function impairment by means of pulmonary function tests. Recommendations of the Committee on Pulmonary Physiology, American College of Chest Physicians. Dis. Chest, *52*:270, 1967.
44. Hyatt, R. E., Schilder, D. P., and Fry, D. L.: Relationship between maximum expiratory flow and degree of lung inflation. J. Appl. Physiol., *13*:331, 1958.
45. Fry, D. L., and Hyatt, R. E.: Pulmonary mechanics: a unified analysis of the relationship between pressure, volume and gasflow in the lungs of normal and diseased human subjects. Am. J. Med., *29*:672, 1960.
46. Hyatt, R. E.: The interrelationships of pressure, flow, and volume during various respiratory maneuvers in normal and emphysematous subjects. Am. Rev. Respir. Dis., *83*:676, 1961.
47. Jordanoglou, J., and Pride, N. B.: Factors determining maximum inspiratory flow and maximum expiratory flow of the lung. Thorax, *23*:33, 1968.
48. ———: A comparison of maximum inspiratory and expiratory flow in health and in lung disease. Thorax, *23*:38, 1968.
49. Hyatt, R. E., and Black, L. F.: The flow-volume curve: a current perspective. Am. Rev. Respir. Dis., *107*:191, 1973.
50. Macklem, P. T.: Current concepts: tests of lung mechanics. N. Engl. J. Med., *243*:339, 1975.
51. Gelb, A. F., and MacAnally, B. J.: Early detection of obstructive lung disease by analysis of maximal expiratory flow-volume curves. Chest, *64*:749, 1973.
52. Black, L. F., Offord, K., and Hyatt, R. E.: Variability in the maximal expiratory flow volume curve in asymptomatic smokers and in nonsmokers. Am. Rev. Respir. Dis., *110*:282, 1974.
53. Gazioglu, K., Condemi, J., Kaltreider, N. L., and Yu, P. N.: Study of forced vital capacity and maximal expiratory flow-volume curves in obstructive lung disease. Am. Rev. Respir. Dis., *98*:857, 1968.
54. Lord, G. P., Gazioglu, K., and Kaltreider, N.: The maximum expiratory flow-volume in the evaluation of patients with lung disease. Am. J. Med., *46*:72, 1969.
55. Carilli, A. D., Denson, L. J., Rock, F., and Malabanan, S.: The flow-volume loop in normal subjects and in diffuse lung disease. Chest, *66*:472, 1974.
56. Shim, C., Corro, P., Park, S. S., and Williams, M. H., Jr.: Pulmonary function studies in patients with upper airway obstruction. Am. Rev. Respir. Dis., *106*:233, 1972.
57. Miller, R. D., and Hyatt, R. E.: Obstructing lesions of the larynx and trachea: clinical and physiological characteristics. Mayo Clin. Proc., *44*:145, 1969.
58. ———: Evaluation of obstructing lesions of the trachea and larynx by flow-volume loops. Am. Rev. Respir. Dis., *108*:475, 1973.
59. Darling, R. C., Cournand, A., and Richards, D. W., Jr.: Studies on the intrapulmonary mixture of gases. III. An open circuit method for measuring residual air. J. Clin. Invest., *19*:609, 1940.
60. DuBois, A. B., *et al.*: A rapid plethysmographic method for measuring thoracic gas volume: a comparison with a nitrogen washout method for measuring functional residual capacity in human subjects. J. Clin. Invest., *35*:322, 1956.
61. Meneely, G. R., *et al.*: A simplified closed circuit helium dilution method for the determination of the residual volume of the lungs. Am. J. Med., *28*:824, 1960.

62. Schaaning, C. G., and Gulsvik, A.: Accuracy and precision of helium dilution technique and body plethysmography in measuring lung volumes. Scand. J. Clin. Lab. Invest., *32*:271, 1973.
63. O'Shea, J., *et al*.: Determination of lung volumes from chest films. Thorax, *25*:544, 1970.
64. Greene, R.: Radiographic measurement of thoracic gas volume. Radiol. Clin. North Am., *9*:63, 1971.
65. Harris, T. R., Pratt, P. C., and Kilburn, K. H.: Total lung capacity measured by roentgenograms. Am. J. Med., *50*:756, 1971.
66. Marmorstein, B. L., and Cianciulli, F. D.: Planimetric measurement of total lung capacity in asthma. Chest, *66*:378, 1974.
67. Boren, H. G., Kory, R. C., and Syner, J. C.: The Veterans Administration–Army cooperative study of pulmonary function. II. The lung volume and its subdivisions in normal men. Am. J. Med., *41*:96, 1966.
68. Dejours, P.: Control of respiration in muscular exercise. *In* Fenn, W. O., and Rahn, H. (eds.): Handbook of Physiology. Section 3: Respiration. Baltimore, Williams & Wilkins, 1964.
69. Fox, S. M. III, Naughton, J. P., and Gorman, P. A.: Physical activity and cardiovascular health. Part II. The exercise prescription: intensity and duration. Mod. Concepts Cardiovasc. Dis., *41*:21, 1972.
70. Pierce, A. K., Taylor, H. F., Archer, R. K., and Miller, W. F.: Responses to exercise training in patients with emphysema. Arch. Intern. Med., *113*:28, 1964.
71. Fox, S. M. III, Naughton, J. P., and Gorman, P. A.: Physical activity and cardiovascular health. Part III. The exercise prescription: frequency and type of activity. Mod. Concepts Cardiovasc. Dis., *41*:25, 1972.
72. Jones, N. L.: Exercise testing in pulmonary evaluation. N. Engl. J. Med., *293*:541, 647, 1975.
73. Wasserman, K., and Whipp, B. J.: Exercise physiology in health and disease. Am. Rev. Respir. Dis., *112*:219, 1975.
74. Armstrong, B. W., Workman, J. N., Hurt, H. H., and Roemich, W. R.: Clinicophysiologic evaluation of physical working capacity in persons with pulmonary disease. Am. Rev. Respir. Dis., *93*:90 (Part I); 223 (Part II); 1966.
75. Mead, J.: Mechanical properties of lungs. Physiol. Rev., *41*:281, 1961.
76. Mead, J., and Whittenberger, J. L.: Physical properties of human lungs measured during spontaneous respiration. J. Appl. Physiol., *5*:779, 1953.
77. Fisher, A. B., DuBois, A. B., and Hyde, R. W.: Evaluation of the forced oscillation technique for the determination of resistance to breathing. J. Clin. Invest., *47*:2045, 1968.
78. Otis, A. B., and Proctor, D. F.: Measurement of alveolar pressure in human subjects. Am. J. Physiol., *152*:106, 1948.
79. DuBois, A. B., Botelho, S. Y., and Comroe, J. H.: A new method for measuring airway resistance in man using a body plethysmograph: values in normal subjects and in patients with respiratory disease. J. Clin. Invest., *35*:327, 1956.
80. Hogg, J. C., Macklem, P. T., and Thurlbeck, W. M.: Site and nature of airway obstruction in chronic obstructive lung disease. N. Engl. J. Med., *278*:1355, 1968.
81. Mead, J., McIlroy, M. B., Selverstone, N. J., and Kriete, B. C.: Measurement of intraesophageal pressure. J. Appl. Physiol., *7*:491, 1955.
82. Milic-Emili, J., Mead, J., Turner, J. M., and Glauser, E. M.: Improved technique for estimating pleural pressure from esophageal balloons. J. Appl. Physiol., *19*:207, 1964.
83. Cherniack, R. M., and Brown, E.: A simple method for measuring total respiratory compliance: normal values for males. J. Appl. Physiol., *20*:87, 1965.
84. Turner, J. M., Mead, J., and Wohl, M. E.: Elasticity of human lungs in relation to age. J. Appl. Physiol., *25*:664, 1968.
85. Schlueter, D. P., Immekus, J., and Stead, W. W.: Relationship between maximal inspiratory pressure and total lung capacity (coefficient of retraction) in normal subjects and in patients with emphysema, asthma, and diffuse pulmonary infiltration. Am. Rev. Respir. Dis., *96*:656, 1967.
86. Milic-Emili, J., Henderson, J. A. M., and Kaneko, K.: Regional distribution of pulmonary ventilation. *In* Cumming, G., and Hunt, L. B. (eds.): Form and Function in the Human Lung. Edinburgh, E. & G. Livingstone, 1968.
87. Craig, D. B., *et al*.: "Closing volume" and its relationship to gas exchange in seated and supine positions. J. Appl. Physiol., *31*:717, 1971.
88. LeBlanc, P., Ruff, F., and Milic-Emili, J.:

Effects of age and body position on "airway closure" in man. J. Appl. Physiol., *28*:448, 1970.
89. Anthonisen, N. R., Danson, J., Robertson, P. C., and Ross, W. R. D.: Airway closure as a function of age. Respir. Physiol., *8*:58, 1969.
90. Fowler, W. S.: Lung function studies. III. Uneven pulmonary ventilation in normal subjects and in patients with pulmonary disease. J. Appl. Physiol., *2*:283, 1949.
91. Brody, A. W., Navin, J. J., Stoughton, R. R., and Barta, F.: Standards and significance for three tests of the distribution of ventilation. The time to equilibration, the forced equilibrating expiration, and the Fowler Single Breath Test. Am. J. Med., *48*:424, 1970.
92. Cournand, A., Baldwin, E. deF., Darling, R. C., and Richards, W., Jr.: Studies on the intrapulmonary mixture of gases. IV. The significance of the pulmonary emptying rate and simplified open circuit measurement of residual air. J. Clin. Invest., *20*:681, 1941.
93. Medina, J. R., Lillehei, J. P., Loken, M. K., and Ebert, R. V.: Use of the scintillation Anger camera and xenon Xe^{133} in the study of chronic obstructive lung disease. J.A.M.A., *208*:985, 1969.
94. Macklem, P. T.: Obstruction in small airways—a challenge to medicine. Am. J. Med., *52*:721, 1972.
95. McFadden, E. R., Jr., and Linden, D. A.: A reduction in maximum mid-expiratory flow rate: a spirographic manifestation of small airway disease. Am. J. Med., *52*:725, 1972.
96. Macklem, P. T.: Workshop on screening programs for early diagnosis of airway obstruction. Am. Rev. Respir. Dis., *109*:567, 1974.
97. Burrows, B.: Early detection of airways obstruction. Chest, *65*:239, 1974.
98. Niewoehner, D. E., Kleinerman, J., and Rice, D. B.: Pathologic changes in the peripheral airways of young cigarette smokers. N. Engl. J. Med., *291*:755, 1974.
99. Bates, D. V.: The prevention of emphysema. Chest, *65*:437, 1974.
100. McFadden, E. R., Kiker, R., Holmes, B., and DeGroot, W. J.: Small airway disease: an assessment of the tests of peripheral airway function. Am. J. Med., *57*:171, 1974.
101. Woolcock, A. J., Vincent, N. J., and Macklem, P. T.: Frequency dependence of compliance as a test for obstruction in the small airways. J. Clin. Invest., *48*:1097, 1968.
102. Mansell, A., Bryan, C., and Levison, H.: Airway closure in children. J. Appl. Physiol., *33*:711, 1972.
103. Hyatt, R. E., and Rodarte, J. R.: "Closing volume," one man's noise—other mens' experiment. Mayo Clin. Proc., *50*:17, 1975.
104. McCarthy, D. S., Spencer, R., Greene, R., and Milic-Emili, J.: Measurement of "closing volume" as a simple and sensitive test for early detection of small airway disease. Am. J. Med., *52*:747, 1972.
105. Buist, A. S., VanFleet, D. L., and Ross, B. B.: A comparison of conventional spirometric tests and the test of closing volume in an emphysema screening center. Am. Rev. Respir. Dis., *107*:735, 1973.
106. Buist, A. S., and Ross, B. B.: Predicted values for closing volumes using a modified single breath nitrogen test. Am. Rev. Respir. Dis., *107*:744, 1973.
107. Buist, A. S.: Early detection of airways obstruction by the closing volume technique. Chest, *64*:495, 1973.

4 Respiratory Function of the Lungs and Blood

Clarence A. Guenter, M.D.

ARTERIAL BLOOD GAS ANALYSIS: THE FINAL YARDSTICK OF OVERALL ADEQUACY OF LUNG FUNCTION

The major function of the lungs is the exchange of oxygen and carbon dioxide. It is convenient that this function can be assessed by measurement of oxygen and carbon dioxide in systemic arterial blood. Techniques for rapid and simple analysis of gases in the blood have become widely available since the early 1960s and have had enormous impact on the diagnosis and treatment of respiratory insufficiency.

Obtaining Arterial Blood

Selection of an Artery. Arterial puncture for sampling of blood has been established as a relatively safe and simple procedure (see list below). Although any artery in the body could conceivably be utilized, the radial, brachial, and femoral arteries are most accessible to percutaneous cannulation.[1,2] Generally, the complications of puncture of the radial artery are less than those of the brachial or femoral artery.

Most major complications of arterial puncture have occurred when the femoral artery has been utilized. In that artery, (a) atherosclerotic plaques may be dislodged, resulting in distal occlusion of the artery; (b) hemorrhage may occur, occasionally dissecting upward retroperitoneally, with major blood loss occurring before it is apparent; and (c) thrombosis at the site of the puncture may result in distal ischemia. These problems are more likely to arise in patients with clinical evidence of atherosclerosis (such as tortuous vessels, aneurysms, or bruits) or in patients with clotting abnormalities. All of these complications are relatively rare when a small needle is used for a single arterial puncture, placed well below the inguinal ligament in the femoral region. In view of the potential for complications, however, the femoral artery should only be used as a last resort.

Requirements for Safe Arterial Blood Sampling

Sterile needle, heparinized syringe
Aseptic technique
Palpable artery
Understanding of the anatomy of the region
Identification of the risk factors
  Hypertension
  Local disease (atherosclerosis, aneurysm)
  Anticoagulants or bleeding diathesis
Compression of artery after puncture

Venous blood is not an acceptable substitute for arterial blood when respiratory function is being assessed. The blood draining the tissues reflects the metabolism of the particular tissue that the vein drains. Mixed venous blood provides useful information regarding net oxygen availability to the body and acid-base balance. "Arterialized" capillary blood can be obtained after warming a capillary bed for approximately 10 minutes, the vasodilation resulting in an increased rate of blood flow that approaches the flow rate of arterial blood. The preferred puncture sites include the heel pad, earlobe, and finger tip.

Although arterialized capillary blood values only approximate arterial blood values, they may be sufficiently accurate for major therapeutic considerations, particularly in infants with inaccessible arteries.[3]

Single puncture of the radial artery is performed readily as follows. The patient is comfortably seated or preferably allowed to lie down (to minimize the likelihood of a vasovagal faint). The forearm is extended, and the wrist is dorsiflexed about 30 degrees. The radial artery should then be carefully palpated proximally from the wrist crease as the artery passes medial to the styloid process of the radius, and for about 2 inches up the forearm. After the course of the artery has been well defined, a needle (21 or 22 gauge) is inserted through the skin approximately 1 inch proximal to the wrist crease (and immediately over the pulsating vessel). The needle is then advanced at an angle almost parallel to the artery, but to a sufficient depth to actually enter the artery (Fig. 4-1). This oblique angle provides a longer vessel for the needle to traverse; it also provides a longer tract, permitting the spasm of the muscle wall to assist in occlusion when the needle has been withdrawn. When the needle enters the artery, a slow but pulsatile flow of blood occurs. Occasionally, the artery is completely traversed, and the needle passes through the opposite wall. When this occurs, if the needle is withdrawn gradually, the tip will again enter the lumen, and blood can then be obtained. When a free flow of definite arterial blood is apparent through the hub of the needle, a 5-ml. heparinized syringe is attached, and blood is withdrawn. When a glass syringe with a well-lubricated barrel is used, the pressure of the blood generally causes the syringe to fill spontaneously. When plastic syringes are used, this generally does not occur. Introducing the needle without the syringe attached permits definite identification of arterial flow. This may not be important in well-oxygenated patients, whose arterial blood is bright red; however, it is particularly important in patients with hypoxemia, whose blue arterial blood may be indistinguishable from the dark color of venous blood.

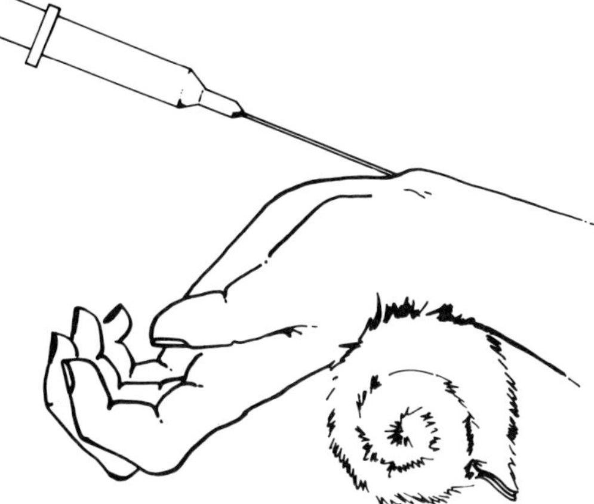

Fig. 4-1. Optimal position for radial artery puncture. Note the extension of the wrist and the angle of entry of the needle.

Many physicians prefer to inject a small amount of topical anesthetic in the skin and infiltrate locally along each side of the arterial wall prior to arterial puncture. This may decrease the pain if multiple punctures are necessary before the artery is entered, but it is just as painful as a single direct arterial puncture performed by a skilled technologist.

The cleaning of the skin need not be elaborate; swabbing with an alcohol sponge generally is as effective for this procedure as for a venipuncture.[4] After withdrawal of the required volume of blood (generally 3 to 5 ml.), any air bubbles should be expressed, the syringe capped, and the sample placed on ice until analysis is carried out. Direct pressure should be applied to the puncture site for at least 3 to 5 minutes, or longer if the patient is anticoagulated or has other bleeding diatheses. The puncture site should be rechecked within 5 minutes after releasing pressure, to be sure that a hematoma is not gradually forming. The swelling of a hematoma is easily apparent at the site of a radial artery puncture. Although hematomas at the site of radial artery puncture rarely cause major complications, they result in disconcerting pain and discomfort. Perhaps every physician should have to experience this. A hematoma in the fascial plane of the wrist rarely may cause median nerve compression. Multiple punctures of an artery can be safely carried out in the course of a day if skill and care are exerted. If multiple samples are required, an indwelling arterial cannula may be desirable.

Insertion of an indwelling arterial cannula into the radial artery may be desirable to provide multiple sequential sampling. This technique is also desirable when acute effects of breath holding or hyperventilation in response to the procedure need to be avoided. The artery is identified and its course determined in the same manner as for a single arterial puncture. The overlying skin is swabbed with alcohol, and an indwelling arterial cannula (of which many commercial varieties are now available) is inserted into the artery. The polyethylene or Teflon sheath is advanced proximally to a secure position well within the lumen of the artery. The cannula may then be attached to a stopcock and may be kept open by flushing intermittently with heparinized saline. Alternatively, a pressure-sensitive valve may be introduced, preventing any flow except during the time of sampling, with intermittent injection of heparin to prevent thrombosis. The cannula may be safely left in position for 24 to 48 hours. The incidence of infection and thrombosis tends to increase with prolonged cannulation.

Complications of single arterial needle punctures are infrequent. In our experience, with more than 10,000 radial arterial punctures performed predominantly by ancillary medical personnel (respiratory technologists and nurses), only two major complications occurred. Both of these consisted of extensive bleeding into the fascial planes of the wrist, with median nerve compression. Paresthesias were transient, relieved after 5 to 7 days. One of these patients had been on anticoagulants.

On the other hand, cannulation of the radial artery frequently results in obstruction to blood flow.[5] As high as 40 per cent of patients who had cannulation of the radial artery developed evidence of thrombosis, as assessed by ultrasonic measurements of flow. All of these patients subsequently had developed full return of blood flow. In view of this rate of vascular occlusion, it is recommended that prior to the insertion of a cannula into the radial artery, flow through the ulnar artery be demonstrated by means of the Allen's test. This test is performed by having the patient make a fist, to drain the palmar vascular bed of blood, then occluding the radial and ulnar arteries by local pressure. The hand is then opened, while the radial and ulnar arteries are occluded. Pressure is first released from the ulnar artery, permitting flow to the hand. The blanching of palmar vascular beds should give place to erythema if the ulnar artery is patent. Although it is not certain that cannulation of the radial artery in the face of an occluded ulnar artery causes complications, the risk is probably increased.[6] Embolization from an indwelling arterial cannula to the pulp spaces of the fingers occurs commonly, but this is generally of minor significance if care is taken in the maintenance of a clot-free arterial cannula.[3,7-9]

It is generally considered reasonable to train respiratory technologists, intensive-care-unit nurses, and pulmonary laboratory technologists to obtain samples of arterial blood, although the medicolegal implications have not been uniformly established.[10,11] A system of training, supervision, and certification of competence must be established in each institution, as for other procedures, to protect the patient.

Processing the Blood. Because arterial blood is deliberately sampled to assess the effects of equilibration of alveolar gas with the blood passing through the lungs, it is of utmost importance that no other gas be permitted contact with the blood. Every effort must be made to prevent air from entering the syringe. A discrete bubble may be expelled immediately, but multiple small bubbles generally cause a modification of blood gases. When air contaminates the sample, the oxygen and carbon dioxide of the blood are altered in the direction of the partial pressures of those gases in air; therefore, the blood Pco_2 decreases, and, in a sample from a normal or hypoxic person, the Po_2 increases.

The sample should be cooled as rapidly

as possible in order to lower the metabolic rate of the erythrocytes and leukocytes, which utilize oxygen and produce carbon dioxide and metabolic acids at sufficiently rapid rates to alter the gas partial pressures and pH. An iced sample, tightly sealed, may be analyzed in 30 to 45 minutes with barely measurable changes, and for as long as 2 hours after sampling with only minor degrees of alteration in the gases.

Diffusion of carbon dioxide and oxygen is sufficiently slow through plastic so that disposable syringes may be used if prompt analysis is available. An exception should be made when collecting blood with high oxygen tension (greater than 300 mm. Hg), because the high pressure gradient between blood and room air increases the rate of diffusion; under this circumstance, glass syringes are preferable.

When the patient is febrile or hypothermic, errors in gas values may be introduced by analyzing the blood at the usual instrument temperature of 37° C. Blood analyzed routinely at 37° C. from a hypothermic patient results in falsely high Po_2 and Pco_2 values and a low pH. Conversely, blood from a hyperthermic patient has low Po_2 and Pco_2 values and a high pH, compared with the true values in vivo. Nomograms have been developed that permit corrections back to the values at the patient's temperature, particularly the pH and the Po_2 values. Such corrections take into account the difference in hydrogen ion concentration with varying temperature, and shifts in the oxyhemoglobin dissociation curve.[12,13] For example, blood analyzed with a normal pH and Pco_2, with a Po_2 of 50 mm. Hg, may reflect a patient Po_2 of 40 mm. Hg if the body temperature is 34° C., or a Po_2 of 62 mm. Hg if the body temperature is 40° C. These changes are even more significant at lower levels of oxyhemoglobin saturation, or when hemoglobin is completely saturated.

Instruments for measuring arterial blood pH, Po_2 and Pco_2 are relatively inexpensive and available in many forms. These instruments should be available in any institution that accepts the responsibility for oxygen therapy, general anesthetics, care of comatose patients, or respiratory care. The mere presence of a technician willing to perform arterial blood gas analysis on an available instrument does not assure a high standard of quality in the analytic technique (see list below). Reliable systems of quality control must be established, yet they are frequently absent in apparently smoothly functioning laboratories.

Pitfalls in Interpretation of Blood Gas Values

Blood from vein or hematoma rather than artery

Patient status not noted (e.g., breathing oxygen, on respirator)

Blood contaminated by air (bubbles or unsealed syringe)

Patient temperature significantly different from 37° C.

Blood stored too long prior to analysis

Analytic error (faulty calibration, handling of specimen, or instrument)

Factors Affecting Arterial Blood Po_2 and Pco_2

The sum of the pressures of each of the gases in the atmosphere equals the total atmospheric pressure. As discussed in Chapter 1, the fraction of the total that each gas represents may be expressed as its *partial pressure*. For example, at sea level, the average barometric pressure is 760 mm. Hg (sometimes expressed as *tension* or *Torr*, according to the Torricelli scale); the amount of oxygen is 20.95 per cent, and the partial pressure of oxygen (Po_2) is 159 mm. Hg. When the air equilibrates with a liquid such as blood, the gas partial pressure in the blood is the same as in the air.

The volume of gas that may be present in a liquid varies with each gas and the specific liquid. The volume of gas in a liquid is determined by (a) the solubility of the gas in the liquid, (b) the partial pressure of the gas, and (c) the presence of additional binding mechanisms in the liquid (e.g., hemoglobin in blood). It is of utmost importance to bear in mind that analysis of blood Po_2 and Pco_2 reflects only the partial

Table 4-1. Mechanisms of Reduced Arterial Po_2

	Arterial Gas Tensions		*Alveolar-Arterial Oxygen Gradient*	
	Pao_2	*$Paco_2$*	*Room Air*	*100% Oxygen*
Reduced atmospheric oxygen (high altitude)	↓	↓	N	N
Alveolar hypoventilation	↓	↑	N	N
Altered intrapulmonary gas exchange				
Regionally decreased ventilation compared with perfusion	↓	↓N or↑	↑	N or↑
Intrapulmonary right-to-left shunt	↓	N or↓	↑	↑
"Diffusion block"	↓	N or↓	↑	N
Anatomical right-to-left shunt (intrapulmonary or intracardiac)	↓	N or↓	↑	↑

pressure of the gases and not the volume. If the solubility and other binding mechanisms are known, relationships between partial pressures and volumes of the gases may be predicted. This extrapolation is frequently useful in medical practice, as long as its limitations are kept in mind.

Arterial blood analysis for Po_2 and Pco_2 primarily reflects the effect of blood coming into contact with gases in the lungs. This analysis of gas exchange in the lungs reflects oxygen delivery to the tissues only if other aspects of the transport system are normal. Abnormalities in oxygen transport are discussed below. The factors that result in arterial hypoxemia are listed in Table 4-1.

Reduced Atmospheric Oxygen. When a normal person is transported from sea level to an altitude of 3,500 feet, his environment changes from a barometric pressure of approximately 760 to approximately 660 mm. Hg. The Po_2 in the inspired air (P_IO_2) decreases from about 159 to 138 mm. Hg. Therefore, air breathed into the terminal air units produces a lower level of alveolar oxygen. Blood perfusing the lungs with this reduced level of oxygen necessarily equilibrates at the lower level, and there is a reduced Po_2 in the arterial blood (see Chap. 1). This mechanism produces predictable decreases in arterial Po_2 whenever environmental Po_2 is reduced. Conversely, when the environmental oxygen is increased (either as a result of oxygen supplements or of hyperbaric environments), the alveolar Po_2 normally increases in a predictable fashion. Because the equilibration of blood with alveolar gas is not perfect, alveolar ventilation is variable, and the transport of oxygen in the blood is complex (the relationship of environmental oxygen to arterial blood oxygen content is not simple, direct, or linear). The normal arterial Po_2 at sea level (P_IO_2 = 159 mm. Hg) is about 90 mm. Hg. At Calgary, Alberta, altitude 3,500 feet (P_IO_2 = 138), arterial Po_2 is about 79 mm. Hg. At sea level, breathing pure oxygen (P_IO_2 = 760), the arterial Po_2 is about 600 mm. Hg.

Changes in inspired oxygen do not affect arterial Pco_2 directly, but may result in altered levels as a result of secondary effects on alveolar ventilation. Generally, hypoxemia stimulates respiration.

Alveolar Ventilation. The next phase of the respiratory pathway that may result in reduced blood oxygen levels is the bellows function of the lung. If ventilation of the alveolar spaces is reduced, the amount of oxygen available to the pulmonary blood is reduced. Consequently, a greater proportion of alveolar oxygen is removed, resulting in a decreased alveolar oxygen partial pressure.

The effects of alveolar hypoventilation are illustrated in Table 4-2. In Subject A, with normal ventilation, the alveolar venti-

Table 4-2. Mechanism of Arterial Hypoxemia in Alveolar Hypoventilation

	Subject A *Normal Ventilation*	*Subject B* *Severe Hypoventilation*
Alveolar ventilation	5 L./min.	2.5 L./min.
Oxygen consumption	250 ml./min.	250 ml./min.
Oxygen content		
Inspired air	210 ml./L. (21% of atmospheric gas)	210 ml./L. (21%)
Alveolar air	160 ml./L. (16% alveolar gas)	110 ml./L. (11%)
Po_2 Alveolar gas	114 mm. Hg (0.16 × 713)*	78 mm. Hg (0.11 × 713)*
Po_2 Arterial blood	95 mm. Hg (approx.)	65 mm. Hg (approx.)

*Corrected for water vapor pressure (47 mm. Hg at 37° C.).

lation is approximately 5 L. per minute. At rest, the oxygen consumption is 250 ml. per minute. Knowing these factors, it is possible to calculate the rate of extraction of oxygen from the air as breathing goes on. The oxygen content (21% of the air) will be 210 ml. per liter of air. Because the subject has 5 L. per minute of alveolar ventilation, he will have to extract 250 ml. per minute from the 5 L. of air, thus extracting 50 ml. per liter. Subtracting 50 ml. from the 210 ml. that are present in air leaves 160 ml. per liter in the alveolar gas (16% of the alveolar gas). Compare this with Subject B, who has severe hypoventilation, with 2.5 L. per minute of alveolar ventilation; it is clear that the same amount of oxygen will have to be extracted from a much smaller amount of air. By the same calculations, one can demonstrate that the oxygen left in the alveolar gas will be 110 ml. per liter, or only 11 per cent. It follows, then, that with less oxygen in the alveolar gas, there will be less oxygen available to the arterial blood, and arterial hypoxemia will result. These figures may now be readily corrected to partial pressures. If the total barometric pressure is 760 mm. Hg, a fixed proportion of this will be composed of water vapor when inside the body at the alveolar level. At body temperature (37° C.), this is 47 mm. Hg. For Subject A, the fraction of oxygen (0.16) times the corrected barometric pressure (713 mm. Hg) will be the Po_2 of the oxygen in the alveoli. The calculated decrease in alveolar Po_2 from 114 to 98 mm. Hg is thus accounted for purely on the basis of alveolar hypoventilation.

Conversely, a hyperventilating subject has an increased alveolar oxygen content and alveolar Po_2, with a resultant rise in arterial Po_2 (see list below). In fact, this is the only mechanism whereby an individual can have an elevated arterial Po_2 without an increased inspired Po_2.

Mechanisms of Increased Arterial Po_2

Hyperventilation (always associated with reduced Pco_2; Po_2 generally at least 20 mm. Hg below inspired Po_2)

Increased environmental oxygen (Po_2 increased in proportion to P_IO_2)

Contamination of blood by air (Po_2 never higher than environmental Po_2)

Changes in alveolar ventilation directly influence the level of carbon dioxide as well. This relationship has been defined as follows:

$$PaCO_2 \cong \frac{0.863\ (CO_2\ \text{production})}{\text{alveolar ventilation}}$$

A decrease in alveolar ventilation, therefore, results in elevated $PaCO_2$, and,

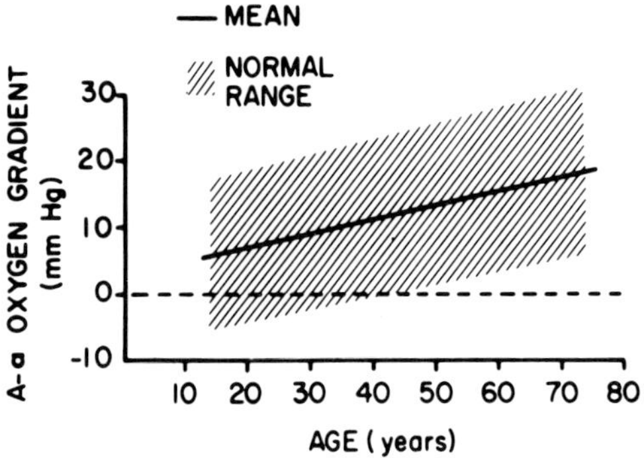

Fig. 4-2. Alveolar-arterial (A-a) oxygen gradient in normal subjects at various ages. Mean value for $P(A\text{-}a)O_2 = 2.5 + 0.21$ (age) in mm. Hg. Shaded areas indicate 2 standard deviations. (Compiled from data in Mellemgaard, K.: The alveolar-arterial oxygen difference: its size and components in normal man. Acta Physiol. Scand., *67*:10, 1966)

conversely, hyperventilation results in reduced arterial Pco_2.

Altered Intrapulmonary Gas Exchange. The most common cause of arterial hypoxemia in patients with pulmonary disease is altered intrapulmonary gas exchange. The elegant mechanism whereby air is distributed throughout the tracheobronchial tree to terminal lung units is discussed below. Ideally, every terminal lung unit that receives air also is serviced by an appropriate allotment of venous blood. In the average alveolus, the ratio of the flow of air to that of blood, at rest is approximately 0.8. Total alveolar ventilation is approximately 4 L. per minute, and the total pulmonary perfusion is approximately 5 L. per minute.

In the ideal alveolus, with appropriate matching of ventilation and perfusion, the blood is fully arterialized, and the Po_2 of the blood leaving the alveolus is virtually the same as the Po_2 of alveolar air. The very thin alveolocapillary wall normally presents no significant barrier to diffusion. Not all alveoli, however, function in this ideal fashion; in fact, the mixed arterial blood has a Po_2 approximately 10 mm. Hg lower than the alveolar Po_2,[14-18] known as the *alveolar-arterial (A-a) gradient*. This is a result of three contributing factors: (a) venous blood that enters pulmonary veins and the left heart (i.e., thebesian veins and bronchial blood flow); (b) anatomical arteriovenous communication in the lungs (these factors normally account for a 2 to 5% shunt, or approximately 50% of the A-a oxygen gradient)[14,15,17]; and (c) mismatching of ventilation in relation to perfusion. The latter mechanism has been estimated to contribute about half of the A-a gradient in normal persons, and the contribution of any of these may be increased in disease.

Even in normal persons, there are marked regional disparities in the distribution of air and blood. For example, in the upright position, while breathing spontaneously at a normal resting volume (functional residual capacity), more air is distributed to the alveoli in the lower lung zones than the upper lung zones.[19,20] There is even significantly more blood distributed to the lower zones, however, than the upper zones, and the proportion of air to blood is greater than 1.0 in the upper zones and less than 0.8 in the lower zones. This general mismatching of air in relation to blood flow results in some alveoli receiving excessive amounts of blood in the lower lung zones, resulting in inadequately available gas; whereas in the upper zones, with an excessive amount of air, the blood is more than fully arterialized, and there is wasted ventilation.

Normal persons probably have increased A-a oxygen gradients with prolonged recumbency.[21] In one study, healthy young men had an increase from 9 mm. Hg to 19 mm. Hg after 10 days of imposed recumbency. This elevated gradient was a result of a decreased arterial Po_2, because the alveolar Po_2 remained normal. The mechanism of the decreased arterial Po_2 was not established but probably relates to mismatched ventilation in relation to perfusion. This was not observed in a shorter study of 24 to 48 hours of recumbency.[22] Furthermore, the A-a gradient is increased with age, as illustrated in Figure 4-2. This, too, is a result of reduced arterial Po_2, probably due to uneven matching of ventilation and perfusion.[23]

The alveoloarterial oxygen gradient is characteristically increased in diseases involving lung parenchyma, pulmonary airways, the pleural space, and the chest wall. As indicated in Table 4-1, when gas exchange is altered, with decreased ventilation compared with perfusion, the arterial Po_2 is reduced, and the alveolar-arterial oxygen gradient is increased while room air is breathed. When these regions are partially ventilated, the administration of 100 per cent oxygen may provide sufficient alveolar oxygen for complete arterialization of blood, with a normal A-a gradient or a slightly increased gradient. This is in contrast to conditions in which there is complete absence of ventilation, resulting in an intrapulmonary right-to-left shunt. Under these circumstances, the administration of 100 per cent oxygen has no effect on the abnormal regions, and a high A-a gradient will be observed.

A diffusion block is characterized by a decrease in the arterial Po_2, with an increased A-a oxygen gradient while room air is breathed. When high oxygen concentrations are administered, the diffusion gradient is unchanged, and the A-a gradient generally falls within the normal range.

An anatomical right-to-left shunt, such as a pulmonary arterial-venous fistula, or an atrial septal defect with reversed shunt has the same gas-exchange characteristics as an intrapulmonary right-to-left shunt which results from a complete lack of ventilation of some lung regions.

In general, the mechanism of the hypoxemia can be defined on the basis of the alveoloarterial oxygen gradient and the response of that gradient to inhalation of 100 per cent oxygen. The arterial Pco_2 is elevated only in alveolar hypoventilation or in severe disturbances of ventilation-perfusion relationships, where some regions of the lung are critically underventilated. All other causes of hypoxemia tend to stimulate ventilation, which results in normal or reduced arterial Pco_2 levels.

Exercise at modest levels is associated with mild hyperventilation and no significant change in the alveolar-arterial oxygen gradient in normal persons. In patients with alveolar hypoventilation due to primary pulmonary disease, the arterial gas abnormalities are generally aggravated. When abnormal intrapulmonary gas exchange is present, exercise produces widely varying effects on arterial blood gases. Patients with regionally decreased ventilation, compared with perfusion, may have arterial Po_2 further reduced, unchanged, or actually improved, depending on the regional effects on ventilation and perfusion during exercise. Patients with "diffusion block" characteristically have further reduced arterial Po_2 as the rate of pulmonary blood flow is increased and the time available for diffusion in the pulmonary capillaries is reduced. Patients with intrapulmonary right-to-left shunts may have variable changes in blood gases during exercise; those with anatomical right-to-left shunts vary with the site and nature of the shunt. Patients with pulmonary arteriovenous fistulas have been reported to have increased, decreased, or unchanged arterial Po_2 with exercise; this is presumably dependent on the balance between flow through the defect and other regions of the lungs. Patients with intracardiac right-to-left shunts generally aggravate their hypoxia during exercise, as a result of reduced systemic vascular resistance, whereas pulmonary arterial pressure is increased.

ASSESSMENT OF INDIVIDUAL COMPONENTS OF THE RESPIRATORY GAS EXCHANGE SYSTEM

The optimal test of respiratory gas exchange would be an analysis of arterial blood gases through the entire spectrum of a person's bodily requirements. If arterial gases were normal, not only in the laboratory while at rest, but also during a full range of physical activity, during sleep, in various body positions, and when exposed to whatever environments the person might find himself in, pulmonary gas exchange would be adequate for clinical purposes. Screening tests of pulmonary function should include the assessment of arterial blood gases at rest and during laboratory-induced exertion. In selected instances, the response to inhaled irritants, to change in posture, or to sleep may be evaluated. If the exercise is well tolerated and if no abnormalities are identified in the gas analysis, further studies are not necessary. On the other hand, if abnormalities are identified, additional studies may be warranted in order to elucidate the underlying mechanism.

ALTERED ENVIRONMENTAL GASES

The effects of altered environmental gases (e.g., at high altitude) have been dealt with in detail in Chapter 1.

ASSESSMENT OF ADEQUACY OF VENTILATION

The arterial Pco_2 is the best criterion for evaluating overall alveolar ventilation. Normally, at sea level, the arterial Pco_2 is maintained in a narrow range, from approximately 38 to 42 mm. Hg. Anxiety with transient hyperventilation, transient breath holding, and other factors that modify the rate of ventilation also modify the gases in the arterial blood. Therefore, measurements should be sought with the person in a "steady state." An increase in arterial Pco_2 above this range (e.g., greater than 45 mm. Hg) indicates alveolar hypoventilation. Conversely, a decrease below 35 mm. Hg indicates alveolar hyperventilation.

Normal Control of Ventilation

In general, the control of ventilation can be classified as follows: (a) neural control: voluntary and involuntary (respiratory center activity, reflexes); (b) chemical control: peripheral chemoreceptors and central chemoreceptors. Figure 4-3 summarizes the interrelationship of these pathways with the respiratory centers.[24]

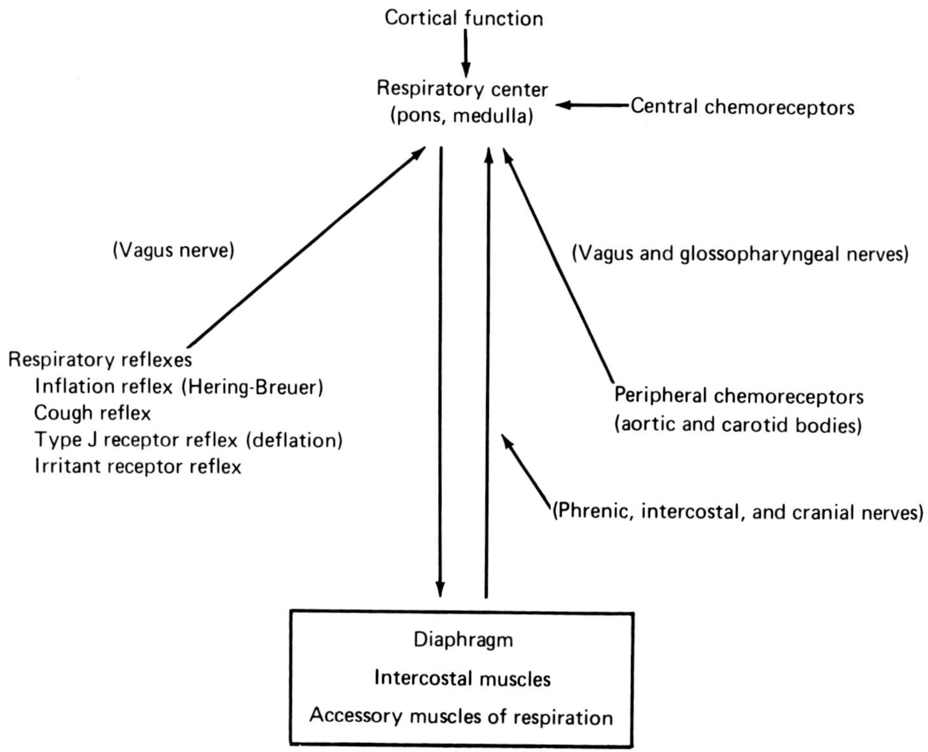

Fig. 4-3. Control of ventilation.

Neural Control

The automatic respiratory control systems arising in the pons and medulla are incredibly complex and involve areas with spontaneous persistent firing and other areas that produce feedback inhibition, eventually resulting in rhythmic stimulation of respiration.[25,26] These rhythmic stimuli are delivered through the spinal cord, the anterior horn cells, and the intercostal and phrenic nerves to the intercostal muscles and diaphragm. Ventilation, then, is proportional to the ventilatory effort. Several reflexes arise from the lung and modify the depth of respiration. The Hering-Breuer reflex is activated by the stretch of receptors in the smooth muscle of airways during inflation. This appears to modify the breathing patterns to decrease the inspiratory force of breathing. Type J receptors located in the juxtacapillary region are activated by lung congestion or microemboli, to cause rapid, shallow breathing. Irritant receptors in the bronchi (between epithelial cells and bronchial walls) are stimulated by irritants, constriction of bronchial smooth muscle, sudden collapse of bronchial walls, atelectasis, and conditions that decrease lung compliance. Stimulation of these receptors appears to cause vagal reflex hyperventilation. None of these reflexes, however, are apparently directly related to the control of blood gases.

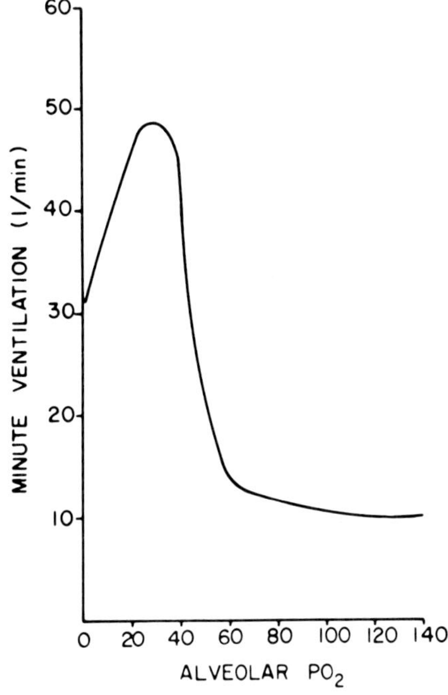

Fig. 4-4. Minute ventilation in response to decreasing inhaled oxygen. These figures from one subject indicate the range of alveolar Po_2 at which maximum respiratory stimulation occurs (approximately 30 mm. Hg). Large variation in maximum ventilatory stimulus is observed from one person to another. Several studies indicate that the ventilation is increased linearly when plotted against decreasing oxygen saturation rather than Po_2. (Compiled from data in Kellog, R. H.: Central chemical regulation of respiration. *In* Fenn, W. O., and Rahn, H. (eds.): Handbook of Physiology. Baltimore, Waverley Press, 1964)

Chemical Control

The chemical control of respiration takes place through peripheral chemoreceptors as well as the central chemoreceptors.

Peripheral Chemoreceptors. The aortic chemoreceptors are comprised of scattered groups of cells located above the aortic arch between the subclavian and common carotid arteries, and below the aortic arch between the aortic arch and the pulmonary artery. The carotid bodies are located near the bifurcation of the common carotid arteries. The blood supply to these groups of chemosensitive cells is from the systemic circulation. The afferent nerve supply is through the glossopharyngeal nerve for the carotid bodies and through the vagus nerve for the aortic chemoreceptors. These chemoreceptors are responsive to three major stimuli: Po_2, Pco_2, and pH.

Hypoxia is a modest ventilatory stimulus, effective only through the peripheral chemoreceptors located in the aortic and carotid bodies. Very mild hypoxic stimulus to respiration can be demonstrated even while room air is breathed at sea level. Further decreases in arterial Po_2 result in progressive stimulation of ventilation, to a maximum ventilatory stimulus around a Po_2 of 30 to 40 mm. Hg (Fig. 4-4). Simultaneously, however, the decreasing level of Po_2 has a suppressant

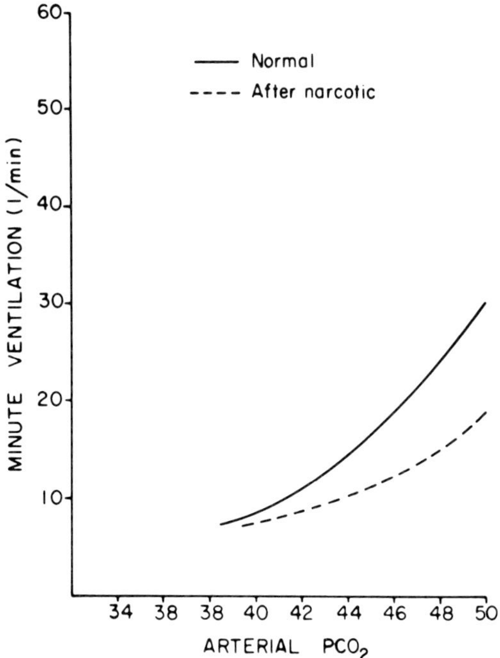

Fig. 4-5. Minute ventilation in response to increasing arterial Pco_2 is plotted for a normal person before and after he received a narcotic drug. Note the attenuated ventilatory response to carbon dioxide after the narcotic. (Compiled from data in Kellog, R. H.: Central chemical regulation of respiration. *In* Fenn, W. O., and Rahn, H. (eds.): Handbook of Physiology. Baltimore, Waverley Press, 1964)

effect on central respiratory mechanisms, and at arterial Po_2 below 20 to 25 mm. Hg, ventilatory suppression takes place. Hypoxia does not cause respiratory stimulation through central mechanisms.[27] Several studies have suggested that the magnitude of the ventilatory response is linearly related to arterial saturation, rather than to Po_2.[28]

An increase in arterial hydrogen ion concentration, or increased CO_2 tension, a decrease in blood flow or increase in blood temperature, also stimulate the peripheral chemoreceptors (Fig. 4-5). A decrease in hydrogen ion concentration, on the other hand, results in decreased stimulus to ventilation. Metabolic acidosis and metabolic alkalosis, when mild, also affect respiration through these chemosensitive areas.

Central Chemoreceptors. The medullary chemoreceptors are predominantly sensitive to changes in hydrogen ion concentration. Increased hydrogen ion concentration results in stimulation of respiration. Reduced hydrogen ion concentration results in inhibition of respiration. The location of the medullary hydrogen ion receptor (about 200 microns below the surface of the brain) makes it somewhat responsive to the characteristics of the perfusing blood, but predominantly responsive to cerebrospinal-fluid hydrogen-ion homeostasis. Normal cerebrospinal fluid pH (7.32) is somewhat more acid than peripheral blood. Furthermore, the buffering capacity of cerebrospinal fluid is substantially less than that of blood, so that rapid changes in the concentration of the highly permeable hydrogen ions result in more profound changes in the spinal fluid than in the blood.[25]

Severe acute metabolic acid-base disturbances and increased levels of carbon dioxide stimulate respiration predominantly through the effect on the chemoreceptors of rapid changes in hydrogen ion concentrations.

Gradual changes in hydrogen ion concentration, due to slow diffusion of organic acids (as may occur in metabolic acid-base disturbances), affect spinal-fluid hydrogen-ion concentration more gradually (Table 4-3). For example, the patient who develops diabetic acidosis has an increase in blood hydrogen ion concentration, which stimulates the peripheral chemoreceptors. This results in increased ventilation and in decreased arterial and spinal fluid CO_2 tension. The cerebrospinal fluid pH shifts in an alkaline direction, modifying the effect of acidosis on the peripheral chemoreceptors. As time progresses, bicarbonate is excreted from the blood and spinal fluid. With the reduced cerebrospinal fluid buffering capacity, the elevated blood hydrogen ion concentration becomes more active in stimulating respiration centrally. This state takes hours to develop. At this point, rapid correction of the metabolic acidosis in the blood would result in decreased stimulus to respiration at the level of the peripheral chemorecep-

Table 4-3. Combined Effect of Peripheral and Central Chemoreceptors in Metabolic Acid-Base Disturbances

Metabolic Event	*Effect Through Peripheral Chemoreceptors*	*Effect Through Central Chemoreceptors*	*Net Effect*
Acidosis (↑ blood [H^+])	↑ Ventilation ↓ Pco_2 blood ↓ Pco_2 C.S.F. ↓ [H^+] in C.S.F.	↓ Ventilation	Mild Hyperventilation; less than predicted from blood pH
This results in ↓ blood and C.S.F. bicarbonate, ↑ C.S.F. [H^+]		↑ Ventilation	Marked hyperventilation
Rapid correction of blood acidosis	↓ Stimulation of ventilation ↑Pco_2 ↑C.S.F. [H^+]	↑ Ventilation	Continued hyperventilation in spite of normal blood [H^+]

tors. If ventilation diminishes, the CO_2 tension increases in the blood and spinal fluid. This results in a further increase in hydrogen ion concentration in the spinal fluid, with a central stimulus to ventilation. This complex system of stimulus and inhibition results in constant modification of individual respiratory control mechanisms. Therefore, the ventilatory stimulus cannot be predicted simply by knowing the peripheral blood status at one point in time. The role of C.S.F. hydrogen ion concentration, and control of mechanisms of C.S.F. bicarbonate levels are currently under active investigation in several laboratories.[29]

Abnormal Ventilation

Causes of Hyperventilation

In the list below, the mechanisms that commonly underlie hyperventilation are itemized. In its florid form, the hyperventilation syndrome is characterized by an acute, transitory episode of gross hypernea, culminating in frank tetany, during an anxiety attack. More commonly, however, a period of anxiety results in intermittent, variable episodes, with one or multiple organ systems involved.[30] The central nervous system symptoms may include faintness, dizziness, impaired concentration, or, rarely, loss of consciousness. Peripheral nervous system symptoms include numbness and tingling of the distal extremities or the perioral regions. Musculoskeletal symptoms range from myalgia to twitching and carpopedal spasm with generalized tetany. Palpitations, tachycardia, and sharp twinges of chest pain are frequent, as is a sense of shortness of breath and chest tightness. Gastrointestinal symptoms may include dysphagia, mouth dryness, abdominal bloating, belching, or flatulence. The degree of tension and anxiety may be overt or only elucidated after considerable exploration. Weakness, chronic fatigue, and insomnia are common features. The mechanism initiating the hyperventilation is not well understood. Central nervous system excitation, increased circulating catecholamines, or inordinate awareness of the breathing act may initially trigger the hyperventilation. Once established, the respiratory alkalosis and its secondary effects on ionized calcium and magnesium result in increased neuromuscular excitability and many of the symptoms listed above. These symptoms in turn probably contribute to the degree of anxiety, thereby perpetuating the cycle (see Table 4-7).

Causes of Hyperventilation

Central nervous system excitation
- Anxiety, neurosis (hyperventilation syndrome)
- Drugs
- Central nervous system disease
- Cerebrospinal fluid acidosis

Peripheral chemoreceptor activation
- Arterial hypoxemia
  - Reduced Po_2
  - ? Reduced arterial oxygen content
- Hypotension
- Fever

Mechanism uncertain
- Exercise
- Pulmonary parenchymal disease

Drugs that increase the state of central nervous system excitation may result in respiratory stimulation as well. These include catecholamines, theophylline, ethamivan, nikethamide, and others. It is not entirely clear whether these drugs increase the responsiveness to normal physiological respiratory stimuli or increase the basic ventilatory drive.[31]

Central nervous system disease may result in a variety of ventilatory patterns.[32] Sustained central neurogenic hyperventilation, characterized by rapid deep ventilation, may occur as a result of discrete dysfunction of the brain stem or tegmentum; however, meningitis, intracranial vascular lesions, and trauma are frequently associated with hyperventilation. Acidosis or hypoxia must be excluded before hyperventilation is attributed to central mechanisms. It is possible that increased sensitivity to carbon dioxide underlies this hyperventilation. Cheyne-Stokes respiration, characterized by periods of cyclical waxing and waning of tidal volume, is commonly associated with intracranial disease. In these patients, the blood gases generally reveal a respiratory alkalosis, even during the apneic phase. This pattern of ventilation is also observed in severe obesity, at high altitudes, and in persons with heart failure. In such persons, hypoxemia, a prolonged lung-to-brain circulation time, and increased carbon dioxide sensitivity may be important causal factors.[25] Apneustic breathing (a prolonged inspiratory cramp), ataxic breathing, yawning, coughing, hiccoughing, apnea, or severe hypoventilation may all result from injuries to the brain stem and generally have a poor prognosis.

Arterial hypoxemia stimulates ventilation as described above. Although the most clearly defined stimulus is a reduction in arterial Po_2, severe sudden reductions in oxygen content (due to anemia) and abnormal oxyhemoglobin transport (such as occurs with carboxyhemoglobin) have been associated with hyperventilation. The maximum increase in ventilation is about three times normal and may be linearly correlated with decreasing oxygen saturation.

Hypotension produces increased ventilation partly through the mechanism of stimulation of carotid baroreceptors; however, it has been suggested that decreased chemoreceptor oxygen supply may play a role.[33]

Fever results in elevated resting ventilation and a marked increase in sensitivity to carbon dioxide.[34,35]

Exercise is associated with hyperventilation, even at work loads that do not result in increased circulating metabolic acids (lactate).[36,37]

Pulmonary parenchymal disease may be associated with hyperventilation, in the absence of any of the above mechanisms. It has been suggested that increased activity of the stretch receptors or the irritant receptors may result in increased stimulation of the respiratory center, with hyperventilation resulting from these mechanical changes. Again, the mechanism whereby this might occur has not been established.

Causes of Hypoventilation

The causes of hypoventilation are well discussed in Chapter 5. The list below outlines the general mechanisms. Decreased central nervous system drive to ventilation may occur as a result of destructive brain stem lesions but most commonly is a result of drugs. Characteristically, general anesthetic are associated with reduction in spontaneous ventilation and attenuated response to elevations of arterial blood Pco_2.[31,38] Recently, it has been recognized that prolonged severe metabolic alkalosis may be associated with cerebrospinal fluid alkalosis and the suppression of spontaneous ventilation.[39-42] In these persons, an increase in cerebrospinal fluid Pco_2 is associated with small increases in hydrogen ion concentration because the CO_2 is buffered by high cerebrospinal fluid bicarbonate levels.

Causes of Hypoventilation

- Decreased ventilatory drive
  - Destructive brain stem lesions
  - Drugs
  - Cerebrospinal fluid alkalosis
  - Denervation of carotid bodies
  - Adaptation to chronic hypoxia
- Neuromuscular disease
  - Spinal cord disease
  - Lower motor neuron lesions
  - Primary muscle disease
  - Decreased transmission at neuromuscular junctions
- Increased work of breathing
  - Chest wall disease
  - Pleural disease
  - Lung disease

Normally, the arterial Po_2 is sufficiently low to stimulate ventilation mildly. When a normal person raises his Po_2 by inhaling oxygen, the resting ventilation decreases. Furthermore, patients who have denervated carotid bodies (a surgical procedure that was temporarily popular in the treatment of asthma) chronically have increased arterial Pco_2, reflecting alveolar hypoventilation.[43,44] These patients have decreased ventilatory responsiveness to both increased Pco_2 and reduced Po_2 in arterial blood.

Chronic hypoxemia, particularly as seen in high-altitude natives or patients with cyanotic congenital heart disease, may be associated with a blunted respiratory drive and decreased ventilation, when compared with normal persons with similar levels of acute hypoxemia.[45]

Neuromuscular disease with paralysis of the respiratory muscles may result in hypoventilation, depending on the severity. Spinal cord transection below the outflow to the phrenic nerves generally permits normal ventilation if there is no associated bronchopulmonary disease; when the transection is above cervical segments C3 to C5, respiration is uniformly inadequate.

In countries where poliomyelitis vaccine is not yet widely disseminated, this disease accounts for a large number of deaths due to respiratory muscle paralysis. In North America, the Guillain-Barré syndrome, with its associated ascending paralysis, is now a more common cause of severe respiratory failure and hypoventilation.

A variety of primary muscular diseases may result in sufficient weakness to prevent adequate ventilation. Decreased transmission at myoneural junctions (such as occurs classically in myasthenia gravis, during the use of muscle relaxant drugs, or, occasionally, as a side effect of aminoglycoside antibiotics such as kanamycin and neomycin) may result in inadequate ventilation.

The practicing physician is most commonly faced with hypoventilation in patients who have an increased work of breathing. Chest wall disease, pleural disease, and a variety of lung diseases that cause an increase in work of breathing may be associated with a decrease in ventilation either at rest or during periods of increased demand, as occurs during exercise. These are discussed in detail in other chapters.

Methods of Assessing Adequacy of Ventilation

The net effects of hypoventilation are a reduction in the mean alveolar concentration of oxygen and an increase in the carbon dioxide, which modify the tensions of gases that equilibrate with the pulmonary capillary blood.

In the normal person, an estimate of mean alveolar gas tensions can be obtained by analyzing a single exhaled breath. The initial exhaled air is from the anatomical dead space; the rest of the exhaled air comes from peripheral lung units. Ideally, assessment of ventilatory adequacy would be done by analysis of these gases from the alveoli. Unfortunately, even in the normal person, the regional distribution of gases is not equal through the lungs, and in the diseased person it is even less uniform, so that expired gas samples do not accurately reflect average alveolar concentrations, particularly in disease. Arterial blood, on the other hand, represents an approximate average of the alveoli and may be used to assess adequacy of ventilation. When the arterial Pco_2 is elevated at rest, during sleep, or during exercise, hypoventilation is established.

Some centers have utilized the technique of having the subject rebreathe air or oxygen from an external reservoir to equilibrate alveolar gas and then assessing the Pco_2 in the reservoir gas at the end of 20 seconds. This so-called rebreathing Pco_2 approximates mixed venous Pco_2 and is approximatley 6 mm. Hg higher than the Pco_2 of alveolar gas in the normal person. The technique requires patient cooperation and is therefore not suited to periods of intense exercise or sleep. It may yield erroneous values during circulatory disturbances that markedly affect mixed venous Pco_2.[46]

Assessment of Ventilatory Drive

Measurement of Impulses to Intercostal and Phrenic Nerves. This is not well suited to analysis in the intact human or experimental animal. Under highly sophisticated experimental conditions, analysis of frequency and intensity of discharge along these nerves permits quantitation of output from the respiratory center. Current research focusing on the application of esophageal leads in assessing phrenic electromyograms has not yet established clinical usefulness.[47]

Analysis of Respiratory Effort. In recent studies, attempts have been made to assess inspiratory effort by occlusion of the airway during the initial portion of the inspiratory phase of respiration.[48] In this way, the muscles that are responsible for expanding the thoracic cage are assumed to be responding directly in proportion to the neurological stimulus and thus reflect output from the respiratory center. The peak pressure generated during the first 0.1 to 0.2 second of inspiration appears to have a quantitative correlation with the ventilatory drive. This test has the advantage of permitting an analysis of ventilatory drive in response to various stimuli, such as exercise, CO_2 breathing, oxygen or hypoxic breathing, and drugs. Furthermore, because it assesses the change in pressure developed over a very small period of time, it is not influenced by an increase in work of breathing due to lung disease. It is probably modified, however, by neuromuscular disease and severe chest wall diseases that interfere with the ability of the bellows to respond to neurological stimuli. These tests are currently being standardized and evaluated with respect to application in a variety of clinical conditions.

Ventilatory Response to Physiological Stimuli. Hypoxia. Figure 4-4 illustrates the ventilatory response commonly seen in normal persons with graded reductions in oxygen.[49,50]

In human subjects, the ventilatory response to hypoxia is best assessed by having the subject breathe graded levels of subatmospheric oxygen (e.g., 14, 12, 10%). Successive decreases in oxygen concentration may be assessed, but in normal persons, oxygen concentrations below 12 per cent may be dangerous because of severe reduction in arterial Po_2. In persons with lung disease, dangerous levels of hypoxemia may be reached at much higher concentrations of inspired oxygen. In diseased persons, concomitant analysis of arterial Po_2 may be necessary, in order to avoid hazardous hypoxemia. Ventilation may be measured by a pneumotachygraph at the mouth, or the gases may be collected in a reservoir or recording spirometer.

Increased Pco_2. Progressively increasing levels of alveolar carbon dioxide may be achieved by one of two methods (Fig. 4-5).

(a) Inhaled carbon dioxide under steady state conditions. A reservoir with a preanalyzed concentration of carbon dioxide (e.g., 5%) may be utilized. The level of oxygen should be at ambient levels, and the ventilatory response to the increased carbon dioxide should be assessed as above. Various gradations of increasing levels of carbon dioxide (e.g., 2%, 5%, 7%) may be evaluated to obtain a carbon dioxide response curve.[49]

(b) Rebreathing technique. When exhaled air is rebreathed from a reservoir, the level of CO_2 in the reservoir gradually rises, producing an increased alveolar and arterial P_{CO_2}. Ventilation may be plotted on a breath-to-breath basis or at set intervals (e.g., 30 seconds), to assess the ventilation at any given level of alveolar carbon dioxide. This technique demonstrates a wide range of ventilatory responsiveness in normal persons.[51,52] Adequate oxygen in the reservoir bag avoids a combination of hypoxic and carbon dioxide stimuli. The technique has been standardized and utilized in a wide variety of clinical conditions.

The wide range of ventilatory response to CO_2 in normal persons makes it particularly difficult to establish a cause for an elevated P_{CO_2} in patients who have a borderline response curve. For example, obesity, obstructive lung disease,[53] and bronchial asthma[54] all have a high incidence of abnormal carbon dioxide response curves. The ventilatory response to CO_2 is improved when acute episodes of respiratory failure with increased work of breathing are alleviated. Several explanations for a low ventilatory response to carbon dioxide have been considered. These persons may have a borderline carbon dioxide responsiveness in their normal state, further suppressed by a period of increased work of breathing. On the other hand, the increased work of breathing may be sufficient to cause a high level of carbon dioxide production, with a biological feedback inhibition of respiratory centers, which results in a decreased respiratory drive.

Assessment of Neuromuscular Function

Neurological or muscular diseases that result in hypoventilation impair the bellows function of the lung. This can be readily identified by simple ventilatory measurements such as the vital capacity or maximum voluntary ventilation. In general, if the vital capacity is more than three times the normal tidal volume for that person, hypoventilation should not occur, at least while at rest.[55]

Assessment of Work of Breathing

Increased resistance to the breathing act may be due to (a) elastic resistance, which accompanies a decreased compliance of the chest wall or lung, or (b) nonelastic resistance, which results from increased airway resistance, tissue viscous resistance, or inertia.

Although these physiological concepts may be of great interest, and although each component can be quantitated by sophisticated techniques, it is unlikely that a detailed breakdown is required for clinical purposes. In most instances where the work of breathing is contributing to a clinically significant degree of hypoventilation, ventilatory function is abnormal, as assessed by the vital capacity, maximum expiratory flow rates, and lung volumes. Under special circumstances, it may be desirable to assess the individual components of resistance in detail (see Chap. 3).

The oxygen cost of breathing is very difficult to assess, because it is impossible to partition the blood flow to respiratory muscles from the rest of the body. The oxygen cost of increasing ventilation above resting levels, however, can be estimated during carbon-dioxide induced hyperventilation, assuming that the subject's only change in energy consumption is due to the work of the respiratory muscles. The normal person appears to utilize 1 to 2 milliliters of oxygen per liter of ventilation, and diseased persons utilize approximately two to ten times this amount.[56,57] With severe obstructive disease, the cost of increasing ventilation may exceed the benefits of increasing the ventilation.

ASSESSMENT OF INTRAPULMONARY GAS EXCHANGE

The factors affecting the ventilatory function of the lungs were reviewed in detail in Chapter 3. The effectiveness of the lung as a gas exchange unit requires more than overall ventilation in appropriate quantities. Regional distribution of that air through each of the peripheral lung units must be exquisitely balanced with the blood flow. Too much air will be wasted by ventilating units in excess of blood flow. On the other hand, too little air fails to arterialize the blood perfusing those units.

Distribution of Ventilation

Regional differences in pleural pressures, along with gravity acting on the lung, result in dependent (lower) lung regions being less expanded than the upper regions of the lung. While breathing at normal resting levels (FRC), there is greater respiratory movement in the dependent regions. In the upright position, then, the lower regions of the lung receive more air per breath than the upper regions of the lung (Fig. 4-6). Patients with respiratory disease may have dramatically impaired regional distribution of ventilation to any size of lung unit. For example, a large pneumothorax, pleural effusion, or total atelectasis of the lung may completely prevent ventilation of a hemithorax. Similarly, conditions affecting smaller portions of the airways, such as obstruction due to secretions or bronchospasm in bronchial asthma, a foreign body, aspiration of foreign material, or pulmonary edema affecting bronchial walls, may all decrease the size of the airway to a given region of the lung and thereby diminish the ventilation to that region. In addition, a partially destroyed lung unit may be hyperinflated, as occurs in emphysema, but may not be ventilated with each breath and therefore may receive inadequate ventilation. In each of these circumstances, ventilation may be reduced, as compared with the pulmonary blood flow, and there will be insufficient ventilation to permit arterialization of the blood flowing through the lung units.[58,59]

Conversely, persons with thromboembolic disease resulting in pulmonary vascular occlusion, or regional spasm of the pulmonary arteries due to hypoxia, or acidosis may have some areas of the lung receiving poor blood supply, compared with the level of ventilation. Such regions of the lung may be relatively overventilated and contribute to wasted ventilation.

Methods of Assessing Regional Ventilation

- Abnormal movement of the chest wall
  - Asymmetrical movement of the thoracic wall
    - Atelectasis
    - Pneumothorax
    - Pleural disease
    - Pneumonia
    - Kyphoscoliosis
    - Chest wall pain
- Reduced diaphragmatic motion
  - Phrenic paralysis
  - Postoperatively
- Auscultation
  - Regional abnormalities of breath sounds
  - Rhonchi (inspiratory or expiratory)
- Chest film
  - Regional hyperlucency
  - Parenchymal disease
  - Abnormal bronchial walls
- Bronchospirometry
- Tests of distribution of inhaled inert gases
  - Single-breath nitrogen washout
  - Multiple-breath nitrogen washout
  - Mixing efficiency (helium)
  - Closing volume
  - Radioisotope inhalation with lung scanning
- Assessment of physiological dead space or alveolar-arterial oxygen gradient

---

The list above shows the methods that may be used to identify abnormalities of regional ventilation. When patients have gross abnormalities, bedside examination may reveal marked changes. With the patient positioned comfortably and symmetrically, unilateral lag of chest wall movement may be the most striking clinical manifestation of atelectasis, pneumothorax, pleural disease, pneumonia, kyphoscoliosis, or localized chest wall disease. Similarly, reduced diaphragmatic motion with respiration may indicate phrenic paralysis or the characteristic decrease in diaphragmatic motion after abdominal surgery. The latter results in re-

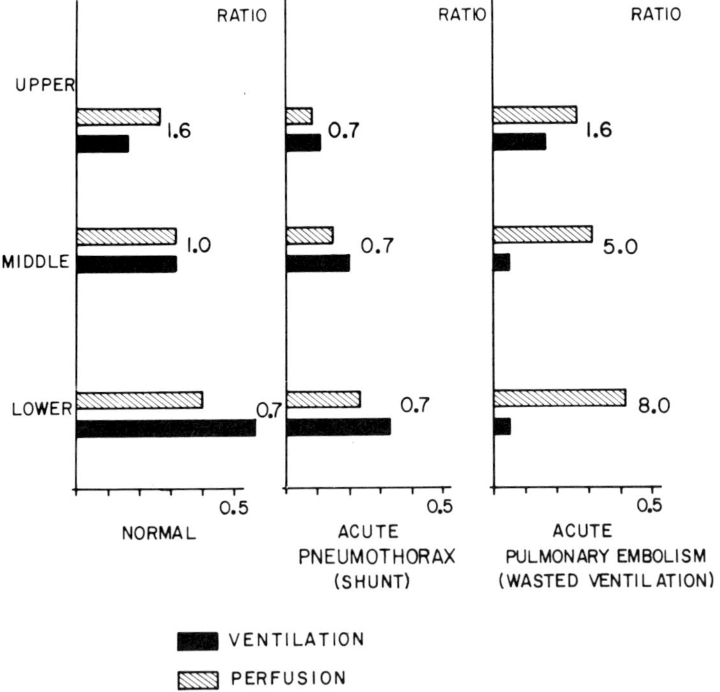

Fig. 4-6. Ventilation-perfusion relationships in the lung. (*Left*) Bar graphs indicate the proportion of normal total ventilation and perfusion for the upper, middle, and lower thirds of the lung. These arbitrary divisions are not precisely quantitative and do not coincide with the physiologically sound division into Zone 1, Zone 2, and Zone 3. As indicated in the text, Zone 1 has no perfusion and would therefore be even higher than the upper zone indicated in this graph. (*Center*) Bar graphs demonstrate the effect of a pneumothorax on ventilation and perfusion in the affected lung. During the acute phase, ventilation would be strikingly reduced. As a compensatory mechanism, the perfusion is eventually also shunted to the opposite lung (which is being ventilated). This takes minutes to hours, however, to become established. As is apparent, perfusion in excess of ventilation in this lung will result in physiological shunt. (*Right*) The third set of graphs demonstrates the effect of a massive pulmonary embolism involving vessels to the middle and lower zones of the lung. Note that the perfusion is strikingly reduced, but ventilation is initially near normal. This, then, will result in wasted ventilation or physiological dead space. Later in the course, the distribution of ventilation and perfusion is affected by more complex factors.

duced ventilation, particularly in the lower lung zones. When motion of the thoracic cage in all its diameters appears to be approximately normal, abnormalities of regional ventilation may still be identified by physical examination. Auscultation frequently demonstrates evidence of underlying airways disease. The dramatically reduced breath sounds in the periphery of the lung in patients with emphysema, the presence of widespread inspiratory and expiratory rhonchi in the asthmatic, terminal expiratory rhonchi in the patient with bronchitis, and the inspiratory rales commonly heard in pulmonary edema all provide sound clinical suspicion of abnormalities of regional distribution of air.

The plain chest film is commonly helpful in identifying abnormalities associated with alterations in regional ventilation. Hyperlucency may indicate the parenchymal destruction of emphysema. Densities indicating parenchymal disease may suggest areas of decreased compliance that will be poorly ventilated. Thickened bronchial walls may indicate airway abnormalities, as in bronchitis or bronchial asthma. Each of these should alert the physician to the possibility of abnormal gas exchange. Some centers take inspiratory and expiratory films, with sequential films during a forced expiratory maneuver. The changes in lung volume measured in specific lobes and in the entire lung fields, particularly in relation to expiratory time, can provide substantial evidence regarding the regional distribution of gases.

Bronchospirometry, a technique that measures the ventilation of each lung by direct cannulation of the bronchi with a tracheal tube, has been less popular since the introduction of indirect and less traumatic tests of distribution of ventilation.[60]

Numerous tests have been designed to assess the evenness of distribution of air in the lungs. These have been discussed in detail in Chapter 3. In symptomatic patients, they are required only to confirm or quantitate clinical impressions. In mild or early disease, these tests may provide the only objective evidence for abnormal function. It is of utmost importance to recognize that all of these tests only indicate abnormalities in ventilation. No assessment of perfusion in relation to the regions of altered ventilation can be obtained by these methods.

Distribution of Perfusion

It is now well established that the patterns of blood flow in the lung can be generally divided into four zones.[59-63] This distribution of blood flow through the lungs is normally predominantly determined by simple pressure relationships as follows.

Zone 1, which is in the apical regions of the lung in the upright position, is too high for the hydrostatic pressure in the pulmonary artery to perfuse. At this level, the pressure in the alveolus (atmospheric) is greater than the pressure in the artery, and consequently the capillaries remain collapsed. This arbitrary zone is, of course, obliterated when the person lies down, or during exercise, when pulmonary artery pressure rises. Furthermore, there is no sharp division between Zone 1 and the next lower zone, because slightly lower regions of the lung have portions of the cardiac cycle during which pulmonary artery pressure is greater than atmospheric, therefore distending the capillaries at least during systole, resulting in small amounts of pulsatile flow.

In the next lower zone, Zone 2, pulmonary artery pressure is greater than atmospheric and therefore greater than the alveolar pressure, and there is a driving pressure for forward flow through the pulmonary capillaries. Progressing to lower regions of the lung, the pulmonary artery pressure increases linearly with the distance, but the alveolar pressure is still atmospheric. Therefore, the hydrostatic driving pressure increases linearly, and blood flow increases proportionately with distance down the lung. This second zone is roughly in the upper portion of the midlung field and again is not sharply demarcated from the next lower zone.

The third zone, representing the lower lung regions, is also characterized by linear increases in blood flow proportionate to the distance down the lung. At this level in the lung, the pulmonary venous pressure and the pulmonary arterial pressure are both greater than atmospheric. Therefore, the driving pressure is determined by pulmonary arterial pressure minus pulmonary venous pressure. Because both pressures increase linearly with descent down the lung, intravascular hydrostatic driving pressure does not explain the progressive increase in blood flow. A more likely explanation is the increase in both arterial and venous pressure, resulting in high intracapillary hydrostatic pressures that produce distention of pulmonary capillaries in this lower zone. In fact, studies of capillary volume have indicated that the capillaries in the apices of the lung are collapsed throughout the cardiac cycle, whereas capillaries in the bases of the lung are widely distended.[59] The progressive increments in blood flow in Zones 2 and 3 are illustrated in the upper, middle, and lower thirds of the lung (Fig. 4-6).

A fourth zone is of little clinical significance at the present time in normal persons. In this small region at the inferior aspect of the lung, flow is limited by interstitial pressure, owing to the effects of gravity on the parenchyma of the lung and pleural pressures, and in this region blood flow is again reduced.

It is clear from this physiological zoning in the lung that changes in alveolar pressure, pulmonary arterial pressure, or pulmonary venous pressure all affect the hydrostatic pressures in the pulmonary vasculature and modify the dustribution of blood flow. Similarly, changes in the person's position modify the dependent region (Zone 3) and the upper region (Zone 1). The zones can be entirely reversed in the normal subject who stands on his head.

Symmetrical changes in the distribution of perfusion are seen in both lungs in patients with elevated venous pressure. For example, patients with mitral stenosis shift the region of maximum blood flow in their lungs from the bottom upward and may do so approximately proportionally to the increase in venous pressure.[64,65] Patients with elevated pulmonary artery pressures also have symmetrically altered perfusion, predominantly characterized by increased perfusion of the apical lung regions and somewhat decreased perfusion in the lower lung regions.[66]

Regional changes in perfusion occur in a number of disease states. Pulmonary embolism results in obstruction of vessels of varying sizes and in various locations, with decreased blood flow beyond the region of the obstruction. A condition that occurs uncommonly, the Swyer-James syndrome, or the Macleod syndrome, is characterized by severe narrowing of one of the pulmonary arteries.[67-69] Transient modifications in pulmonary vascular tone, due to hypoxia, acidosis, or perhaps inflammation, may result in regional deficits of perfusion, and patients with destructive changes of emphysema characteristically lose blood supply to areas of the lung.[70] Ventilation is less evenly distributed in the older age groups.[71] Whenever these lung regions continue to be ventilated out of proportion to the lung blood flow, the ventilation is wasted.

The list below summarizes the methods of evaluating regional distribution of perfusion. Here the physical examination is not nearly as rewarding as when evaluating ventilation. The physical examination is helpful only in those circumstances where modified flow results in turbulence with the production of murmurs. Consequently, the continuous murmur heard in the region of a pulmonary arteriovenous fistula or the systolic murmurs heard peripherally in the lung with peripheral pulmonary artery stenosis may draw attention to these uncommon abnormalities of regional distribution of perfusion. The chest film may be somewhat more helpful, because striking decreases in vascularity are seen with pulmonary embolism, and increased vascularity is seen with acute elevations in pulmonary venous pressure or in high pulmonary blood flow, as noted in congenital left-to-right shunts. The nodular densities seen in pulmonary arteriovenous fistulas generally require additional evidence, such as angiography, to confirm the nature of the lesion.

Methods of Assessing Regional Perfusion

Auscultation
- Continuous murmur with pulmonary A-V fistula
- Systolic murmurs with pulmonary artery stenosis

Chest film
- Decreased vascularity (pulmonary embolism)
- Increased vascularity (congenital left-to-right shunt)
- Nodular densities (pulmonary A-V fistulas)

Bronchospirometry

Tests of distribution of blood flow
- Intravenous, inert, insoluble isotopic gases with lung scanning
- Intravenous isotope-labeled macroaggregates with lung scanning
- Pulmonary angiography

Assessment of physiological dead space or alveolar-arterial oxygen gradients

In general, definitive demonstration of abnormal regional distribution of blood in the lungs is dependent on more sophisticated techniques. Bronchospirometry permits estimation of blood flow by analyzing the oxygen uptake and carbon dioxide release of a lung that is ventilated. Lung scanning by use of radioisotopes may be performed following injection of gaseous isotopes that are insoluble and that cross the alveolar membrane into alveolar tissues in the lungs. Appropriately timed counting of radioactivity over the lungs permits imaging.[60] Clinically, more commonly macroaggregated proteins are labeled with isotopes and injected intravenously. They are distributed wherever blood flow goes in the lung, trapped in pulmonary capillaries, and emit their radioactivity. Lung tissues may then be mapped according to the amount of radioactivity in the capillaries. Regions with decreased radioactivity indicate decreased blood flow. This technique is particularly applicable to the study of the microcirculation of the lung, but as might be expected, only fairly large lung units can be analyzed; terminal lung units cannot be identified individually by this technique. Pulmonary angiography is useful when identifying the structure of the large vessels and, if sequentially performed, can demonstrate approximately where blood flow is distributed. Large abnormalities in the amount of blood flow can be estimated from the density of the radiopaque dye.

Determinants of Pulmonary Artery Pressure

The factors that result in elevated pulmonary artery pressure are indicated in the list below.[72-77] In general, these can be classified according to the well-known formula that describes the interrelationships of flow, driving pressures, and resistance:

$$\text{resistance} = \frac{\text{driving pressure}}{\text{flow}}$$

For the majority of blood flow, in the pulmonary vascular bed, the driving pressure equals the pulmonary artery pressure minus the pulmonary venous pressure. Therefore, the formula can be rearranged as follows:

$$\text{resistance} = \frac{\text{pulmonary artery pressure} - \text{pulmonary venous pressure}}{\text{flow}}$$

or: pulmonary artery pressure = [resistance × flow] + pulmonary venous pressure.

Factors Affecting Pulmonary Artery Pressure

- Increased pulmonary blood flow
  - Exercise
  - Fever
  - Congenital heart disease with left-to-right shunts
- Increased pulmonary venous pressure
  - Left ventricular failure
  - Mitral valve disease
  - Pulmonary vein thrombosis
- Increased pulmonary vascular resistance
  - Vasospasm
    - Hypoxia
    - Hypercapnia
    - Acidosis
    - Histamine
    - Angiotensin
    - ? Serotonin
    - ? Vasoactive peptides
    - ? Prostaglandins ($F_{2\alpha}$)
  - Vascular wall hypertrophy
    - Long-standing hypoxia
    - Long-standing increase in PA pressure
  - Perivascular edema
  - Vascular thromboemboli
  - Destruction of vascular bed
    - Emphysema
    - Fibrosis
    - Surgical resection

It is apparent that any factors which increase pulmonary blood flow, pulmonary vascular resistance, or pulmonary venous pressure will produce elevated pulmonary artery pressures. The pulmonary vascular bed is very distensible, and consequently increased pulmonary blood flow accounts for only small changes in pulmonary artery pressure. Exercise that results in a two- to threefold increase in pulmonary blood flow increases the pulmonary artery pressure only to a small degree. Further increases in

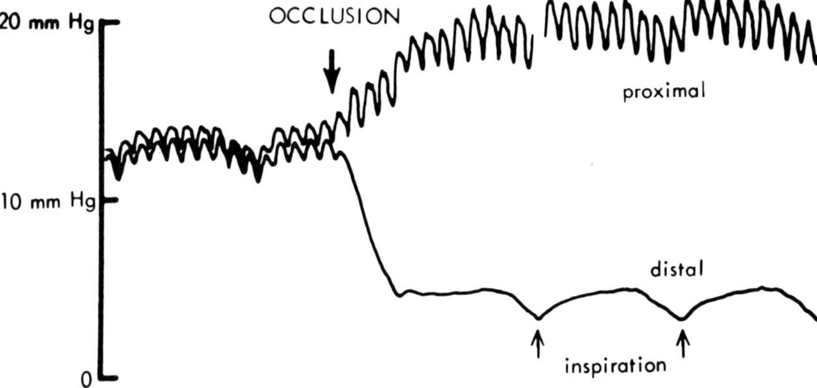

Fig. 4-7. Effect of occlusion of one pulmonary artery on pulmonary-artery pressure. The graph demonstrates the pressure in the pulmonary artery proximal and distal to an inflatable balloon. At the time of occlusion, the pressure distal to the balloon drops to the pressure in the pulmonary veins and left atrium. The pressure proximal to the balloon rises because of the reduced total vascular bed. The mean increase in pressure demonstrated here, from 12 to 18 mm. Hg, is a normal pulmonary-artery-pressure response to doubling the blood flow to the lung. Because the pulmonary-artery pressure did not double, the pulmonary vascular resistance in the perfused lung has decreased to accept the additional blood flow.

the rate of flow, however, result in a striking increase in pulmonary artery pressure.

Blood flow through a given lung can also be increased by occlusion of the artery to the opposite lung. When this is done by inflation of a balloon catheter positioned in one of the pulmonary arteries, the pressure in the artery perfusing the opposite lung rises to a slight degree (Fig. 4-7). As is apparent, this small rise in pressure that occurs with the relatively large rise in blood flow must be associated with an actual drop in pulmonary vascular resistance. This is generally attributed to recruitment of additional vessels that may not have been perfused or to distention of vessels in this relatively compliant vascular system. Patients with more rigid vascular beds due to disease (as occurs with sustained pulmonary hypertension, chronic obstructive lung disease, and diffuse pulmonary parenchymal disease) no longer have the same compliant pulmonary vascular bed, and their pulmonary artery pressure rises much more quickly during exercise or times of increased cardiac output. The increase in pulmonary artery pressure that results from increased pulmonary venous pressure is seen characteristically in patients with left ventricular failure or mitral valve disease. During the early phase, the rise of pulmonary artery pressure is approximately proportionate to the rise in pulmonary venous pressure.

The above mechanisms of increasing pulmonary pressure are readily evaluated. A more comprehensive understanding of pulmonary vascular physiology is required to elucidate the mechanisms of increased vascular resistance. In general, this may be caused by vasospasm, vascular wall hypertrophy as a result of long-standing vasospasm, perivascular edema, vascular thrombi or emboli, or destruction of the vascular bed by parenchymal disease. Of this group of causes, those which are physiologically reversible bear additional consideration. Alveolar hypoxia,[76-78] hypercapnia, and acidosis[79,80] are common causes of pulmonary hypertension during episodes of acute respiratory failure. Many times, however, the above mechanisms are not so clearly active,[81] and numerous other factors affecting pulmonary vasomotor

Table 4-4. Comparison of Responses of Systemic and Pulmonary Vascular Beds

Vasoactive Factor	*Systemic*	*Pulmonary*
Hypoxia	Dilates	Constricts
Acidosis	Dilates	Constricts
Hypercapnia	Dilates	Constricts
Theophylline	Dilates	Dilates
Isoproterenol	Dilates (β adrenergic)	Dilates
Angiotensin	Constricts	Constricts
Histamine	Dilates	Constricts

tone have been well documented. Histamine, serotonin, and various prostaglandins have all been incriminated at one time or another, but none of these has been clearly demonstrated to be the specific mechanism of pulmonary vasomotor changes in a given disease. It is to be hoped that active investigation in this area will clarify additional factors that are clinically important.[73,82-86] Finally, increased blood viscosity (particularly at hematocrits above 55 and under conditions of high pulmonary blood flow) may raise the resistance to perfusion.[87,88]

It is noteworthy that several factors affecting the pulmonary circulation have quite different effects on the systemic circulation, as itemized in Table 4-4.

The administration of oxygen, theophylline, isoproterenol, or acetylcholine may result in reduced pulmonary vascular resistance in persons in whom it was elevated. This evidence of reversibility may be particularly important when planning therapy. Prolonged administration of oxygen may further reduce pulmonary vascular resistance in those whose primary problem is related to hypoxia. These factors are discussed in detail in Chapter 13.

The vasospasm that takes place in pulmonary vessels during hypoxia seems teleologically appropriate in the fetus, where blood should be shunted to the systemic circulation. Furthermore, if the ductus arteriosus remains patent, increased pulmonary vascular resistance in the neonate may modify the degree of shunting of systemic blood through the pulmonary circulation. In the adult, the advantages of diminished blood flow through lung regions that are not ventilated (and have a low Po_2) are also apparent. This diminishes the amount of wasted perfusion or shunt-like effect in the lung and thereby permits diseased regions of the lung to autoregulate the impact on oxygen exchange in the lungs. The generalized vasoconstriction that occurs in persons with respiratory failure or at high altitude, however, cannot be rationalized to the same degree.

Effects of Abnormalities of Regional Ventilation or Perfusion on Gas Exchange

Decreased Ventilation in Relation to Perfusion

When ventilation is reduced in relation to perfusion, blood flowing through these areas of the lungs will leave without adequate exposure to respiratory gases and will be partially venous. This has the same effect as an anatomical shunt. Most diseases that affect the airways do not affect the vasculature of the lungs in precisely the same location or to the same degree; therefore, a wide variety of airway diseases result in some regions with ventilation decreased in relation to perfusion. Such persons generally have arterial hypoxemia.

The presence of arterial hypoxemia raises concern regarding regional hypoventilation (Fig. 4-8). This can be further defined by calculation of the alveoloarterial gradient. The average alveolar Po_2 can be calculated by using the alveolar gas equation as follows.[89]

$$\underset{\text{unknown}}{\underset{\downarrow}{P_AO_2}} = \underset{\text{known}}{\underset{\downarrow}{P_IO_2}} - \underset{\text{measured}}{\underset{\downarrow}{P_ACO_2}} \left[F_IO_2 + \underset{\text{correcting factor}}{\underset{\downarrow}{\frac{1 - F_IO_2}{R}}}\right]$$

The partial pressure of inspired oxygen (P_IO_2) can be calculated as outlined in Chapter 1. The partial pressure of alveolar CO_2 is almost identical to arterial Pco_2, and thus they can be used interchangeably. The

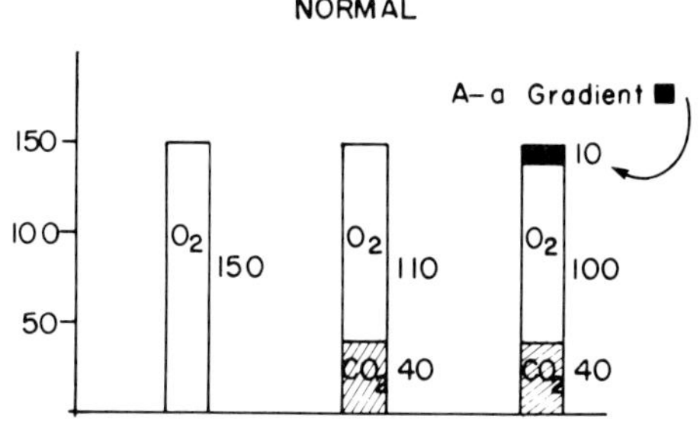

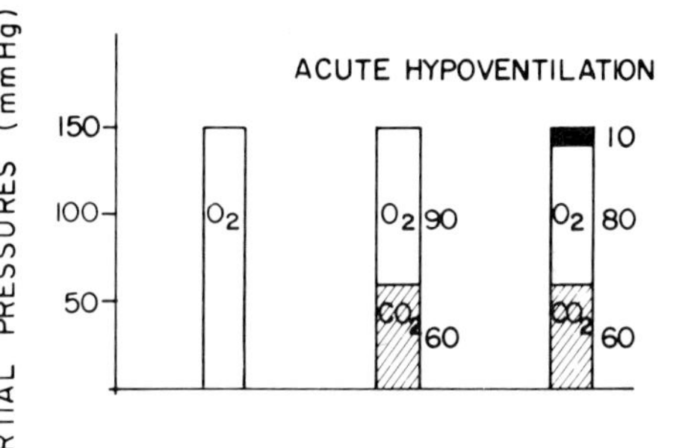

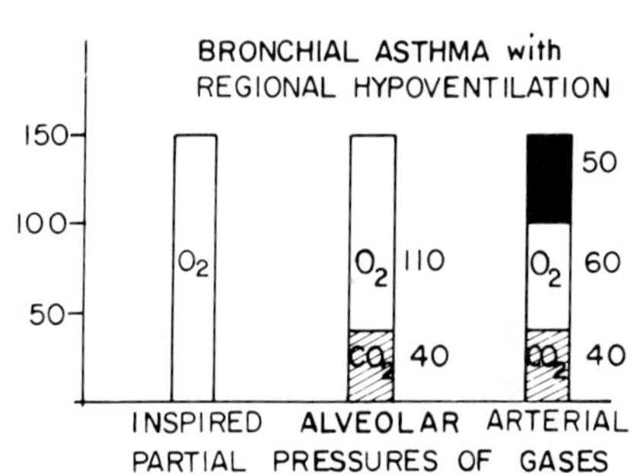

Fig. 4-8. Alveolar-arterial oxygen gradient. (*Top*) Bar graph demonstrates the normal gas partial-pressure relationships in inspired, alveolar, and arterial compartments, respectively. At sea level, the inspired oxygen (corrected for water vapor pressure) is 150 mm. Hg. As the air is inhaled, the gas partial pressures in the alveolus must add up to barometric pressure. Because nitrogen is neither utilized nor produced by the body, the partial pressure of nitrogen is approximately the same in the alveolus as in the inspired air. When the respiratory quotient is 1, the oxygen removed from the alveolus equals the carbon dioxide delivered to the alveolus (i. e., if 40 mm. Hg of oxygen are removed, 40 mm. Hg of carbon dioxide will be added). Because alveolar carbon dioxide is approximately equal to the arterial carbon dioxide, the inspired Po_2 minus the arterial Pco_2 equals the alveolar Po_2, and the alveolar Po_2 minus the arterial Po_2 equals the alveoloarterial gradient. Although under highly controlled conditions this gradient is less than 10 in most normal subjects, when these crude calculations are used, a range of up to 20 should probably be accepted as normal. (*Center*) Graph demonstrates the effect of a high arterial (and alveolar) Pco_2 on alveolar Po_2. This patient with acute hypoventilation cannot possibly have an arterial Po_2 greater than 90; with a gradient of 10, his arterial Po_2 is 80. This, then, is a normal gradient in spite of a reduced arterial Po_2. (*Bottom*) Graph demonstrates a patient with a normal arterial (and alveolar) Pco_2, a normal alveolar Po_2, but an unusually low arterial Po_2. The alveolar Po_2 (110) is 50 mm. higher than the arterial Po_2, indicating a very high alveoloarterial gradient. Simple construction of these plots for hypoxic patients permits reasonably accurate delineation of the mechanism of reduced arterial Po_2. When the arterial Po_2 is reduced as a result of high altitude, the inspired Po_2 would be less than 150 mm. Hg, and each subsequent compartment would reflect this reduced inspired oxygen.

correcting factor is introduced because of the variation in tension of alveolar gases under conditions with different respiratory quotients. The effect of the respiratory quotient on alveolar gases was discussed in Chapter 1. This can be determined simply by measuring oxygen consumption and carbon dioxide production. The average respiratory quotient is 0.8. For clinical purposes, this equation can be simplified to:

$$P_AO_2 = P_IO_2 - \frac{PaCO_2}{0.8}$$

Furthermore:

$$\text{A-a gradient} = P_AO_2 - P_aO_2$$

Then one can calculate the alveoloarterial oxygen gradient by subtracting this alveolar gas Po_2 from the measured arterial Po_2. For practical clinical purposes, gradients greater than 20 mm. Hg are abnormal. In the older age groups, perhaps 25 mm. Hg should be considered abnormal (Fig. 4-2).

Additional tests to elucidate the mechanism of an increased alveolar-arterial gra-

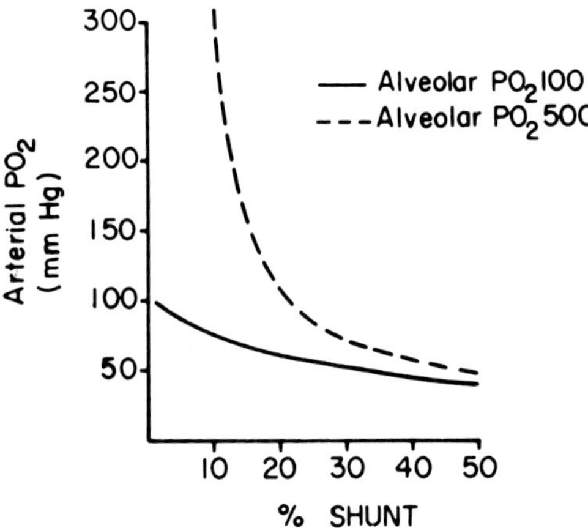

Fig. 4-9. Effect of true physiological shunt on arterial Po_2. This figure demonstrates the magnitude of shunt required to produce various levels of arterial Po_2, breathing room air (alveolar Po_2 100) or breathing 75 per cent oxygen (alveolar Po_2 500). Note that an arterial Po_2 less than 50 mm. Hg, with a normal alveolar Po_2, indicates approximately 30 per cent physiological shunt. When breathing high concentrations of inspired oxygen, the Po_2 is regularly greater than 100, except where the shunt is quite large (greater than 20%). (Adapted from Pontoppidan, H., Geffin, B., and Lowenstein, E.: Acute respiratory failure in the adult. N. Engl. J. Med., *287*:743, 1972)

dient may be directed at understanding whether the region is underventilated (but still ventilated) or has a "true physiological shunt" (perfused areas of the lung that are totally without ventilation).[90] If there is some (although inadequate) ventilation, the administration of oxygen to the inhaled air may dramatically improve the oxygen available to the pulmonary capillary blood flow, and the arterial Po_2 will approach normal values. When there is a complete absence of ventilation, as may occur with atelectasis, administration of increased inhaled oxygen will not improve the arterialization of blood in that region of the lung, and the arterial blood Po_2 value will remain much lower than that predicted for the inspired oxygen. The list below shows factors that affect the A-a gradient.[90]

Factors That Influence the Alveolar-Arterial Oxygen Gradient

Right-to-left shunt

Inspired oxygen levels (ventilation-perfusion inequalities have a greater role at lower inspired Po_2)

Mixed venous oxygen content

Oxygen consumption (through its effect on mixed venous oxygen content)

Cardiac output (through its effect on arteriovenous oxygen difference)

Position of the oxyhemoglobin dissociation curve

It is impossible to tell from this data whether a high A-a gradient on 100 per cent oxygen is due to an anatomical intracardiac or intrapulmonary shunt or merely to blood flowing through regions of the lung that are totally without ventilation.

The easiest way to quantitate such a true physiological shunt is to have the patient inhale 100 per cent oxygen until all the nitrogen is washed out of the lungs. At this point, the alveolar Po_2 equals barometric pressure minus arterial Pco_2 minus water vapor pressure. At sea level, this would be 760 − 40 − 47, or 673, mm. Hg.[90]

The deficiency of oxygen exchange can be estimated from this alveoloarterial gradient and expressed as a quantitative shunt. In normal man at rest, the portion of blood "shunted" ranges from 2 to 5 per cent of the cardiac output. A 50 per cent shunt is compatible with life only if the person is breathing nearly 100 per cent oxygen. Figure 4-9 illustrates the effect of increasing inspired oxygen tensions on the A-a gradient with different degrees of shunt. The following parameters permit quantitation of the shunt.[89,90]

$$\frac{\text{shunt blood flow}}{\text{cardiac output}} = \frac{\text{arterial oxygen content} - \text{pulmonary venous oxygen content}}{\text{systemic venous oxygen content} - \text{pulmonary venous oxygen content}}$$

Application of this shunt calculation in detail requires measurement of cardiac output, mixed venous oxygen content, arterial oxygen content, and the assumption that pulmonary venous blood is ideally oxygenated.[89] If inhalation of 100 per cent oxygen does not raise the arterial Po_2 above 100 mm. Hg, the shunt is greater than 20 per cent.

Precise localization of the area of shunt (e.g., anatomical vascular or pulmonary parenchymal) may require cardiac catheterization or angiography.

Increased Ventilation in Relation to Perfusion

Under normal circumstances, ventilation of the nasal passages, oropharynx, trachea, and bronchi, down to the gas-exchanging units, has been termed the *anatomical dead space*. This dead space ventilation is "wasted." When peripheral lung units contribute to wasted ventilation, this is in excess of the anatomical dead space, and the entire functional dead space has been termed the *physiological dead space*.

The physiological dead space can be readily measured during normal breathing. The following equation indicates the components that must be known:

$$\text{dead space ventilation} = \frac{(\text{arterial } Pco_2 - \text{expired } Pco_2) \times \text{minute ventilation}}{\text{arterial } Pco_2}$$

This simply requires measurement of arterial Pco_2, collection of timed samples of expired air, calculation of minute ventilation, and analysis of the expired gas for carbon dioxide. When the rate of respiration is known, this may be converted to dead space per breath.[89] (Dividing minute ventilation by the respiratory rate yields tidal volume; dividing dead space ventilation by the tidal rate yields dead space per breath.) Dead space is normally increased approximately proportionally to body size and tidal volume. The ratio of physiological dead space (per breath) to tidal volume permits an estimate of the wasted ventilation. In general, this ratio should not exceed 0.3 in normal persons.

The techniques of assessing the alveoloarterial oxygen gradient and the physiological dead space are useful in establishing functionally significant ventilation-perfusion inequalities. (See also Chap. 5.)

Diffusion Across the Alveolocapillary Membranes

Normally, blood perfusing the pulmonary capillaries is in contact with aerated alveoli long enough to permit almost complete equilibration of gases. In fact, carbon dioxide diffuses readily, so that the major portion of diffusion is completed within the first 20 per cent of the transit time through the pulmonary capillary. Oxygen, on the other hand, is only 95 per cent equilibrated within the first 30 per cent of the time the blood is in the capillary. The rate of diffusion of oxygen may decrease when the alveolocapillary membrane is thickened, thus increasing the length of the diffusion path. When the time required for equilibration exceeds the time available in the capillary, the blood leaving the capillary is incompletely arterialized. In view of the very rapid diffusion of carbon dioxide, this does not influence arterial Pco_2 significantly. It is apparent, then, that in a patient with an increased barrier to diffusion, anything that speeds up the rate of blood flow through the pulmonary capillary consequently shortens the time for equilibration and amplifies the degree of hypoxia. Consequently, hypoxia that results from a diffusion block is always worse during exercise, fever, and other circumstances with an increased rate of pulmonary blood flow. At present, there is no widely accepted technique for assessing the rate of diffusion as such. Although the rate of diffusion might be easily calculated if the lung were composed of a single alveolus, analysis of gas exchange throughout millions of terminal lung units becomes much more complex. Methods have been established for calculating the diffusing capacity of oxygen, but these are not readily applicable clinically.[89]

The most popular methods use the rate of transfer of carbon monoxide. Carbon monoxide is readily measurable; its diffusion characteristics are approximately comparable to those of oxygen; and it is bound by hemoglobin, as is oxygen. Therefore, many of the factors involved in oxygen transfer are comparable to those of carbon monoxide. Two general methods have been developed for the assessment of carbon monoxide "diffusion capacity."[91] Steady-state techniques assess the average rate of transfer of tracer amounts of carbon monoxide from inhaled air to the blood, over a period of several minutes. The amount of carbon monoxide inhaled minus the amount exhaled indicates the amount that has been transferred. Estimates of the alveolar carbon monoxide partial pressure then permit calculations of the amount of carbon monoxide transferred per mm. Hg partial pressure of carbon monoxide, per minute. Single-breath techniques require an inhalation of tracer amounts of carbon monoxide with a timed period of breath holding, during which carbon monoxide is transferred to pulmonary capillary blood. Although the principles are similar, these single-breath techniques generally estimate higher levels of carbon monoxide diffusing capacity than do steady-state techniques. In fact, neither of these methods measures the diffusion characteristics of the alveolocapillary membrane as such. Both methods are affected by regional distribution of ventilation, alveolocapillary surface area, pulmonary vascular back pressure of carbon monoxide (which may be present as a result of environmental pollution or smoking), pulmonary capillary blood flow, alveolar oxygen partial pressures, hemoglobin of the perfusing blood, and other factors. Thus, although the diffusing capacity is characteristically reduced in patients with diffuse interstitial disease from any cause, it is also reduced in patients with pneumonectomy, pulmonary emphysema with parenchymal destruction, pulmonary embolic disease with widespread vascular occlusion, pulmonary vascular disease associated with connective-tissue disorders, and conditions that severely alter ventilation-perfusion relationships.

There is no pure test for diffusion, and it has not yet been established that a clinical situation exists in which a barrier to diffusion alone is responsible for abnormalities of gas exchange. Diseases in which the diffusing capacity is most consistently abnormal are listed below. Tests of diffusing capacity may have their greatest value in following the course of certain diseases sequentially.

Conditions Commonly Associated with Reduced Diffusion Capacity*

Diffuse interstitial disease
- Pulmonary edema
- Interstitial pneumonia
- Lung fibrosis

Reduced lung volume

Parenchymal destruction (emphysema)

Reduced pulmonary vascular bed (thromboembolism)

Pulmonary resection

*Anemia and carboxyhemoglobin may result in low values not related to the lung.

TRANSPORT OF OXYGEN AND CARBON DIOXIDE TO THE TISSUES

Oxygen Transport to the Tissues

Arterial Oxygen Content. The cardiac output of an average person at rest is about 5 L. per minute. The body oxygen consumption is approximately 250 ml. per minute. Therefore, the requirement of oxygen by the tissues is approximately 5 ml. per 100 ml. of blood flow per minute. During strenuous exertion, the cardiac output may rise to 20 L. per minute and the oxygen consumption to 2,500 ml. per minute. At this level, the requirement of oxygen by the tissues is approximately 12.5 ml. per 100 ml. of blood flow. To provide the requirements during exercise, the arterial blood must contain at least 12.5 ml. of oxygen. Because the body is unable to function at very low levels of blood oxygen, additional reserve oxygen is carried. In fact, the arterial blood contains approximately 20 ml. of oxygen per 100 ml. of blood.

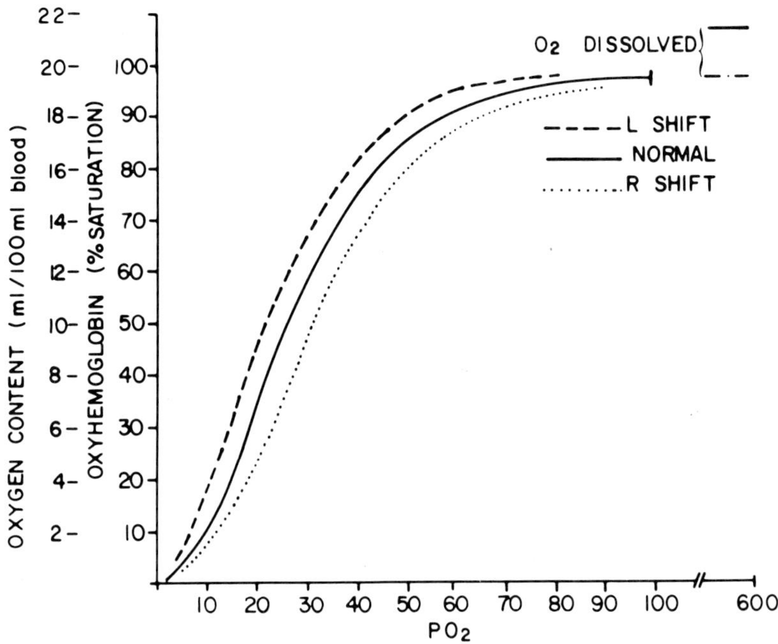

Fig. 4-10. Oxyhemoglobin dissociation curve. The oxygen content increases in proportion to the oxyhemoglobin saturation. When the hemoglobin is 95 per cent saturated ($Po_2 > 80$), further increases in Po_2 produce small increases in oxygen content. Increasing the Po_2 from 100 to 600 results in a small additional increase in oxygen content (about 1.8 ml./100 ml., almost all in dissolved form). As the Po_2 is reduced from arterial blood values (80 to 100) to mixed venous values (about 40), the saturation is reduced from 97 per cent to 70 per cent. This permits a high oxygen content in the venous blood in spite of a relatively low extracting partial pressure at the tissue level. As discussed in the text, factors that shift the curve to the right facilitate the unloading of oxygen, and factors that shift the curve to the left facilitate the loading of oxygen. For example, normal blood provides an oxygen content of 15 ml. per 100 ml. of blood with a Po_2 of 40; the curve shifted 5 mm. to the right provides 15 ml. of oxygen at a Po_2 of 46; the curve shifted 5 mm. to the left provides 15 ml. of oxygen at a Po_2 of 36. Factors that determine the position of the curve are listed in Table 4-5.

The solubility of oxygen in plasma at body temperature is low (0.3 ml. dissolved in 100 ml. per 100 mm. Hg partial pressure of oxygen). Therefore, only about 0.3 ml. of oxygen is carried in the dissolved state. The remainder of the oxygen is carried in combination with hemoglobin. Normal hemoglobin, when fully saturated, binds with 1.39 ml. of oxygen per gram. A person with a normal hemoglobin value of 14 to 15 g. per 100 ml. of blood has a potential binding capacity of approximately 20 ml.

The list below summarizes the factors that determine the transport of oxygen to the tissues. The oxygen content of the arterial blood is not the only important factor.

The Oxygen Transport System

- Oxygen content of arterial blood, determined by:
  - Po_2 (dependent on pulmonary gas exchange)
  - Hemoglobin content
  - Hemoglobin affinity for oxygen
    - physiological variables
    - abnormal hemoglobin
- Blood flow to tissues
  - Cardiac output
  - Regional distribution
- Tissue factors
  - Vascularity
  - Diffusion characteristics
  - Intracellular mechanisms

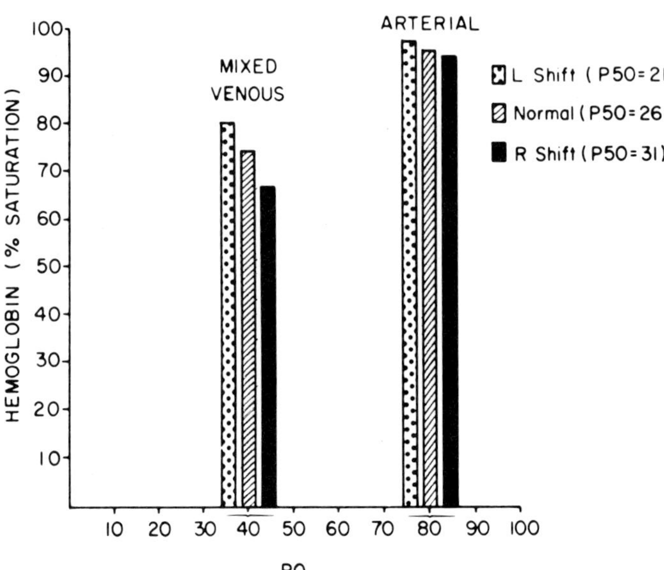

Fig. 4-11. Bar graph demonstrates oxygen content at the mixed venous level and at the arterial level for a normal curve (P_{50} equals 26 mm. Hg), for a right-shifted curve (P_{50} equals 31 mm. Hg), and for a left-shifted curve (P_{50} equals 21 mm. Hg). Note that when the arterial Po_2 is normal, the major effect is on the unloading of oxygen. If the arterial Po_2 is less than 60 mm. Hg, these changes in hemoglobin affinity for oxygen affect the uptake of oxygen in the lungs almost as much as the unloading in the tissues (see Fig. 4-10).

Total blood flow to the tissues, regional distribution of blood flow in the tissues, and numerous poorly defined tissue factors are also important.

Hemoglobin is bound to oxygen in a relationship that is peculiarly suited to the body's wide range of physiological requirements. The relationship of dissolved plasma oxygen (Po_2) to the hemoglobin-bound oxygen is curvilinear (Fig. 4-10). The affinity of hemoglobin for oxygen permits almost complete saturation at the level of the pulmonary capillary ($Po_2 \cong 100$), with the release of about 30 per cent of this oxygen in the tissues, as reflected in mixed venous blood (Po_2 approximately 40). The precise chemical reactions of oxygen with hemoglobin have been actively explored, and changes in configuration of the oxygenated hemoglobin molecule have been compared to the reduced state.[92] Under normal circumstances, the relationship of hemoglobin affinity for oxygen to the partial pressure of oxygen in the plasma is highly predictable. The affinity of hemoglobin for oxygen is popularly defined by the Po_2 required to produce 50 per cent saturation. This so-called P_{50} is readily measured by modern technology.[93-95] At sea level, in normal persons, it is approximately 26 mm. Hg, with more than 95 per cent of the population having values between 24 and 28 mm. Hg. Increased affinity for oxygen results in a shift of the curve to the left and a decrease in the P_{50}. Decreased affinity for oxygen results in a shift of the curve to the right or an increase in the P_{50} (Figs. 4-10, 4-11) Table 4-5 lists the factors that influence the affinity of hemoglobin for oxygen.

Cyclic circulation from the tissues to the lungs is associated with blood changes that affect oxygen's affinity for hemoglobin, improving both the unloading of oxygen in the tissues and the loading of oxygen at the pulmonary capillary level. As the blood flows through the tissues, carbon dioxide is delivered to the blood. The carbon dioxide combines with hemoglobin to produce carbamino groups, resulting in decreased affinity of hemoglobin for oxygen. This results in greater release of oxygen at the tissue level. The delivery of metabolic acids to the blood results in a further decrease in pH, with further reduction of affinity of hemoglobin for oxygen. Both these factors facilitate the release of oxygen at the tissue level. When the blood returns to the pulmonary capillary, carbon dioxide is diffused to the alveolus and exhaled. This results in a rise in pH, with a resultant increase in affinity for oxygen and im-

Table 4-5. Factors Affecting Hemoglobin Affinity for Oxygen

Physiological Factors Affecting Persons With Normal Erythrocytes		
	Increased Affinity (↓P_{50}) (Shift of the curve to left)	*Decreased Affinity* (↑P_{50}) (Shift of the curve to right)
pH	Increased	Decreased
Pco_2	Decreased	Increased
Temperature	Decreased	Increased
2,3-DPG	Decreased Stored blood Acidosis Phosphate depletion	Increased Alkalosis Hypoxemia Phosphate retention (renal failure)
Other Factors		
	Decreased 2,3-DPG binding to hemoglobin	
	Fetal hemoglobin	
	Acquired abnormalities of hemoglobin Carboxyhemoglobin Methemoglobin	
	Abnormalities of erythrocytes that affect hemoglobin affinity for oxygen	
	Enzyme abnormalities Pyruvate kinase excess Hexokinase deficiency	 Pyruvate kinase deficiency
	Abnormal hemoglobins Rainier, Bart's, H, Yakima, Capetown, Chesapeake, Kempsey, Hiroshima, Little Rock	 Kansas, Seattle, S

proved uptake at the pulmonary capillary level. Similarly, highly metabolically active tissues have a higher temperature, which results in decreased affinity of hemoglobin for oxygen and improved release of oxygen. Under these circumstances, the alveolar air has a somewhat lower temperature, permitting improved uptake of oxygen at the alveolar level. For each of these circumstances, it can be readily understood how the changes in hemoglobin affinity for oxygen are advantageous for tissue oxygenation.

Other factors that result in modified hemoglobin affinity for oxygen are not so obviously beneficial. For example, chronic hypoxemia (as a result of pulmonary disease, high altitude, or congestive heart failure) may be associated with reduced affinity of hemoglobin for oxygen. This seems reasonable as an adaptive mechanism to improve oxygen unloading; however, most of these states are also associated with reduced arterial blood Po_2, and reduced pulmonary capillary oxygen loading may cancel out any benefits of im-

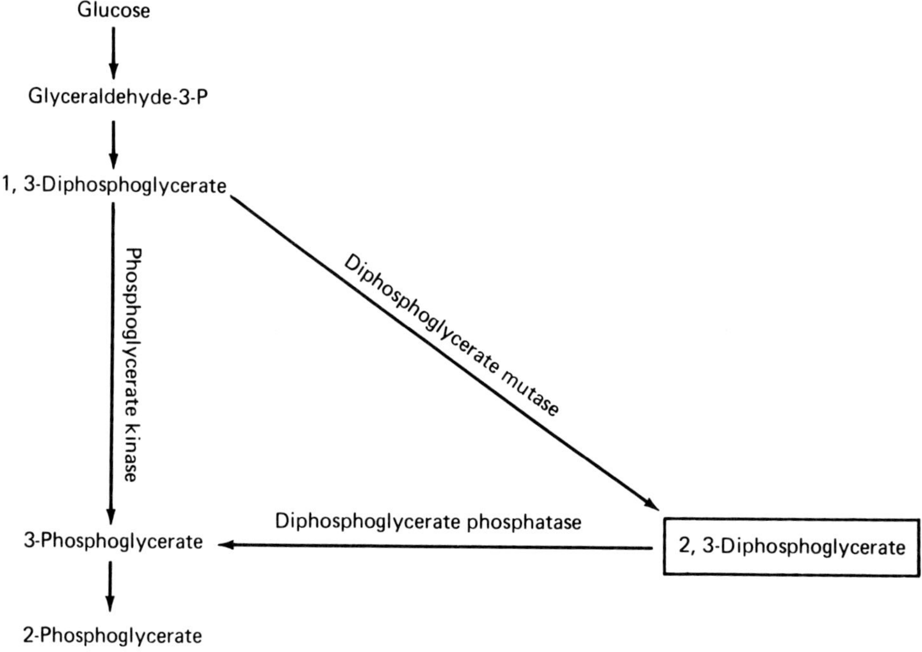

Fig. 4-12. Chemical pathway involved in the production of erythrocyte 2,3-diphosphoglycerate.

proved unloading of oxygen at the tissue level.[96-98]

In recent years, a great deal of interest has focused on the intracellular organic phosphate, 2,3-diphosphoglycerate (2,3-DPG), which apparently enters the hemoglobin molecule, modifying its affinity for oxygen.[99-101] Increased levels of 2,3-DPG are associated with reduced affinity for oxygen, and decreased levels of intraerythrocytic 2,3-DPG are associated with increased affinity for oxygen. 2,3-DPG is predominantly, if not solely, produced in erythrocytes (Fig. 4-12), and numerous factors affect the production of intraerythrocytic 2,3-DPG, as listed in Table 4-5. Several clinical situations are associated with marked changes in 2,3-DPG. Uremia, characteristically associated with elevated circulating phosphate levels, is associated with high levels of 2,3-DPG and reduced affinity of hemoglobin for oxygen.[102,103] This may be an advantage in terms of tissue oxygen delivery, because these patients are generally severly anemic. Chronic hypoxemia is associated with increased 2,3-DPG and reduced affinity of hemoglobin for oxygen.[92,104] In other situations, the effects on oxygen delivery to tissues may, in fact, be detrimental. For example, in sustained metabolic acidosis seen during the development of diabetic acidosis, the hemoglobin affinity for oxygen is reduced (with improved tissue release of oxygen) as a result of the decreased pH. Subsequently, as the acidosis inhibits production of 2,3-DPG, the hemoglobin affinity for oxygen is increased, resulting in reduced unloading of oxygen at the tissue level.[94] Similarly, massive transfusions of stored blood with high oxygen affinity may measurably impair oxygen delivery.[105-109]

Cardiac Output and Tissue Perfusion. Normally, the cardiac output is regulated at least in part by the tissue oxygen requirements.[110] Exercise, fever, hyperthyroidism, and anxiety are all associated with elevated cardiac output. This increase in blood flow is generally distributed to the most metabolically active tissue. There is no easy way to assess the cardiac output at the bedside. Clinical clues include warm, well-perfused skin; good urinary output; a normal pulse pressure suggestive of normal stroke volume and heart rate; and normal sensorium. Laboratory techniques for measuring cardiac output include indicator dilution techniques (which involve intravascular injections and blood sampling), assessment of ventricular stroke volume by ultrasound, radioisotope angiography with measurement of stroke volume, and the Fick method.

Direct sampling of arteriovenous differences, use of flow meters, or isotope angiography may be used to assess the regional distribution of blood flow to various organs.

The distribution of blood within the microcirculation of various organs is more elusive, and no clinically available technique provides an accurate assessment of tissue oxygenation or blood flow. Research techniques involving isotope angiography or tissue diffusion of isotopes can be utilized to identify the regions of decreased or increased tissue blood flow. Recently, attempts have been made to assess tissue oxygenation by oxygen electrodes or tissue sampling probes. Although these techniques now have limited clinical applicability, they may eventually be refined to provide additional information regarding distribution of oxygen in the body tissues.[111-113]

Critical Levels of Tissue Oxygenation. At the present time, the minimum oxygen delivery to tissues without producing adverse effects has not been established. Furthermore, no precise information regarding the most critical vascular beds is available.[98] Studies carried out to establish the critical level of jugular venous Po_2, below which manifestations of abnormal cerebral function would occur, have generally indicated potential danger below a Po_2 of 20, but this has not been uniformly confirmed.[114,115] Evidence of anaerobic metabolism and metabolic acidosis may occur in some conditions, with a mixed venous Po_2 as high as 30; whereas, in other circumstances, in normal persons, the arterial Po_2 may be below that level, with no evidence of major tissue dysfunction. Presumably, these differences reflect alterations in regional blood flow to critical tissues.

The importance of oxygen delivery must be considered in the light of specific organ requirements. It has been calculated[98] that the kidney extracts oxygen under normal circumstances to produce an average arteriovenous difference of 1.7 volumes per cent. The heart, on the other hand, extracts 13 volumes per cent. Therefore, a decrease in arterial oxygen content (as a result of a reduced Po_2 or severe anemia) to half of the normal value would mean that the heart would not be able to extract sufficient oxygen, even though the kidney would still have reserves. The heart, therefore, would have to either increase its blood flow or decrease the oxygen consumption. In normal persons, blood flow is readily increased. Furthermore, the effects of tissue CO_2 and metabolic acids in the heart capillary would promote oxygen release through reduced hemoglobin affinity for oxygen (to a greater degree than would occur in the kidney capillaries). Differential distribution of blood flow, favoring brain over skeletal muscles, has been well demonstrated.[115] Diseased persons may not have normal ability to redistribute blood flow or increase cardiac output, and simple extrapolations of known arterial oxygen transport mechanisms may be misleading.

When hypoxia is severe, clinical evidence of decreased tissue oxygenation may become important. Some organs, such as the brain, may demonstrate loss of function. A decrease in aerobic glycolysis results in reduced oxygen consumption, increased production of lactic acid, and measurable metabolic acidosis.[116-120] This is reviewed in Chapter 1, in relation to the effects of high altitude.

It is appropriate, then, to make every effort to ensure adequate oxygen delivery by the known transport mechanisms until a clearer assessment of the critical levels of oxygenation of specific tissues becomes possible.

Methods of Assessing the Oxygen Transport System. Table 4-6 lists the methods in

Table 4-6. Methods of Assessing the Oxygen Transport System

Clinical Features	
Dyspnea	
Abnormal organ function (e.g., mental function)	
Hyperventilation	
Cyanosis	
Laboratory Analysis	
Component	*Method of Assessing*
Dissolved oxygen	Po_2 (blood gas electrodes)
Oxygen carrying capacity	Oxygen content of fully saturated blood
Hemoglobin	Hb (clinical laboratory)
Hemoglobin affinity for oxygen	P_{50} (blood gas electrodes, tonometer, spectrophotometer, for assessing oxyhemoglobin)
Oxygen content, oxygen capacity	Van Slyke chemical analysis, Lexington instruments polarographic technique
Oxyhemoglobin saturation	Oxygen content/oxygen capacity
Carboxyhemoglobin	Spectrophotometer
Meth- or sulfhemoglobin	Spectrophotometer
Cardiac output	Fick method, indicator dilution technique
Regional perfusion	Difficult Individual organ blood flow
Tissue oxygen levels	None clinically available Tissue Po_2 electrode under investigation Mixed venous Po_2

common clinical use for estimating oxygen delivery to the tissues. Clinical methods are notoriously unreliable except when hypoxia is severe. Dyspnea is generally mild in conditions resulting in hypoxia, when compared with conditions that increase the work of breathing. Hyperventilation may be present but is also nonspecific. When abnormal organ function occurs, it is a late manifestation of hypoxia. Cyanosis can be helpful when present, but is frequently misleading whether present or absent.[121] This bluish discoloration is best sought for in vascular capillary beds of nails, conjunctivae, lips, and tongue.

Causes of Cyanosis

Increased unoxygenated hemoglobin in capillaries
- Decreased arterial Po_2 (generally less than 55 mm. Hg)
- Mildly reduced arterial Po_2 with polycythemia
- Normal arterial Po_2 with severe reduction in blood flow (shock)
- Hemoglobinopathy (e.g., Kansas)

Abnormal hemoglobin pigment
- Methemoglobin
- Sulfhemoglobin

Other pigmentation
- Argyria
- Hemochromatosis

Cyanosis has been described to occur when the capillary content of reduced hemoglobin exceeds 5 g./100 ml. This may occur when arterial hemoglobin is unsaturated or when tissue extraction is high. When the extremities demonstrate cyanosis but central tissues such as the tongue and conjunctiva do not (peripheral cyanosis), the cause may be reduced peripheral perfusion with increased tissue oxygen extraction. When central and peripheral tissues are cyanosed (central cyanosis), it generally indicates unsaturated arterial hemoglobin (see list above). Rarely, hemoglobinopathies with severely reduced oxygen affinity have been reported to cause cyanosis in spite of a normal Po_2. More commonly, the altered color characteristics of sulfhemoglobin or methemoglobin result in central cyanosis. These generally result from reactions to drugs or chemicals, although congenital methemoglobinemia has been reported.[110]

Equally important are the conditions associated with severe hypoxemia in which cyanosis may not be present (see list below). With anemia, as is now commonly seen in patients in chronic renal dialysis programs, total hemoglobin values of 3 to 5 g./100 ml. of blood are not uncommon. In spite of severely reduced arterial oxygen delivery commonly associated with a low arterial Po_2, these persons are rarely, if ever, cyanosed. Carboxyhemoglobin is red, similar to oxyhemoglobin, and, therefore, fatal carbon monoxide poisoning does not produce cyanosis. In patients with fever and peripheral vasodilatation, the high capillary blood flow may reduce oxygen extraction and minimize otherwise apparent cyanosis. Finally, cosmetics have frequently masked the underlying cyanosis of the lips and nail beds. The examination for cyanosis is not complete until several vascular beds have been examined.

Conditions With Severe Hypoxia Without Cyanosis

Reduced circulating hemoglobin (anemia)

Abnormal hemoglobin (carboxyhemoglobin)

Systemic vasodilatation with rapid blood flow

Abnormal pigmentation

Of the laboratory techniques available, measurement of arterial Po_2, hemoglobin, arterial oxyhemoglobin saturation, and, in some hospitals, an estimate of the oxyhemoglobin dissociation curve are in most common use. Most clinicians must make an assessment of cardiac output and regional distribution of perfusion on clinical grounds. Mixed venous Po_2 may be helpful in following a specific patient, although no fixed level has been established

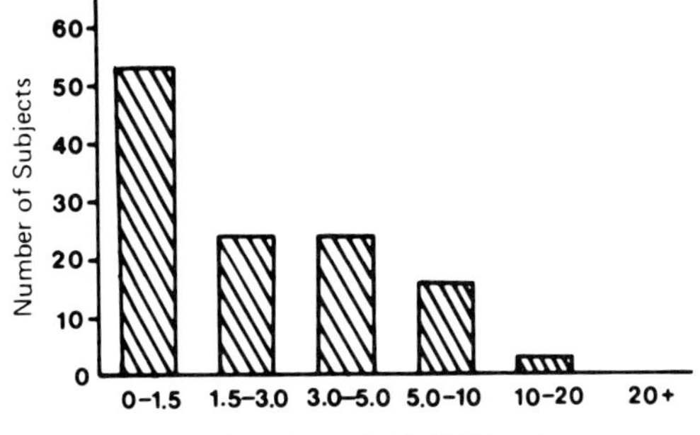

Fig. 4-13. Carboxyhemoglobin levels in patients during routine pulmonary-function tests. One hundred and twenty-one consecutive patients who were evaluated in the clinical pulmonary-function laboratory in the Foothills Hospital in Calgary, Alberta, had carboxyhemoglobin determinations. Note the large number who had carboxyhemoglobin levels greater than 3 per cent (levels considered to have significant effect on patients with cardiopulmonary disease). Most of these elevated values could be directly attributed to tobacco smoking; several nonsmokers had been exposed to urban environmental pollution.

to be helpful. Additional information about oxygen delivery can be obtained by knowing the patient's temperature, blood pH, amount of carboxyhemoglobin, and evidence of other factors affecting the oxyhemoglobin dissociation curve. Recently, increased concern about the adverse effects of moderate amounts of carboxyhemoglobin has resulted in more common use of this analysis (Fig. 4-13).

Carbon Dioxide Transport

Approximately 200 ml. of carbon dioxide are removed per minute from the tissues at rest, and 2,000 ml. are removed per minute during exhaustive exercise. As is true for oxygen, the solubility of carbon dioxide in plasma provides a negligible amount of transport. Carbon dioxide produced in the mitochondria is diffused through the cytoplasm to interstitial spaces and then into the blood (Fig. 4-14). In the blood, the carbon dioxide diffuses through the plasma, where some is dissolved or is bound to

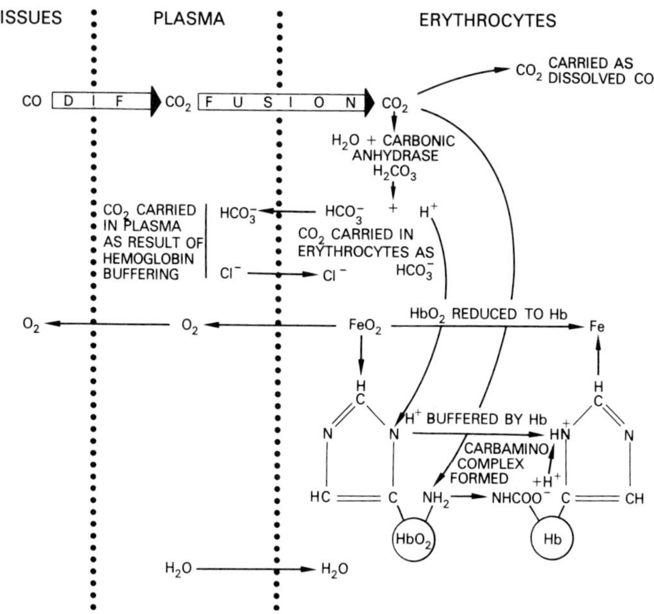

Fig. 4-14. Carbon dioxide transport. Note that carbon dioxide diffuses from cells and tissues through plasma into erythrocutes. Here it is dissolved, bound to reduced hemoglobin as carbamino groups, or hydrated to carbonic acid. This dissociates to produce bicarbonate, which may diffuse into the plasma. When the blood reaches the alveolar level, the entire process is reversed, and the diffusion is in the direction of the alveolus rather than the tissues. (Davenport, H. W.: The ABC of Acid-Base Chemistry. ed. 6. Chicago, University of Chicago Press, 1974)

plasma proteins as carbamino groups. Most of it, however, diffuses into the erythrocyte, where the enzyme carbonic anhydrase facilitates hydration of the carbon dioxide to form carbonic acid:

$$CO_2 + H_2O \underset{\text{carbonic anhydrase}}{\rightleftarrows} H_2CO_3$$

The carbonic acid then dissociates to some degree, producing free hydrogen ions and bicarbonate. Some bicarbonate then diffuses out of the erythrocyte into the plasma, thereby reducing the concentration in the erythrocyte. This takes place according to standard laws of concentration gradients. Because this results in a net increase in negatively charged ions in the plasma, an additional transfer of negatively charged ions must take place into the cell; and chloride generally moves intracellularly.[122,123] In addition, the carbon dioxide may combine with the protein of reduced hemoglobin to form carbamino groups.

The majority of carbon dioxide, then, is transported from the tissues to the lungs in the form of bicarbonate in the plasma or as carbamino groups in the erythrocytes.[122,123] When the blood reaches the lungs, carbon dioxide is diffused from the plasma into the alveolar air, along diffusion gradients. In the lungs, the entire process that occurred in the tissues is reversed; in the presence of carbonic anhydrase, the carbon dioxide is quickly released from carbonic acid, and plasma and erythrocyte bicarbonate levels are decreased. Furthermore, in the presence of oxygen, hemoglobin binds to oxygen, eliminating carbamino groups. The cyclic unloading of carbon dioxide at the alveolar level is therefore facilitated by the loading of oxygen, and the uptake of carbon dioxide at the tissue level is facilitated by the release of oxygen.[124]

As with oxygen, the carbon dioxide blood transport mechanisms normally function with substantial reserves, so that in circumstances of decreased rate of blood flow or increased metabolic activity, adequate transport is available. Abnormalities of the carbon dioxide transport system have not been incriminated as a mechanism of symptoms. Most studies have concentrated on the role of oxygenation in regional tissue metabolism rather than on the role of carbon dioxide removal. Consequently, at the present time, metabolic effects of regional tissue hypercapnia are not considered to be clinically significant. This entire area, however, has not been investigated adequately. It is quite clear that major acidosis in the systemic venous bed, as seen in shock, can be largely attributed to increased carbon dioxide in venous blood, caused by low circulatory rates. When regional perfusion is strikingly impaired, severe tissue acidosis might be expected, even though the arterial blood may have a normal or nearly normal pH and Pco_2. In general, however, carbon dioxide transport is most commonly a clinical problem when alveolar ventilation is abnormal.

Respiratory Aspects of Acid-Base Balance

Relationship of Respiratory Gases to Acid-Base Balance in Blood. In body fluids, as in classical chemistry, a fluid with increased hydrogen ion concentration is acidic; one with decreased hydrogen ion concentration is basic. The major respiratory factor controlling hydrogen ion concentration in the blood is the amount of carbonic acid, which is directly proportional to the dissolved carbon dioxide, which is proportional to the Pco_2. The following formula describes the relationships:

$$H_2O + CO_2 \rightleftarrows H_2CO_3 \rightleftarrows H^+ + HCO_3^-$$

An increase in carbon dioxide results in a shift of the equation to the right, forming more carbonic acid that will dissociate and form more hydrogen ions. Because bicarbonate is a weak base, this results in increased acidosis. Whenever the Pco_2 is increased, there are increased hydrogen ions. Whenever the Pco_2 is decreased, there are decreased hydrogen ions. Unfortunately, the practice of clinical medicine has been complicated by the concept of pH. This concept, apparently well founded in the laws of physics,[125-127] requires use of the inverse logarithm (log) of the hydrogen ion concentration. This complex relationship is described in the Henderson-Hasselbalch equation:

$$pH = pK + \log \frac{[HCO_3]}{[H_2CO_3]} \text{ or}$$

$$pH = 6.10 + \log \frac{[HCO_3^-]}{0.0301\ Pco_2}$$

Normally, the ratio of bicarbonate to carbonic acid is approximately 20 to 1; when Pco_2 is introduced into the equation, it is apparent that an increase in Pco_2 reduces the ratio of bicarbonate to carbonic acid and thereby reduces the pH.

The concentration of bicarbonate is controlled by metabolic processes, and the Pco_2 by alveolar ventilation. Therefore, metabolic acid-base disturbances affect the numerator, and the respiratory acid-base disturbances affect the denominator.

Acute or severe changes in hydrogen ion concentration (and pH) are generally detrimental to the body. Because the process of cellular metabolism produces thousands of milliequivalents (mEq.) of hydrogen each day, elaborate mechanisms are available to control the concentration. Buffer systems in the body act immediately to modify the hydrogen ion concentration. These include phosphates, sulfates, reduced hemoglobin, and proteins. Respiratory responses are early, increasing or decreasing the ventilation to blow off or retain carbon dioxide as required. Finally, the control of bicarbonate levels through renal excretion or conservation takes hours or days to become effective.

Changes in pH that result from changes in Pco_2 can be predicted with reliability. Nomograms have been established to permit ready calculation.[122,126,128] The precise quantitative interrelationship of hydrogen ion concentration and dissolved CO_2 observed in blood in vitro is somewhat modified in vivo. Consequently, recent studies have attempted to quantitate the pH-Pco_2 relationships in vivo in a variety of acid-base disorders.[129,130] Fig. 4-15 is a compilation of much of this data.

Respiratory Alkalosis. Hyperventilation results in a decrease in the level of dissolved carbon dioxide (and consequently carbonic acid) in the blood, a reduced hydrogen ion concentration, and an increase in pH. Values for pH that are above 7.45 may be accepted as indicating clinically significant alkalemia. When the hyperventilation persists, as occurs at high altitude

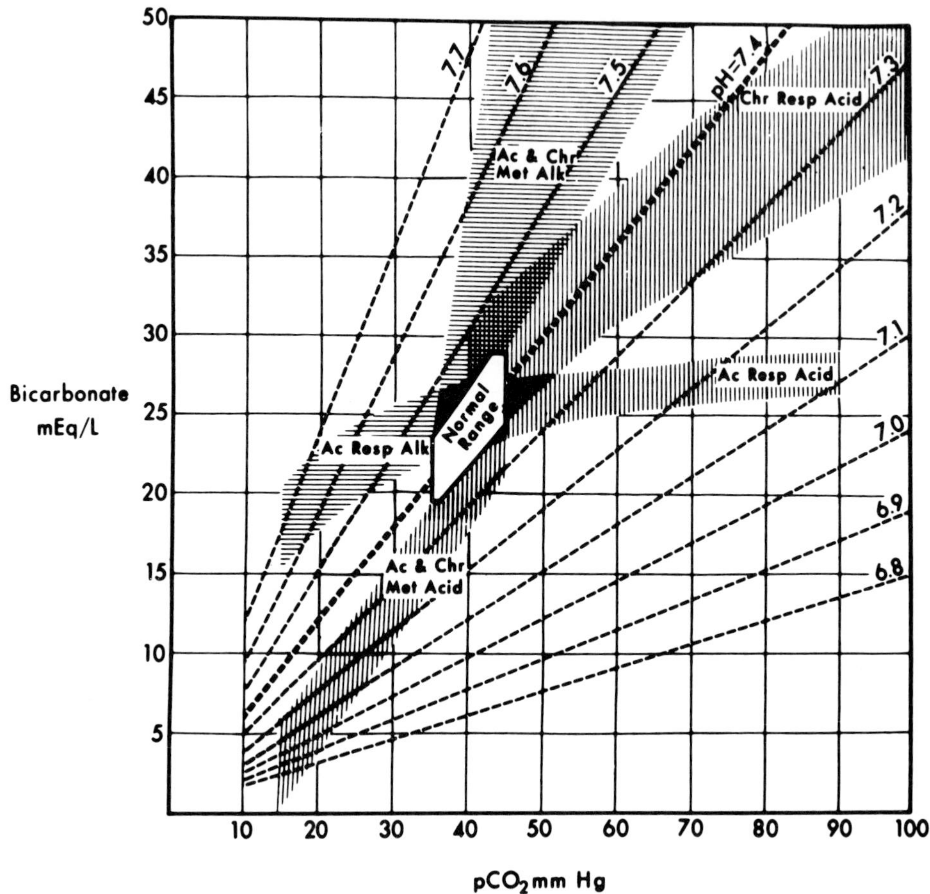

Fig. 4-15. Nomogram for acid-base disturbances in vivo. This graph displays the quantity and direction of changes in pH, Pco_2, and bicarbonate in a variety of metabolic and respiratory acid-base disorders. The shaded areas represent the range of variability observed in selected populations with pure acid-base disorders as designated. In general, patients whose values lie outside of the "significance bands" have mixed acid-base disturbances. *Ac* indicates acute; *Chr* indicates chronic; *Alk*, alkalosis; *Met*, metabolic. (Arbus, G. S.: An in vivo acid-base nomogram for clinical use. Can. Med. Assoc. J., *109*:291, 1973)

or with chronic hypoxemia, there is compensatory excretion of bicarbonate by the kidneys, which results in maintenance of the pH near normal. Under these circumstances, the pH generally ranges from 7.40 to 7.45. This is called a *compensated respiratory alkalosis*.

Respiratory alkalosis may be symptomatic when there is a substantial elevation in pH (alkalemia). In general, this requires pH levels greater than 7.50 to 7.55. Blood pH values greater than 7.70 are rarely tolerated for prolonged periods. The physiological effects and clinical manifestations of respiratory alkalosis are summarized in Table 4-7.

Respiratory Acidosis. Hypoventilation leads to elevated dissolved carbon dioxide (and consequently carbonic acid) in the blood. If this occurs acutely, there is a dramatic decrease in pH. A small increase in bicarbonate occurs acutely in response

Table 4-7. Respiratory Alkalosis

Physiological Effects	*Clinical Manifestations*
Nervous System	
Decreased cerebral blood flow	Anxiety, numbness and tingling, seizures, lightheadedness
Increased excitability	
Increased neuromuscular irritability	
Renal and Metabolic	
Chloride retention and bicarbonate excretion	Carpopedal spasm; Increased reflexes
Decreased ionized serum calcium and magnesium	Chvostek's and Trousseau's signs
Increased production of lactic acid	
Increased catecholamine release	
Cardiovascular	
Systemic vasoconstriction	Palpitations; Arrhythmias
Tachycardia	
Increased myocardial irritability	
Respiratory	
Bronchoconstriction	Dyspnea

to the elevated carbon dioxide (about 3 mEq. of bicarbonate per liter when the arterial P_{CO_2} is increased to 90 mm. Hg). Therefore, the pH change in vivo is approximately equal to that predicted in blood in vitro.[131] With chronic hyperventilation, bicarbonate is retained and thereby buffers the effects of CO_2 on pH. Therefore, dramatic increases in blood bicarbonate may be expected in chronic hypercapnia (Fig. 4-15).

Symptoms in respiratory acidosis are also related to the change in pH more than the change in P_{CO_2}.[132] The physiological effects and clinical manifestations of respiratory acidosis are summarized in Table 4-8. They are minor at a pH of about 7.30, increasing at pH values below 7.25, and marked at pH values as low as 7.10. With rare exceptions, pH values below 6.90 in arterial blood are sustained for only short periods of life.

Interpretation of Acid-Base Disturbances. As listed in Table 4-9, simple acid-base disturbances are readily understood. Increased pH indicates alkalemia; decreased indicates acidemia. Alkalosis or acidosis refer to the acid-base derangement, even if the H^+ has been buffered or compensated for. When acidosis is caused by respiratory mechanisms, the P_{CO_2} is elevated. When acidosis is caused by metabolic mechanisms, the bicarbonate is reduced. When alkalosis is caused by respiratory mechanisms, the P_{CO_2} is reduced; when metabolic, the bicarbonate is increased.

After the primary derangement has been established, compensatory mechanisms become active. The mechanisms of compensation for respiratory acid-base disturbances are metabolic. Therefore, the patient with chronic hyperventilation has a reduced bicarbonate; the patient with chronic hypoventilation, increased bicarbonate. Chronic or compensated acid-base disturbances always represent mixed mechanisms.[128-132] Many laboratories report various computed values reflecting bicarbonate concentration. Base excess, the most popular of these, reflects the total available buffer base and is expressed in milliequivalents per liter. This takes into account alterations in bicarbonate that are directly related to increased or decreased P_{CO_2}, as well as varying hemoglobin concentrations. The clinician can generally utilize base excess or bicarbonate equally well if a nomogram such as Figure 4-15 is understood.

Difficulties in the interpretation of acid-base disturbances arise when (as occurs so commonly in very ill patients) mixed factors are active.[133] Under these circumstances, clinical information that documents loss of hydrogen ions, loss of bicarbonate, or recent dramatic change in status may permit the conclusion that met-

Table 4-8. Respiratory Acidosis

Physiological Effects	*Clinical Manifestations*
Central Nervous System	
Dilated cerebral vessels → increased cerebrospinal fluid pressure	Headache, dyspnea, somnolence, psychosis, papilledema, focal neurological signs, neuromuscular irritability (asterixis) may progress to frank coma
Depresses cortical function	
Stimulates respiratory centers (medulla and carotid bodies)	Hyperventilation
Renal and Metabolic	
Increased H^+, → transfer of H^+ into cells and K^+ out. Thus early increased serum K^+, subsequent increased excretion of K^+	None significant
Increased H^+, → excretion of Cl^- and reabsorption of bicarbonate	
Serum HCO_3 gradually increased	
No definitely known effects on major metabolic function or enzyme systems	
Cardiovascular	
Decreased myocardial contractility	
Increased or decreased irritability	Heart Failure
Decreased responsiveness to catecholamines	Arrhythmias
Systemic vascular dilatation	Pulmonary hypertension
Pulmonary vascular and bronchial smooth muscle contraction	

Table 4-9. Acute and Chronic Acid-Base Disturbances

	P_{CO_2}	*pH*		HCO_3^-	
		Acute	*Chronic*	*Acute*	*Chronic*
Respiratory alkalosis (hyperventilation)	↓	↑	↑ ⟷	⟷	↓
Respiratory acidosis (hypoventilation)	↑	↓	↓ ⟷	⟷	↑
Metabolic acidosis	⟷ ↓	↓	↓ ⟷	↓	↓
Metabolic alkalosis	⟷ ↑	↑	↑ ⟷	↑	↑

Table 4-10. Mechanisms of Metabolic Acidosis

Mechanisms	*Clinical Conditions*
Increased production of acids	
Ketones, beta hydroxybutyric	Diabetes mellitus
	Starvation
Lactic acid	Shock, severe hypoxia
	Drugs (phenformin, INH overdose, salicylate overdose, alcohol)
	Idiopathic
Decreased excretion of acids	
Reduced tubular hydrogen ion excretion	Pyelonephritis, multiple renal diseases
Reduced glomerular filtration	Drugs (carbonic anhydrase inhibitors)
Exogenous acids	NH_4Cl infusions

abolic and respiratory factors are present. A common example in respiratory medicine is the patient with chronic obstructive pulmonary disease and chronic hypercapnia who presents with a nearly normal pH (e.g., 7.43) and increased Pco_2 (e.g., 58). This patient has an alkalosis that at first glance is not respiratory. Closer observation and historical information may permit the conclusion that, in fact, he chronically has an even greater Pco_2 (e.g., 65), but he transiently hyperventilated at the time of sampling of the arterial blood, thus changing the pH from 7.38 to 7.43. Nomograms are not helpful in coming to a specific diagnostic conclusion; however, Figure 4-15, which incorporates the broad range of changes in pH, Pco_2, and bicarbonate in pure acid-base disturbances, permits a judgment regarding the presence of multiple factors.

A common problem in the interpretation of acid-base disturbances relates to the mechanisms of unsuspected metabolic acidosis. When the pH is low, the Pco_2 normal or low (due to compensatory hyperventilation), and the bicarbonate low, numerous mechanisms must be considered. Table 4-10 lists the causes of metabolic acidosis that should be considered.

REFERENCES

1. Petty, T. L., Bigelow, D. B., Levine, B. E.: The simplicity and safety of arterial puncture. J.A.M.A., *195*:693, 1966.
2. Mortensen, J. D.: Clinical sequelae from arterial needle puncture, cannulation and incision. Circulation, *35*:1118, 1967.
3. Shapiro, B. A.: Clinical Application of Blood Gases. Chicago, Year Book Medical Publishers, 1973.
4. Gardner, R. M., Schwartz, R., Wong, H. C., and Burke, J. P.: Percutaneous indwelling radial artery catheters: risk of thrombosis and infection. N. Engl. J. Med., *290*:1227, 1974.
5. Bedford, R. F., and Wollmann, H.: Complication of percutaneous radial-artery cannulation: an objective prospective study in man. Anesthesiology, *38*:228, 1973.
6. Greenhow, D. E.: Incorrect performance of Allen's test: ulnar-artery flow erroneously presumed inadequate. Anesthesiology, *37*:356, 1972.
7. Matthews, J. I., and Gibbons, R. B.: Embolization complicating radial artery puncture. Ann. Intern. Med., *75*:87, 1971.
8. Michaelson, E. D., and Walsh, R. E.: Osler's node: a complication of prolonged arterial cannulation. N. Engl. J. Med., *283*:472, 1970.

9. Lowenstein, E., Little, J. W., and Hing, H. L.: Prevention of cerebral embolization from flushing radial artery cannulas. N. Engl. J. Med., *285*:1414, 1971.
10. Lindesmith, L. A., Winga, E. R., Goodnough, D. E., and Paradise, R. A.: Arterial punctures by inhalation therapy personnel. Chest, *61*:83, 1972.
11. Sackner, M. A., Avery, W. G., and Sokolowski, J.: Arterial punctures by nurses. Chest, *59*:97, 1971.
12. Kelman, G. R., and Nunn, J. F.: Nomograms for correction of blood Po_2, Pco_2, pH, and base excess for time and temperature. J. Appl. Physiol., *21*:1484, 1966.
13. Severinghaus, J. W.: Blood gas calculator. J. Appl. Physiol., *21*:1108, 1966.
14. Bristow, G. K., and Kirk, B. W.: Venous admixture and lung water in healthy subjects over 50 years of age. J. Appl. Physiol., *50*:552, 1971.
15. Lenfant, C.: Measurement of ventilation/perfusion distribution with alveolar-arterial differences. J. Appl. Physiol., *18*:1090, 1963.
16. Raine, J. M., and Bishop, J. M.: A-a difference in oxygen tension and physiological dead space in normal man. J. Appl. Physiol., *18*:284, 1963.
17. Mellemgaard, K.: The alveolar-arterial oxygen difference: its size and components in normal man. Acta Physiol. Scand., *67*:10, 1966.
18. Cole, R. B., and Bishop, J. M.: Effect of varying inspired oxygen tension on alveolar-arterial oxygen tension difference in man. J. Appl. Physiol., *18*:1043, 1963.
19. West, J. B., and Collery, C. T.: Distribution of blood flow and ventilation-perfusion ratio in the lung, measured with radioactive CO_2. J. Appl. Physiol., *15*:405, 1960.
20. Bryan, A. C., *et al.*: Factors affecting regional distribution of ventilation and perfusion in the lung. J. Appl. Physiol., *19*:395, 1964.
21. Cardus, D.: Oxygen alveolar-arterial tension difference after ten days recumbency in man. J. Appl. Physiol., *23*:934, 1967.
22. Trimble, C., Smith, D. E., Cook, T. I., and Trummer, M. J.: The effect of supine bedrest upon alveolar-arterial oxygen gradients and intrapulmonary shunting in normal man. J. Thorac. Cardiovasc. Surg., *63*:873, 1972.
23. Holland, J., Milic-Emili, J., Macklem, P. T., and Bates, D. V.: Regional distribution of pulmonary ventilation and perfusion in elderly subjects. J. Clin. Invest., *47*:81, 1968.
24. Guz, A.: Regulation of respiration in man. Annu. Rev. Physiol., *37*:303, 1975.
25. Mitchell, R. A.: Control of respiration in pathophysiology—altered regulatory mechanisms. *In* Frohlich, E. D. (ed.): Pathophysiology: Altered Regulatory Mechanisms in Disease. ed. 2. Philadelphia, J. B. Lippincott, 1976.
26. Wang, S. C., and Ngai, S. H.: General organization of central respiratory mechanisms. *In* Fenn, W. O., and Rahn, H. (eds.): Handbook of Physiology. Section 3. Respiration. Volume I, Chapter 20. Baltimore, Waverley Press, 1964.
27. Watt, J. G., Dumke, P. R., and Comroe, J. H., Jr.: Effects of inhalation of 100 percent and 14 percent oxygen upon respiration of unanesthetized dogs before and after chemoreceptor denervation. Am. J. Physiol., *138*:610, 1943.
28. Rebuck, A. S., and Woodley, W. E.: Ventilatory effects of hypoxia and their dependence on Pco_2. J. Appl. Physiol., *38*:16, 1975.
29. Hasan, F. M., and Kazemi, H.: Dual contribution theory of regulation of CSF HCO_3^- in respiratory acidosis. J. Appl. Physiol., *40*:559; 1976.
30. Lewis, B. I.: The hyperventilation syndrome. Ann. Intern. Med., *38*:918, 1953.
31. Lambertson, C. J.: Effects of drugs and hormones on the respiratory response to carbon dioxide. *In* Fenn, W. O., and Rahn, H. (eds.): Handbook of Physiology. Section 3. Respiration. Volume I, Chapter 22. Baltimore, Waverley Press, 1964.
32. Plum, F., and Posner, J. (eds.): The Diagnosis of Stupor and Coma. ed. 2. p. 25. Philadelphia, F. A. Davis, 1972.
33. Comroe, J. H., Jr.: The peripheral chemoreceptors. *In* Fenn, W. O., and Rahn, H. (eds.): Handbook of Physiology. Section 3. Respiration. Volume I, Chapter 23. Baltimore, Waverley Press, 1964.
34. Cunningham, D. J. C., and O'Riordan, J. L. H.: The effect of a rise in the temperature of the body on the respiratory response to carbon dioxide at rest. J. Exp. Physiol., *42*:329, 1957.
35. Moser, K. M., Perry, R. B., and Luchsinger, P. C.: Cardiopulmonary consequences of pyrogen induced hyperpyrexia in man. J. Clin. Invest., *42*:626, 1963.

36. Asmussen, E., and Nielsen, M.: Studies on the regulation of respiration in heavy work. Acta Physiol. Scand. *12*:171, 1947.
37. Weil, J. V., *et al.*: Augmentation of chemosensitivity during mild exercise in normal man. J. Appl. Physiol., *33*:813, 1972.
38. Weil, J. V., McCullough, R. E., Kline, J. S., and Sodal, I. E.: Diminished ventilatory response to hypoxia and hypercapnia after morphine in the normal man. N. Engl. J. Med., *292*:1103, 1975.
39. Perez, G. F.: Hypercapnia during iatrogenically induced metabolic alkalosis. Chest, *65*:108, 1974.
40. Lifschitz, M. D., Brasch, R., Cuomo, A. J., and Menn, S. J.: Marked Hypercapnia secondary to severe metabolic alkalosis. Ann. Intern. Med., *77*:405, 1972.
41. Heineman, H. O., and Goldring, R. M.: Bicarbonate and the regulation of respiration. Am. J. Med., *57*:361, 1974.
42. Jarboe, T. M., Penman, R. W., and Luke, R. G.: Ventilatory failure due to metabolic alkalosis. Chest, *61* [Suppl]: 61, 1972.
43. Wade, J. G., *et al.*: Effect of carotid endarterectomy on carotid chemoreceptors and baroreceptor function in man. N. Engl. J. Med., *282*:833, 1970.
44. Davidson, J. T., *et al.*: Role of the carotid bodies in breath holding. N. Engl. J. Med., *290*:819, 1974.
45. Edelman, N. H., *et al.*: The blunted ventilatory response to hypoxia in cyanotic congenital heart disease. N. Engl. J. Med., *282*:405, 1970.
46. Campbell, E. J. M., and Howell, J. B. L.: Rebreathing method for measurement of mixed venous Pco_2. Br. Med. J., *2*:630, 1962.
47. Lourenco, R. V.: Diaphragm activity in obesity. J. Clin. Invest., *49*:170, 1970.
48. Whitelaw, W. A., Derenne, J. P., and Milic-Emili, J.: Occlusion pressure as a measure of respiratory center output in conscious man. Respir. Physiol., *23*:181, 1975.
49. Kellog, R. H.: Central chemical regulation of respiration. *In* Fenn, W. O., and Rahn, H. (eds.): Handbook of Physiology. Section 3. Respiration. Volume I, Chapter 20. Baltimore, Waverley Press, 1964.
50. Kronenberg, R., *et al.*: Comparison of three methods for quantitating respiratory response to hypoxia in man. Respir. Physiol., *16*:109, 1972.
51. Read, D. J. C.: A clinical method for assessing the ventilatory response to carbon dioxide. Aust. Ann. Med., *16*:20, 1967.
52. Rebuck, A. S., Jones, N. L., and Campbell, E. J. M.: Ventilatory response to exercise and to CO_2 rebreathing in normal subjects. Clin. Sci., *43*:861, 1972.
53. Cherniack, R. M., and Snidal, D. P.: The effect of obstruction to breathing on the ventilatory response to CO_2. J. Clin. Invest., *35*:1286, 1956.
54. Rebuck, A. S., and Read, J.: Patterns of ventilatory response to carbon dioxide during recovery from severe asthma. Clin. Sci., *41*:13, 1971.
55. Pontoppidan, H., Geffin, G., and Lowenstein, E.: Acute respiratory failure in the adult. N. Engl. J. Med., *287*:743, 1972.
56. Levison, H., and Cherniack, R. M.: Ventilatory cost of exercise in chronic obstructive pulmonary disease. J. Appl. Physiol., *25*:21, 1968.
57. Otis, A. B.: The work of breathing. *In* Fenn, W. O., and Rahn, H. (eds.): Handbook of Physiology. Section 3. Respiration. Volume II, Chapter 17. Baltimore, Waverley Press, 1964.
58. West, J. B.: Respiratory Physiology. p. 51. Baltimore, Williams & Wilkins, 1974.
59. ———: Ventilation/Blood Flow and Gas Exchange. ed. 2. Oxford, Blackwell Scientific Publications, 1970.
60. Ball, W. C., Stewart, P. B., Newsham, L. G. S., and Bates, D. V.: Regional pulmonary function studied with xenon^{133}. J. Clin. Invest., *41*:519, 1962.
61. West, J. B., Dollery, C. T., and Naimark, P.: Distribution of blood flow in isolated lung: relation to vascular and alveolar pressures. J. Appl. Physiol., *19*:713, 1964.
62. Anthonisen, N. R., and Milic-Emili, J.: Distribution of pulmonary perfusion in erect man. J. Appl. Physiol., *21*:760, 1966.
63. Hughes, J. M. B., Glazier, J. B., Maloney, J. E., and West, J. B.: Effect of interstitial pressure on pulmonary blood flow. Lancet, *1*:192, 1967.
64. Hughes, J. M. B., Glazier, J. B., Rozenzweig, D. Y., and West, J. B.: Factors determining the distribution of pulmonary blood flow in patients with raised pulmonary venous pressure. Clin. Sci., *37*:847, 1969.
65. Ritchie, B. C., Schauberger, G., and Staub, N.: Inadequacy of perivascular edema hypothesis to account for distribution of pulmonary blood flow in lung edema. Circ. Res., *24*:807, 1969.

66. Berglund, E., Malmberg, R., and Simonsson, B. G.: Effect of body position on regional lung perfusion at normal and elevated pulmonary pressures. Scand. J. Respir. Dis., *48*:208, 1967.
67. Swyer, P. R., and James, G. C. W.: A case of unilateral pulmonary emphysema. Thorax, *8*:133, 1953.
68. Macleod, W. M.: Abnormal transradiancy of one lung. Thorax, *9*:147, 1954.
69. Bates, D. V., Macklem, P. T., and Christie, R. V.: Respiratory Function in Disease. p. 201. Philadelphia, W. B. Saunders, 1971.
70. Welch, M. H., *et al.*: The lung scan in alpha$_1$ antitrypsin deficiency. J. Nucl. Med., *10*:687, 1969.
71. Holland, J., Milic-Emili, J., Macklem, P. T., and Bates, D. V.: Regional distribution of pulmonary ventilation and perfusion in elderly subjects. J. Clin. Invest., *47*:81, 1968.
72. Cournand, A. F.: Pulmonary circulation. Its control in man, with some remarks on methodology. Am. Heart J., *54*:172, 1957.
73. Fishman, A. P., and Hecht, H. H. (eds.): The Pulmonary Circulation and Interstitial Space. Chicago, University of Chicago Press, 1969.
74. Harris, P., and Heath, D.: The Human Pulmonary Circulation, Its Form and Function in Health and Disease. London, E. & S. Livingstone, 1962.
75. Brody, J. S., Stemmler, E. J., and DuBois, A. B.: Longitudinal distribution of vascular resistance in the pulmonary arteries, capillaries and veins. J. Clin. Invest., *47*:783, 1968.
76. Lopez-Majano, V., *et al.*: Effect of regional hypoxia on the distribution of pulmonary blood flow in man. Circ. Res., *18*:550, 1966.
77. Hauge, A.: Hypoxia and pulmonary vascular resistance. The relative effects of pulmonary arterial and alveolar Po_2. Acta Physiol. Scand., *76*:121, 1969.
78. Abraham, A. S., *et al.*: Factors contributing to the reversible pulmonary hypertension of patients with acute respiratory failure studied by serial observations during recovery. Circ. Res., *24*:51, 1969.
79. Kilburn, K. H., Asmundsson, T., Britt, R. C., and Cardon, R.: Effects of breathing 10 per cent carbon dioxide on the pulmonary circulation of human subjects. Circulation, *39*:639, 1969.
80. Ferrer, M. I.: Disturbances in the circulation in patients with cor pulmonale. Bull. N.Y. Acad. Med., *41*:942, 1965.
81. Housley, E., Clarke, S. W., Hedworth-Whitty, R. B., and Bishop, J. M.: Effect of acute and chronic acidemia and associated hypoxia on the pulmonary circulation of patients with chronic bronchitis. Cardiovasc. Res., *4*:482, 1970.
82. Nakano, J., and Cole, B.: Effects of prostaglandins E_1 and $F_{2\alpha}$ on systemic, pulmonary, and splanchnic circulations in dogs. Am. J. Physiol., *217*:222, 1969.
83. Hyland, J. W., *et al.*: Behavior of pulmonary hypertension produced by serotonin and emboli. Am. J. Physiol., *205*:591, 1963.
84. Brody, J. S., and Stemmler, E. J.: Differential reactivity in the pulmonary circulation. J. Clin. Invest., *47*:800, 1968.
85. Aviado, D. M.: The Lung Circulation. Oxford, Pergamon Press, 1965.
86. Bergofsky, E. H.: Mechanisms underlying vasomotor regulation of regional pulmonary blood flow in normal and disease states. Am. J. Med., *57*:378, 1974.
87. Murray, J. F., Karp, R. B., and Nadel, J. A.: Viscosity effects on pressure-flow relations and vascular resistance in dogs' lungs. J. Appl. Physiol., *27*:336, 1969.
88. Agarwal, J. B., Paltoo, R., and Palmer, W. H.: Relative viscosity of blood at varying hematocrits in pulmonary circulation. J. Appl. Physiol., *29*:866, 1970.
89. Comroe, J. H., *et al.*: The Lung: Clinical Physiology and Pulmonary Function Tests. ed. 2. Chicago, Year Book Medical Publishers, 1962.
90. Pontoppidan, H., Geffin, B., and Lowenstein, E.: Acute respiratory failure in the adult. N. Engl. J. Med., *287*:743, 1972.
91. Bates, D. V., Macklem, P. T., and Christie, R. V.: Respiratory Function in Disease: An Introduction to the Integrated Study of the Lung. ed. 2. Philadelphia, W. B. Saunders, 1971.
92. Harkness, D. R.: The regulation of hemoglobin oxygenation. Adv. Intern. Med., *17*:189, 1972.
93. Edwards, M. J., and Martin, R. J.: Mixing techniques for oxygen hemoglobin equilibrium and Bohr effect. J. Appl. Physiol., *21*:1898, 1966.
94. Bellingham, A. J., DeHer, J. C., and Lenfant, C.: Regulatory mechanisms of hemoglobin oxygen affinity in acidosis and alkalosis. J. Clin. Invest., *50*:700, 1971.
95. Bellingham, A. J., and Lenfant, C.: Hemoglobin affinity for oxygen determined by oxygen-hemoglobin dissociation analyzer and mixing technique. J. Appl. Physiol., *30*:903, 1971.

96. Rand, P. W., *et al.*: Responses to graded hypoxia at high and low 2,3-diphosphoglycerate concentrations. J. Appl. Physiol., *34*:827, 1973.
97. Lenfant, C., Torrance, J. D., and Reynafarje, C.: Shift of the O_2-Hb dissociation curve at altitude: mechanism and effect. J. Appl. Physiol., *30*:625, 1971.
98. Klocke, R. A.: Oxygen transport and 2,3-diphosphoglycerate (DPG). Chest, *62*:79S, 1972.
99. Benesch, R., and Benesch, R. E.: Intracellular organic phosphates as regulators of oxygen release by hemoglobin. Nature, *221*:618, 1967.
100. Brewer, G. J., and Eaton, J. W.: Erythrocyte metabolism: interaction with oxygen transport. Science, *171*:1205, 1971.
101. Thomas, H. M., *et al.*: The oxyhemoglobin dissociation curve in health and disease, role of 2,3-DPG. Am. J. Med., *57*:331, 1974.
102. Raich, P. C., Rodriguez, J. M., Desai, J. N., and Shahidi, N. T.: Effect of hemodialysis on erythrocyte 2,3-diphosphoglycerate in patients with uremia. Am. J. Med. Sci., *265*:147, 1973.
103. Szwed, J. J., *et al.*: Effect of hemodialysis on oxygen-hemoglobin affinity in chronic uremics. Chest, *66*:278, 1974.
104. Brewer, G. J.: 2,3-DPG and erythrocyte oxygen affinity. Annu. Rev. Med., *25*:29, 1974.
105. McConn, R., and Derrick, J. B.: The respiratory function of blood: transfusion and blood storage. Anesthesiology, *36*:119, 1972.
106. Herman, C. M., Rodkey, F. L., Valeri, C. R., and Fortier, N. L.: Changes in the oxyhemoglobin dissociation curve and peripheral blood after acute red cell mass depletion and subsequent red cell mass restoration in baboons. Ann. Surg., *174*:734, 1971.
107. Shafer, A. W., Tague, L. L., Welch, M. H., and Guenter, C. A.: 2,3-diphosphoglycerate in red cells stored in acid-citrate-dextrose and citrate-phosphate-dextrose: implications regarding delivery of oxygen. J. Lab. Clin. Invest., *77*:430, 1971.
108. Riggs, T. E., Shafer, A. W., and Guenter, C. A.: Acute changes in oxyhemoglobin affinity: effects on oxygen transport and utilization. J. Clin. Invest., *52*:2660, 1973.
109. Papadopoulos, M. D., Morrow, G., and Oski, F. A.: Exchange transfusion in the newborn infant with fresh and "old" blood: the role of storage on 2,3-diphosphoglycerate, hemoglobin-oxygen affinity, and oxygen release. J. Pediatr., *79*:898, 1971.
110. Frohlich, E. D. (ed.): Pathophysiology: Altered Regulatory Mechanisms in Disease. ed. 2. Philadelphia, J. B. Lippincott, 1976.
111. Brantigan, J. W., Perna, A. M., Gardner, T. J., and Gott, V. L.: Intramyocardial gas tensions in the canine heart during anoxic cardiac arrest. Surg. Gynecol. Obstet., *134*:67, 1972.
112. Brantigan, J. W., Gott, V. L., and Martz, M. N.: A teflon membrane for measurement of blood and intramyocardial gas tensions by mass spectroscopy. J. Appl. Physiol., *32*:276, 1972.
113. Wilson, G. J., *et al.*: Mass spectrometry for measuring changes in intramyocardial Po_2 and Pco_2. *In* Bicher, H. I., and Duane, F. B. (eds.): Oxygen Transport to Tissue: Instrumentation, Methods, and Physiology. New York, Plenum, 1973.
114. Boysen, G., *et al.*: On a critical lower level of cerebral blood flow in man with particular reference to carotid surgery. Circulation, *49*:1023, 1974.
115. Larson, C. P., Jr., Ehrenfeld, W. K., Wade, J. G., and Wylie, E. J.: Jugular venous oxygen saturation as an index of adequacy of cerebral oxygenation. Surgery, *62*:31, 1967.
116. Edelman, N. H., *et al.*: The effect of impairment of O_2 delivery on the aerobic metabolism of brain and skeletal muscle. Chest, *61*:49S, 1972.
117. Henderson, A. R.: Biochemistry of hypoxia: current concepts. I. An introduction to biochemical pathways and their control. Br. J. Anaesth., *41*:245, 1969.
118. McDowall, D. G.: Biochemistry of hypoxia: current concepts. II. Biochemical derangements associated with hypoxia and their measurement. Br. J. Anaesth., *41*:251, 1969.
119. Peretz, D. I., *et al.*: The significance of lacticacidemia in the shock syndrome. Ann. N.Y. Acad. Sci., *119*:1133, 1965.
120. Cain, S. M.: Relative rates of arterial lactate and oxygen-deficit accumulation in hypoxic dogs. Am. J. Physiol., *224*:1190, 1973.
121. Comroe, J. H., Jr., and Bothello, S.: The unreliability of cyanosis in the recognition of arterial anoxemia. Am. J. Med. Sci., *214*:1, 1947.
122. Davenport, H. W.: The ABC of Acid-Base Chemistry. ed. 6. Chicago, University of Chicago Press, 1974.

123. Dejours, P.: Respiration. New York, Oxford University Press, 1966.
124. Siggaard-Andersen, O., and Garby, L.: The Bohr effect and the Haldane effect. Scand. J. Clin. Lab. Invest., *31*:1, 1973.
125. Davis, R. P., Log, I., and Gibbs, A.: Ion view of acid-base balance. Am. J. Med., *42*:159, 1967.
126. Lennon, E. J., and Lemann, J., Jr.: Defense of hydrogen ion concentration in chronic metabolic acidosis. A new evaluation of an old approach. Ann. Intern. Med., *65*:265, 1966.
127. Hills, A. G., and Reid, E. L.: pH defended—is it defensible? Ann. Intern. Med., *65*:1150, 1966.
128. Siggaard-Andersen, O. Blood acid-base alignment nomogram. Scand. J. Clin. Lab. Invest., *15*:211, 1963.
129. ———: An acid-base chart for arterial blood with normal and pathophysiological reference areas. Scand. J. Clin. Lab. Invest., *27*:239, 1971.
130. Arbus, G. S.: An in vivo acid-base nomogram for clinical use. Can. Med. Assoc. J., *109*:291, 1973.
131. Brackett, N. C., Cohen, J. J., and Schwartz, W. B.: Carbon dioxide titration curve of normal man: effect of increasing degrees of acute hypercapnia on acid-base equilibrium. N. Engl. J. Med., *272*:6, 1965.
132. Brackett, N. C., Jr., Wingo, C. F., Muren, O., and Solano, J. T.: Acid-base response to chronic hypercapnia in man. N. Engl. J. Med., *280*:124, 1969.
133. Welt, L. G.: Acidosis and alkalosis. *In* Wintrobe, M. M., *et al.* (eds.): Principles of Internal Medicine. ed. 7. New York, McGraw-Hill, 1974.

Index

Numerals in italics indicate a figure.